The Compressed Spinal Cord

Editor

MICHAEL G. FEHLINGS

NEUROSURGERY
CLINICS OF NORTH AMERICA

www.neurosurgery.theclinics.com

Consulting Editors
RUSSELL R. LONSER
DANIEL K. RESNICK

October 2026 • Volume 37 • Number 4

ELSEVIER

1818 Market Street • Suite 3323 • Philadelphia, Pennsylvania, 19103-2899

http://www.theclinics.com

NEUROSURGERY CLINICS OF NORTH AMERICA Volume 37, Number 4
October 2026 ISSN 1042-3680, ISBN-13: 978-0-443-47400-2

Editor: Stacy Eastman
Developmental Editor: Akshay Samson

Publishing Office: *Neurosurgery Clinics of North America* (ISSN 1042-3680) is published quarterly by Elsevier Inc., 1818 Market Street, Philadelphia, PA 19103, United States. Periodicals postage paid at New York, NY and additional mailing offices. USA POSTMASTER: Send address changes to *Neurosurgery Clinics of North America*, Elsevier Customer Service Department, 3251 Riverport Lane, Maryland Heights, MO 63043, USA. Months of issue are January, April, July, and October. Subscription prices are $474.00 per year (US individuals), $509.00 per year (Canadian individuals), $590.00 per year (international individuals), $100.00 per year (US students), $255.00 per year (international students), and $100.00 per year (Canadian students). For institutional access pricing please contact Customer Service via the contact information below. International air speed delivery is included in all *Clinics* subscription prices. All prices are subject to change without notice. Orders, claims, and journal inquiries: Please visit our Support Hub page https://service.elsevier.com for assistance.

Reprints. For copies of 100 or more, of articles in this publication, please contact the Commercial Reprints Department, Elsevier Inc., 360 Park Avenue South, New York, NY 10010-1710. Tel. 212-633-3874; Fax: 212-633-3820; E-mail: reprints@elsevier.com.

Neurosurgery Clinics of North America is covered in *MEDLINE/PubMed (Index Medicus), EMBASE/Excerpta Medica, and Current Contents/Clinical Medicine (CC/CM).*

Contributors

CONSULTING EDITORS

RUSSELL R. LONSER, MD
Professor and Chair, Department of Neurological Surgery, The Ohio State University Wexner Medical Center, Columbus, Ohio, USA

DANIEL K. RESNICK, MD, MS
Professor and Vice Chairman, Program Director, Department of Neurosurgery, University of Wisconsin-Madison School of Medicine and Public Health, Madison, Wisconsin, USA

EDITOR

MICHAEL G. FEHLINGS, MD, PhD, FRCSC, FACS, FRSC, FCAHS
Professor, Division of Neurosurgery and Spine Program, Department of Surgery, University of Toronto; Robert Campeau Family Foundation/ Dr. C.H. Tator Chair in Brain and Spinal Cord Research at UHN, Senior Consultant Neurosurgeon and Clinician Scientist, Krembil Brain Institute, Toronto Western Hospital, University Health Network, Toronto, Ontario, Canada

AUTHORS

BIZHAN AARABI, MD
Professor, Department of Neurosurgery, University of Maryland School of Medicine, Baltimore City, Maryland, USA

RAMAN ABBASPOUR, BSc, MEng
Research Assistant, Temerty Faculty of Medicine, Institute of Biomedical Engineering, University of Toronto, Toronto, Ontario, Canada

NOORI AKHTAR-DANESH, PhD
Associate Professor, Faculty of Health Sciences, McMaster University, Hamilton, Ontario, Canada

MOHAMMED ALI ALVI, MD, MS
Division of Neurosurgery and Spine Program, Department of Surgery, Institute of Medical Science, University of Toronto, Clinical Research Scientist, Researcher, Division of Neurosurgery, Krembil Neuroscience Centre, Toronto Western Hospital, University Health Network, Toronto, Ontario, Canada

YAW ANTWI-YEBOAH, MBBS, BSc, FRCS
Senior Spine Fellow, Department of Neurosurgery, Oxford University Hospitals NHS Foundation Trust, Oxford, United Kingdom

EDOARDO MARIA BARBIERI, MD
Neurosurgery Resident, University of Milan, Milan, Italy

JOSHUA I. CHALIF, MD, PhD
Neurosurgery Resident, Department of Neurosurgery, Mass General Brigham and Harvard Medical School, Boston, Massachusetts, USA

YOUSSEF CHEDID, MD, MBBS, BSc (Hons)
Division of Neurosurgery, Department of Clinical Neurosciences, University of Cambridge, ST1 Neurosurgery, Department of

Clinical Neurosciences, Cambridge University Hospitals NHS Foundation Trust, Cambridge, United Kingdom

TIMOTHY CHRYSSIKOS, MD, PhD
Assistant Professor, Department of Neurosurgery, University of Maryland School of Medicine, Baltimore City, Maryland, USA

FRANCESCO COSTA, MD
Head of Spine Neurosurgery Unit, Department of Neurosurgery, Fondazione IRCCS Istituto Neurologico Carlo Besta, Professor, University of Milan, Milan, Italy

BENJAMIN M. DAVIES, BSC, MPhil, MRCS
Specialist Registrar, Division of Neurosurgery, Department of Clinical Neurosciences, University of Cambridge, Cambridge, United Kingdom

MOUAD ELGANGA, BSc
Research Assistant, Temerty Faculty of Medicine, University of Toronto, Toronto, Ontario, Canada

MICHAEL G. FEHLINGS, MD, PhD, FRCSC, FACS, FRSC, FCAHS
Professor, Division of Neurosurgery and Spine Program, Department of Surgery, University of Toronto; Robert Campeau Family Foundation/ Dr. C.H. Tator Chair in Brain and Spinal Cord Research at UHN, Senior Consultant Neurosurgeon and Clinician Scientist, Krembil Brain Institute, Toronto Western Hospital, University Health Network, Toronto, Ontario, Canada

LAURA GANAU
Medical Student, School of Medicine, University of Cagliari, Cagliari, Sardinia, Italy

MARIO GANAU, MD, PhD, MBA, LLM, FEBNS, FRCSEd, FFSTEd, FACS
Consultant Neurosurgeon, Department of Neurosurgery, Oxford University Hospitals NHS Foundation Trust, Nuffield Department of Clinical Neurosciences, University of Oxford, Oxford, United Kingdom; BAU International University Batumi, Batumi, Georgia

TELEALE F. GEBEYEHU, MD
Post-Doctoral Spine Research Fellow, Department of Neurological Surgery, Thomas Jefferson University, Philadelphia, Pennsylvania, USA

JAMES D. GUEST, MD, PhD, FAANS
The Miami Project to Cure Paralysis, Miller School of Medicine, Professor, Department of Neurological Surgery, University of Miami Miller School of Medicine, Miami, Florida, USA

JAMES S. HARROP, MD, MSHQS
Professor of Neurosurgery and Spine Division Head, Department of Neurological Surgery, Thomas Jefferson University, Philadelphia, Pennsylvania, USA

NADER HEJRATI, MD, PhD
Spinal Neurosurgeon, Department of Neurosurgery and Spine Center, HOCH Health Ostschweiz, St Gallen, Switzerland; Faculty of Medicine, University of Basel, Basel, Switzerland

SHINTARO HONDA, MD, PhD
Postdoctoral Research Fellow, Division of Genetics and Development, Krembil Brain Institute, University Health Network, Toronto, Ontario, Canada

NICCOLÒ INNOCENTI, MD
Neurosurgeon, Spine Neurosurgery Unit, Department of Neurosurgery, Fondazione IRCCS Istituto Neurologico Carlo Besta, Milan, Italy

ASHMAL S. KABANI, MD
Post-Doctoral Spine Research Fellow, Department of Neurological Surgery, Thomas Jefferson University, Philadelphia, Pennsylvania, USA

SO KATO, MD, PhD
Associate Professor, Department of Orthopeadic Surgery, The University of Tokyo, Tokyo, Japan

ANASTASIA KELLER, PhD
Assistant Professor, Department of Neurological Surgery, University of California, San Francisco, California, USA

MARK R. KOTTER, MD, MPhil, PhD
Research Professor, Division of Neurosurgery, Department of Clinical Neurosciences, University of Cambridge, Cambridge, United Kingdom

SHEKAR N. KURPAD, MD, PhD
Professor, Department of Neurosurgery, Medical College of Wisconsin, Milwaukee, Wisconsin, USA

SEBASTIAN A. LARES, BSc
Researcher, The Miami Project to Cure Paralysis, Miller School of Medicine, Miami, Florida, USA

ADAM LEIBOLD, MD, MSc
Spine Fellow, Department of Neurological Surgery, Thomas Jefferson University, Philadelphia, Pennsylvania, USA

GIANFRANCO K.I. LIGAROTTI, MD
Consultant Neurosurgeon, Aerospace Medical Institute of Milan "A. Mosso", Italian Air Force, Milan, Italy

DO H. LIM, BA
Research Assistant, Department of Neurosurgery, Medical College of Wisconsin, Milwaukee, Wisconsin, USA

YI LU, MD, PhD
Spine Fellowship Program Director, Department of Neurosurgery, Mass General Brigham and Harvard Medical School, Boston, Massachusetts, USA

NADINE MANSOUR, MD, MPH, PhD
Postdoctoral Fellow, Departments of Neurosurgery and Biomedical Engineering, University of Minnesota, Minneapolis, Minnesota, USA

ALLAN R. MARTIN, MD, PhD, FRCSC
Associate Professor, Program Director, Vice Chair, Department of Neurological Surgery, University of California, Davis, Sacramento, California, USA

LUCA MATTIOLI, MD
Neurosurgery Resident, University of Milan, Milan, Italy

ELIO MAZZAPICCHI, MD
Neurosurgery Resident, University of Milan, Milan, Italy

EMMANUEL O. MENSAH, MD
Postdoctoral Research Fellow, Department of Neurosurgery, Mass General Brigham and Harvard Medical School, Boston, Massachusetts, USA

FAUZIYYA MUHAMMAD, MD, PhD
Instructor, Department of Neurosurgery, University of Oklahoma Health Campus, Oklahoma City, Oklahoma, USA

NARIHITO NAGOSHI, MD, PhD
Assistant Professor, Department of Orthopaedic Surgery, Keio University School of Medicine, Shinjuku-ku, Tokyo, Japan

NICOLE OSSANDÓN-PINO, MSc
Professor, Neuroimmunology and Regeneration of the Central Nervous System Unit, Biomedical Science Research Laboratory, Department of Basic Sciences, Faculty of Medicine, Universidad Católica de La Santísima Concepción, Neuromet Group, Universidad Católica de La Santisima Concepción, Concepción, Chile

ANN PARR, MD, PhD
Professor, Department of Neurosurgery, University of Minnesota, Minneapolis, Minnesota, USA

KARLO M. PEDRO, MD
Assistant Professor, Division of Neurosurgery and Spine Program, Department of Surgery, Institute of Medical Science, University of Toronto, Assistant Professor, Division of Neurosurgery, Krembil Neuroscience Centre, Toronto Western Hospital, University Health Network, Toronto, Ontario, Canada

LARA PRISCO, MD, MSc, MPH
Consultant, Neuro-Anaesthesia and Intensive Care Medicine, Department of Anaesthesia, Oxford University Hospitals NHS Foundation Trust, Nuffield Department of Clinical Neurosciences, University of Oxford, Oxford, United Kingdom

RAJIV SAIGAL, MD, PhD, FAANS
Associate Professor, Department of Neurological Surgery, University of California, San Francisco, California, USA

MARK JUN SHAH-OSTROWSKI, BM, BCh
Foundation Doctor, Department of Neurosurgery, Oxford University Hospitals NHS Foundation Trust, Oxford, United Kingdom

ZACHARY A. SMITH, MD
Professor, Department of Neurosurgery, University of Oklahoma Health Campus, Oklahoma City, Oklahoma, USA

MUHAMMAD SULMAN, BS
Medical Student, School of Medicine, University of California, Davis, Sacramento, California, USA

OCTAVIAN VATAVU, MD
Neurosurgery Resident, University of Milan, Milan, Italy

ADITYA VEDANTAM, MD
Associate Professor, Department of Neurosurgery, Medical College of Wisconsin, Milwaukee, Wisconsin, USA

PIA M. VIDAL, PhD
Associate Professor, Neuroimmunology and Regeneration of the Central Nervous System Unit, Department of Basic Sciences, Faculty of Medicine, Biomedical Science Research Laboratory, Neuromet Group, Universidad Católica de La Santisima Concepción, Concepción, Chile

BRENDON WANG, BA
Research Assistant, Department of Neurosurgery, Medical College of Wisconsin, Milwaukee, Wisconsin, USA

JEFFERSON R. WILSON, MD, PhD
Associate Professor, Division of Neurosurgery and Spine Program, Department of Surgery, University of Toronto, Neurosurgeon, Division of Neurosurgery, Department of Surgery, St. Michael's Hospital, Toronto, Ontario, Canada

ZHEQING ZHANG, BA
Medical Student, Department of Neurosurgery, Oxford University Hospitals NHS Foundation Trust, Oxford, United Kingdom

CARL M. ZIPSER, MD, MA
Senior Neurologist, Department of Neurology and Neurophysiology, Balgrist University, Spinal Cord Injury Center, Balgrist University Hospital, University of Zurich, Zurich, Switzerland

Contents

Degenerative cervical myelopathy (DCM) is a chronic spinal cord disorder caused by progressive compression leading to ischemia, cell death, inflammation, demyelination, and network reorganization. Unlike traumatic injury, DCM evolves over time, producing distributed pathology across the neuraxis and adaptive but limited neuroplastic responses. Functional deficits arise from both reversible axonal dysfunction and irreversible degeneration, creating a time-sensitive window for intervention. Surgical decompression remains the primary treatment, enabling partial recovery through restoration of perfusion and plasticity. Adjunctive strategies, including neuroprotection, neuromodulation, and remyelination therapies, with rehabilitation, represent promising approaches to enhance recovery by targeting residual neural circuits and the evolving repair environment.

Traumatic and nontraumatic spinal cord injury including degenerative cervical myelopathy, produce heterogeneous neurologic and functional deficits that are incompletely captured by traditional outcome measures. This review summarizes widely used clinician-reported and patient-reported instruments across quality of life, functional independence, and global and focal neurologic assessment, highlighting limitations such as ceiling/floor effects, incomplete domain coverage, and variable responsiveness. Emerging approaches—including batteries of complementary assessments, hybrid measures, digital health tools, imaging biomarkers, and neurophysiology—offer improved sensitivity and multidimensional assessment. Standardized core outcome sets may improve clinical management, reduce reporting heterogeneity, and improve comparability across studies.

Spinal cord injury (SCI) is a complex and heterogeneous condition associated with substantial neurologic disability, functional impairment, and socioeconomic burden. Artificial intelligence (AI) and machine learning are increasingly being applied throughout the SCI care continuum to improve diagnosis, imaging analysis, prognostication, phenotyping, and therapeutic decision-making. Unsupervised learning approaches further support data-driven patient phenotyping and personalized rehabilitation strategies. Emerging applications also extend to regenerative medicine, where AI may optimize patient selection, monitor neural repair, and enhance therapeutic integration. Collectively, these advances support a transition toward precision, data-driven, and individualized SCI management.

Central cord syndrome (CCS) is the most common incomplete traumatic spinal cord injury; however, it remains poorly defined, with no consensus diagnostic criteria, an ambiguous and variable clinical presentation, and significant overlap with other incomplete spinal cord injuries. The available evidence indicates that CCS is

NEUROSURGERY CLINICS OF NORTH AMERICA

FORTHCOMING ISSUES

January 2027
Pituitary Neuroendocrine Tumors
Daniel M. Prevedello, *Editor*

April 2027
Enhanced Navigation, Image Guidance, and Robotics in Spine Surgery
Nicholas Theodore and Michael Y. Wang, *Editors*

July 2027
Trigeminal Neuralgia
Raymond F. Sekula, *Editor*

RECENT ISSUES

July 2026
Intramedullary Spinal Cord Tumors
George I. Jallo and Nir Shimony, *Editors*

April 2026
Decompressive Craniectomy
Shelly D. Timmons and Patrick J. Belton, *Editors*

January 2026
Update on Lumbar Spondylolisthesis: Who, Why, and How
Zoher Ghogawala, *Editor*

Preface

Pathophysiology and Management of the Compressed Spinal Cord: From Molecule to Man

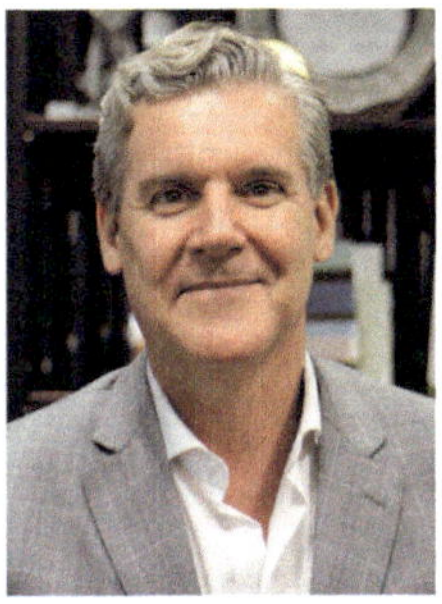

Michael G. Fehlings, MD, PhD, FRCSC, FACS
Editor

When Elsevier first invited me to guest edit an issue focused on the compressed spinal cord for their prestigious *Neurosurgery Clinics of North America* series, I was hesitant to take on the assignment. I was the Editor of two recent Elsevier textbooks, one on spinal cord injury and one covering degenerative cervical myelopathy, published in 2022 and 2023, respectively, and was not sure the world needed another resource so soon.

However, when I began to consider the large volume of exciting and impactful research that has been produced on the topic of spinal cord compression in the past five years alone, I was energized to work with Elsevier and the *Neurosurgery Clinics of North America* series to showcase these developments. Selecting the topics and authors to include was no easy feat, as we have brilliant minds located on every continent working tirelessly to further our understanding of this complex topic. I am confident that the 16 articles included here represent areas of critical importance to the field, written by leading authorities and showcasing cutting-edge science. Of note, this text emphasizes the synergy between traumatic and nontraumatic spinal cord injury, which is a concept that is being increasingly embraced by the international community.

Projects like these highlight that we are living in an exciting era for studying spinal cord conditions, with high-quality research being published almost daily by talented researchers and clinicians around the world.

The Compressed Spinal Cord issue provides a contemporary picture of recent advancements in our understanding and care of spinal cord compression that are relevant to neurosurgeons, orthopedic surgeons, physiatrists, allied health professionals, researchers, clinical and scientific trainees, policy makers, and, most importantly, individuals living with spinal cord compression and their families.

With articles written by some of the biggest names in the field, this issue begins by highlighting the shifting demographics of spinal cord injury, the pathobiology of spinal cord compression, and how artificial intelligence is rapidly reshaping the diagnosis and treatment of these conditions. Central cord injury and degenerative cervical myelopathy are also discussed at length, with recent advancements, such as clinical practice guidelines and trajectory-based analyses, changing how we approach these conditions. The Compressed Spinal Cord issue then transitions to topics such as radiomics, advanced microstructural MRI, neuroprotection, surgical approaches, genetics, biomarkers, neuromodulation,

Neurosurg Clin N Am 37 (2026) xiii–xiv
https://doi.org/10.1016/j.nec.2026.07.001

regenerative approaches, and novel outcome measures. Importantly, each of these topics has witnessed significant advancement in the past few years, with numerous clinical trials and large studies being discussed in these sections. The issue concludes by looking toward the future and where the field is going. In the near future, I anticipate that the integration of precision imaging, artificial intelligence–based assessment, circuit-level neuromodulation, and biologically informed stem cell–based interventions will shift care toward personalized treatment paradigms that improve neurologic and functional outcomes.

I trust this issue of *Neurosurgery Clinics of North America* will become a valuable resource to those who are passionate about improving outcomes for those living with spinal cord compression. I encourage everyone working in the field to be optimistic, passionate, curious, and relentless in their pursuit of improving treatment—even small gains have a dramatic impact on patients' lives.

DISCLOSURES

The author has no relevant disclosures.

Michael G. Fehlings, MD, PhD, FRCSC, FACS
Toronto Western Hospital
University Health Network
Toronto, Ontario, Canada

E-mail address:
michael.fehlings@uhn.ca

Introduction to Evolving Concepts Related to Spinal Cord Compression

Mouad Elganga, BSc[a], Raman Abbaspour, BSc, MEng[a,b],
Mohammed Ali Alvi, MD, MS[c,d,e], Karlo M. Pedro, MD[c,d,e],
Michael G. Fehlings, MD, PhD, FRCSC, FRSC, FCAHS[a,c,d,e,*]

KEYWORDS

- Spinal cord compression • Degenerative cervical myelopathy • Quantitative MRI • Dynamic MRI
- Radiomics • Machine learning • Precision medicine • Neuroprotection

KEY POINTS

- Spinal cord compression is no longer considered a static lesion but a dynamic, multifactorial disorder integrating ischemia, barrier disruption, neuroinflammation, demyelination, and remote tract injury.
- Degenerative cervical myelopathy, the most common cause of nontraumatic spinal cord dysfunction in adults, provides the principal clinical model for characterizing these mechanisms.
- Chronic compression's biological footprint extends beyond the compressed segment, with microstructural and morphometric abnormalities rostral and caudal to the lesion and corresponding cortical changes.
- Quantitative and dynamic MRI, automated morphometrics, radiomics, and machine learning are augmenting conventional scores and qualitative MRI to stage severity and predict outcomes.
- Trajectory-based imaging biomarkers, such as longitudinal change in noncompressed cross-sectional area, may flag deterioration risk early, enabling individualized decompression timing and adjunctive therapy selection.

INTRODUCTION: REFRAMING SPINAL CORD COMPRESSION AS A DYNAMIC, SYSTEMS-LEVEL DISORDER

Spinal cord compression represents a final common pathway shared by a heterogeneous group of traumatic and nontraumatic disorders, including degenerative spinal disease, neoplasia, infection, inflammatory conditions, and acute traumatic injury. For most of the twentieth century, compression was conceptualized as a fundamentally mechanical problem in which bony, discogenic, or ligamentous structures encroached upon the spinal canal, deformed the cord, and produced neurologic dysfunction in proportion to the degree and duration of narrowing.[1–3] This formulation gave rise to a familiar set of geometric metrics, including antero-posterior canal diameter, the Pavlov ratio, and the maximum spinal cord compression (MSCC) index, which translated the cord–canal interface into reproducible, surgically actionable numbers.[4] It also supported a clinical

[a] Temerty Faculty of Medicine, University of Toronto, Toronto, Ontario, Canada; [b] Institute of Biomedical Engineering, University of Toronto, Toronto, Ontario, Canada; [c] Division of Neurosurgery & Spine Program, Department of Surgery, University of Toronto, Toronto, Ontario, Canada; [d] Institute of Medical Science, University of Toronto, Toronto, Ontario, Canada; [e] Division of Neurosurgery, Krembil Neuroscience Centre, Toronto Western Hospital, University Health Network, Toronto, Ontario, Canada
* Corresponding author. Toronto Western Hospital, 399 Bathurst Street, Suite 4WW-449, Toronto, Ontario M5T 2S8, Canada.
E-mail address: Michael.fehlings@uhn.ca

Neurosurg Clin N Am 37 (2026) 453–467
https://doi.org/10.1016/j.nec.2026.05.010

Abbreviations	
AP	antero-posterior
AUC	area under the curve
BSCB	blood–spinal cord barrier
CSA	compressed cross-sectional area
DCM	degenerative cervical myelopathy
DTI	diffusion tensor imaging
IBSI	Image Biomarker Standardization Initiative
IL	interleukin
MCID	minimum clinically important difference
mJOA	modified Japanese Orthopaedic Association
MSCC	maximum spinal cord compression
MT	magnetization transfer
NDI	Neck Disability Index
NH-DCM	Natural History of Mild Degenerative Cervical Myelopathy
PCS	Physical Component Summary
RMSE	root mean squared error
TNF-α	tumor necrosis factor-alpha

algorithm in which decompression was indicated when the canal was sufficiently narrow and the patient was sufficiently symptomatic.

The mechanical paradigm explained much of the clinical phenotype, but not all of it. Patients with marked radiographic compression were sometimes neurologically stable for years, while others with apparently modest stenosis deteriorated rapidly. Recovery after technically successful decompression varied considerably and could not be reliably predicted from imaging or clinical scores alone.[4–6] The discordance between geometry and biology pointed to dimensions of disease that static MRI could not capture: spinal cord compression is a heterogeneous, biologically active process that evolves over time and frequently extends beyond the level of maximum cord deformation (**Fig. 1**).[4,7]

Within the broader spectrum of compressive pathology, degenerative cervical myelopathy (DCM) has emerged as the most informative clinical model for examining these limitations. DCM is an overarching term encompassing cervical spondylotic myelopathy, ossification of the posterior longitudinal ligament, ossification of the ligamentum flavum, and degenerative disc and ligamentous disease, all of which converge upon chronic mechanical compression of the cervical spinal cord.[1,2] DCM is the most common cause of nontraumatic spinal cord impairment in adults, and its prevalence is expected to rise in parallel with population aging.[1,7–9] Imaging-based studies further suggest that asymptomatic cord compression is common in older individuals and that a substantial proportion of these patients will progress to clinically evident myelopathy over time.[10]

The clinical course of DCM is markedly heterogeneous. Some patients deteriorate during conservative management; others remain stable for years; and others decline acutely after seemingly minor cervical trauma. Traditional tools, including the modified Japanese Orthopaedic Association (mJOA) scale, the Nurick grade, the Neck Disability Index (NDI), and qualitative T2-weighted MRI, offer only blunt resolution of this spectrum and are notably insensitive in mild disease.[11–13] The AO Spine RECODE-DCM initiative has identified earlier diagnosis, validated outcome measurement, and improved prognostication as the highest research priorities for the field, underscoring the inadequacy of historical assessment paradigms.[14,15]

This article brings together expert perspectives on traumatic and nontraumatic compression of the spinal cord and addresses epidemiology, pathobiology, central cord injury, mild DCM, neuroprotection, decompression strategy, perfusion, regenerative therapies, and outcome measurement in granular detail. We frame spinal cord compression as a dynamic, biologically active disorder in which mechanical injury triggers vascular, inflammatory, and neurodegenerative cascades extending beyond the visible epicenter, and in which diagnosis and prognosis are shifting from snapshot description toward quantitative, individualized trajectory prediction.[16]

MECHANISTIC EVOLUTION: FROM STATIC COMPRESSION TO DYNAMIC NEUROBIOLOGY

Classical Mechanical Paradigm

The classical mechanical paradigm holds that progressive narrowing of the spinal canal by spondylotic, discogenic, or ligamentous changes produces direct deformation of the cord, with the severity of myelopathy varying as a function of the degree and duration of compression.[1–3] Within this framework, geometric metrics derived from sagittal and axial MRI—antero-posterior canal diameter, Pavlov ratio, and MSCC—became the dominant biomarkers of disease severity and the principal triggers for surgical intervention.[17] This formulation is intuitive, reproducible, and surgically actionable, and it remains foundational to contemporary practice. However, a purely geometric interpretation can neither account for the well-recognized observation that the cross-sectional area of the cord, the degree of canal stenosis, and the integrity of the spinal cord parenchyma

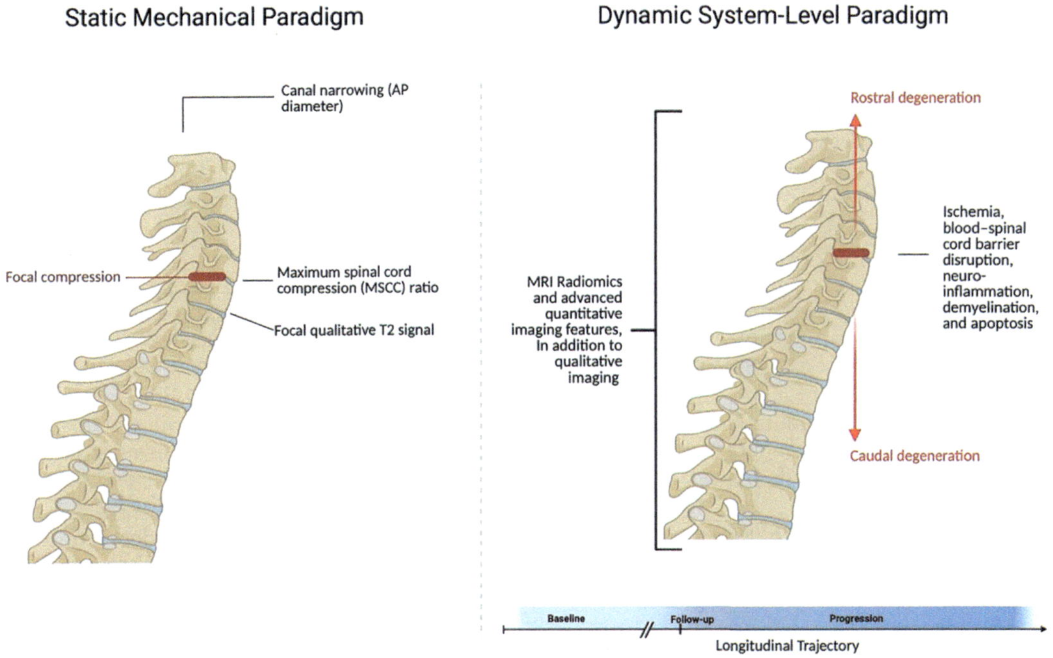

Fig. 1. Evolution from a static mechanical to a dynamic system-level paradigm of spinal cord compression. The traditional model conceptualizes degenerative cervical myelopathy primarily as a focal mechanical disorder, emphasizing canal narrowing, antero-posterior diameter, maximum spinal cord compression ratio, and qualitative T2 signal change at the site of compression. The evolving system-level paradigm incorporates the biological consequences of chronic compression, including ischemia, blood–spinal cord barrier disruption, neuroinflammation, demyelination, apoptosis, as well as rostral and caudal degeneration beyond the compression epicenter. Advanced quantitative MRI, radiomics, and longitudinal imaging trajectories may therefore complement conventional qualitative imaging by capturing both focal injury and distributed cord degeneration over time. AP, antero-posterior; MSCC, maximum spinal cord compression. (*Created in* BioRender. Lab, F. (2026) https://BioRender.com/ikid3ig.)

are imperfectly correlated with neurologic deficit nor explain why a substantial subset of patients with apparently mild radiographic compression progress to severe myelopathy, while others with high-grade stenosis remain asymptomatic for years.[4–6] These limitations necessitate more biologically informative biomarkers that complement the geometry of compression (**Table 1**).

Vascular and Ischemic Mechanisms

It has long been recognized that the pathobiology of compression is closely linked to disturbances of cord perfusion. Macrovascular compromise, particularly involving the anterior spinal artery and its radicular contributions arising from the vertebral and segmental arteries, has been implicated in central cord ischemia and may explain the clinical predilection of certain compressive lesions for the corticospinal tracts.[3,18,19] More importantly, chronic experimental compression has been shown to produce a sustained reduction in intraparenchymal spinal cord blood flow, with consequent ischemic injury to neurons and oligodendrocytes that is disproportionate to the magnitude of mechanical deformation alone.[5,16,19] At the microvascular level, capillary rarefaction, endothelial dysfunction, and disruption of the vascular basement membrane have been demonstrated in both human cervical spinal cord specimens and rodent models of progressive compression, and these changes appear to persist throughout the compressed segment and into adjacent regions.[19,20]

Closely related to these vascular changes is the loss of blood–spinal cord barrier (BSCB) integrity. Increased BSCB permeability has been documented in chronic compressive myelopathy and is accompanied by extravasation of plasma proteins, infiltration of peripheral immune cells, and exacerbation of local edema and neuroinflammation.[19,21] Importantly, BSCB disruption may persist into the chronic phase of compression and has recently been shown to recover, at least in part, after surgical decompression, a finding that supports the role of BSCB integrity as a potentially modifiable contributor to disease progression rather than a fixed structural feature.[22]

Table 1
Traditional versus evolving paradigms in spinal cord compression

Domain	Traditional Paradigm	Evolving Paradigm	Clinical Implication
Disease nature	Static, focal mechanical lesion	Dynamic, multifactorial systems disorder integrating mechanical, vascular, inflammatory, and neurodegenerative processes	Counseling reflects biological complexity, not anatomy alone
Spatial distribution	Confined to maximally compressed level	Global cord involvement; remote rostral and caudal degeneration; supraspinal network effects	Imaging and outcome assessment should sample beyond the epicenter
Imaging	Qualitative T2 MRI; canal diameter; MSCC	Dynamic MRI; DTI/MT/T2*; automated morphometrics; radiomics; machine learning	Quantitative biomarkers refine severity, predict outcome, and detect occult disease
Clinical assessment	mJOA, Nurick, and NDI	Multimodal assessment integrating imaging, electrophysiology, PROMs, and digital measures	Improved detection of mild disease and longitudinal change
Prognostication	Group-level linear models; baseline snapshot	Individualized, machine-learning-based, trajectory-driven predictions	Patient-specific risk stratification supports earlier or delayed intervention
Treatment	Binary surgery vs observation; mJOA-threshold-driven	Personalized timing of decompression with neuroprotective and regenerative adjuncts	Precision medicine matches the right intervention to the right biological stage

Abbreviations: AMPA, α-amino-3-hydroxy-5-methyl-4-isoxazolepropionic acid; AP, anteroposterior; CCL2, C-C motif chemokine ligand 2; DTI, diffusion tensor imaging; MMP-2, matrix metalloproteinase-2; mJOA, modified Japanese Orthopaedic Association; MSCC, maximum spinal cord compression; MT, magnetization transfer; NDI, Neck Disability Index; NMDA, N-methyl-D-aspartate; PROMs, patient-reported outcome measures; RISCIS, Riluzole in Spinal Cord Injury Study; RL, right-left; SF-36, 36-Item Short Form Health Survey; T2*, T2-star–weighted imaging.

Comparison across domains of disease conceptualization, spatial distribution, imaging, clinical assessment, prognostication, and treatment, illustrating the shift from anatomy to biology, snapshot to trajectory, and binary to precision-based decision-making.

Neuroinflammation and Immune Activation

The recognition that chronic compression generates a unique neuroinflammatory response has further reframed the pathobiology of spinal cord compression. Persistent activation of microglia, polarization of macrophage phenotypes, and accumulation of activated peripheral immune cells at the compression site have been demonstrated in both rodent models and human cervical spinal cord specimens.[19,20,23] Cytokine cascades involving tumor necrosis factor-alpha (TNF-α), interleukin (IL)-1β, IL-6, and chemokines such as CCL2 have been implicated in propagating the inflammatory response and recruiting peripheral leukocytes through the disrupted BSCB.[19,23] In addition, matrix metalloproteinases, particularly MMP-2 and MMP-9, have been shown to participate in tissue remodeling, demyelination, and ongoing BSCB breakdown.[19,23] Together, these findings indicate that chronic compression engages an inflammatory program that is biologically continuous with that observed in traumatic spinal cord injury and that contributes to ongoing parenchymal injury independent of the primary mechanical insult.

Cellular Injury and Neurodegeneration

At the cellular level, the persistent ischemic and inflammatory milieu generated by chronic compression activates several injury pathways that converge upon neuronal and oligodendroglial cell death. In both human cervical spinal cord specimens and a rodent model, Fas-mediated apoptosis contributes substantially to neuronal and oligodendroglial loss in chronic compressive myelopathy, and pharmacologic inhibition of this pathway is neuroprotective.[24] TNF-α signaling, caspase activation, and downstream apoptotic effectors have been shown to participate in the progressive cell death observed within and adjacent to the compression site.[19,23] Oligodendrocyte loss is a particularly consequential feature of this cascade, as these cells are the principal myelinating cells of the central nervous system and their loss results in demyelination of long ascending and descending tracts, which is poorly compensated by endogenous remyelination.[19] Glutamate excitotoxicity, mediated through NMDA and AMPA-kainate receptors and amplified by ATP-dependent ion-pump dysfunction, has additionally been implicated in the progressive injury of both gray and white matter compartments.[19] Histologically, the cumulative effects of these processes are evident as gliosis, cavity formation, degeneration of the lateral and ventral corticospinal tracts, interneuronal loss, and atrophy of the anterior horns with motoneuronal depletion, a constellation that defines the neuroanatomic signature of chronic compressive myelopathy.[4,20]

Dynamic Compression and Biomechanics

In addition to the static and biological mechanisms described earlier, dynamic biomechanical injury is increasingly recognized as an important contributor to the pathogenesis of spinal cord compression. Repetitive flexion-extension at unstable or hypermobile motion segments may impose mechanical strain upon a cord already compromised by stenosis, generating microtrauma that is too subtle to be recognized as a discrete event but that accumulates over time.[25] Stretch-associated injury has been described as a complementary mechanism in cervical spondylotic myelopathy, in which longitudinal cord tension generated by altered alignment and dentate-ligament tethering acts in concert with focal compression to produce neurologic injury.[25] Kinematic and dynamic MRI studies have shown that flexion and extension can unmask cord compression that is occult on neutral imaging in a clinically meaningful proportion of symptomatic patients, supporting the inclusion of dynamic acquisition protocols in selected diagnostic workflows.[26,27] Moreover, recent quantitative research has demonstrated that the cord itself moves substantially during routine motion within the canal and that abnormalities of this motion correlate with disease severity in DCM.[28] Dynamic compression, therefore, reframes biomechanics not as a static geometric problem but as a time-varying mechanical input to a biologically active tissue.

PATHOPHYSIOLOGICAL PROGRESSION: BEYOND THE COMPRESSION EPICENTER

Local versus Global Spinal Cord Injury

Clinical and surgical attention has historically been focused on the maximally compressed level because that is where the lesion is mechanically most visible and surgically most actionable. Increasingly, however, neuroimaging and neuropathological evidence suggests that injury is not confined to the epicenter. Prior voxel-based analyses have demonstrated reductions in white matter, gray matter, and posterior column cross-sectional area above the level of stenosis in cervical spondylotic myelopathy, accompanied by reductions in fractional anisotropy in posterior columns and lateral corticospinal tracts.[29] Subsequent study tracking microstructural changes along the entire cord axis in DCM has shown that compromise can extend rostrally to the brainstem and caudally to the lumbosacral enlargement.[30,31] Importantly, our own unpublished morphometric analyses have revealed that, even outside the maximally compressed segment, patients with severe myelopathy demonstrate reductions in cross-sectional area, antero-posterior diameter, and right–left diameter relative to those with mild and moderate disease, a pattern consistent with global rather than purely focal cord involvement.

Remote Degeneration and Network Effects

These remote changes are best understood as a combination of Wallerian degeneration of axons disconnected from their cell bodies, trans-synaptic degeneration through compromised neural circuits, and secondary atrophy of supraspinal targets.[29–31] Brain imaging studies in DCM have demonstrated gray matter volume changes in primary motor and sensory cortices as well as in the corticospinal projection from the brainstem, paralleling the spinal findings and indicating that compressive disease produces network-level effects extending well beyond the cervical cord.[30,31] Functionally, these network changes may help to explain the persistence of disability after technically adequate decompression, the asymmetry between recovery of upper and lower extremity function, and the apparent ceiling on neurologic recovery in patients with long-standing severe disease. A patient with apparent single-level compression may, therefore, harbor an injury footprint that spans multiple cord segments and supraspinal networks, with implications for both clinical assessment and surgical expectation-setting.

Temporal Evolution of Injury

The biology of compression also evolves over time. Acute compression, encountered in traumatic injury, central cord syndrome, or rapid deterioration of pre-existing DCM, is dominated by hemorrhage, edema, and acute ischemic injury, and the molecular response is closely allied to that observed in traumatic spinal cord injury.[4,18,19] Chronic compression layers in fibrotic, gliotic, demyelinating, and atrophic changes that may stabilize, progress in a stepwise manner after subclinical events such as minor trauma, or decline continuously.[4,20] Natural history data suggest that 20% to 62% of conservatively managed patients with myelopathy deteriorate over 3 to 6 years, but precisely identifying which patients will deteriorate, and on what timeline, has remained elusive.[32]

Recent unpublished longitudinal data from the authors' group, examining serial T2-weighted morphometrics in patients with mild DCM enrolled in the ongoing Natural History of Mild Degenerative Cervical Myelopathy (NH-DCM) study, suggest that the rate of change of noncompressed cross-sectional area (CSA) differentiates conservatively managed patients who deteriorate from those who remain stable. In this analysis, deteriorating patients lost approximately 0.43 mm^2 per year remote from the main compression site ($P = .013$; Cohen's $d = -1.76$), whereas stable patients did not exhibit a measurable decline. This observation reinforces the idea that the biologically informative signal in compressive myelopathy is not confined to the lesion epicenter, and longitudinal change in remote cord regions may carry prognostic information that single-timepoint imaging fails to capture.

ADVANCES IN DIAGNOSIS: FROM QUALITATIVE IMAGING TO QUANTITATIVE BIOMARKERS

Clinical Assessment Limitations

Clinical staging in DCM continues to rely heavily on the mJOA score, the Nurick grade, and patient-reported instruments such as the NDI. The mJOA categorizes patients as having mild ($\geq$15), moderate (12–14), or severe ($\leq$11) disease, and these categories anchor current management guidelines.[11,33] However, these instruments suffer from well-recognized limitations, including ceiling effects in mild disease, insensitivity to early deterioration, observer dependence, modest reproducibility across cultural and language settings, and limited ability to discriminate between focal hand dysfunction and gait impairment of comparable severity.[10–13] Indeed, patients with mJOA scores of 17 or 18 may already harbor substantial cord injury that is detectable only on quantitative imaging, and the minimum clinically important difference (MCID) of approximately 1 point in mild disease leaves little dynamic range with which to track progression or response to treatment.[12] Such constraints limit the granularity with which traditional clinical instruments can describe the biology of compression and inform individualized care.

Conventional MRI: Strengths and Limitations

Conventional T2-weighted MRI is the universal standard for diagnosing cord compression and remains essential for surgical planning. Intramedullary T2 hyperintensity, canal narrowing, and visible cord deformation are reliably identifiable, and signal characteristics correlate broadly with clinical severity and surgical outcome.[5,34] However, conventional sequences encode tissue state qualitatively. They do not quantify microstructural integrity, do not differentiate edema from gliosis from demyelination, and provide limited insight into cord dynamics.[34] Multicenter analyses have further shown that MRI-defined compression severity is a strong driver of surgical decision-making despite a relatively weak correlation with clinical disease severity, underscoring the need for biomarkers that more directly reflect parenchymal injury.[6]

Dynamic MRI

Dynamic MRI, performed in flexion and extension or under axial load, addresses one of the principal blind spots of conventional imaging. A recent systematic review demonstrates that dynamic MRI consistently reveals cord compression that is occult on neutral imaging, redefines stenosis severity in a meaningful proportion of patients, and may alter surgical planning by identifying levels of motion-dependent contact that would otherwise be left unaddressed.[26] Comparative study has further shown that combining static and dynamic acquisitions improves the characterization of cervical myelopathy and may prompt reconsideration of the operative plan in selected patients.[27] Whether dynamic MRI should be incorporated into routine DCM workup remains debated; protocol heterogeneity, variable definitions of dynamic compression, and the risk of overcalling clinically irrelevant extension findings all argue for selective rather than indiscriminate use.[26,28] In practice, dynamic imaging is most informative when neutral MRI underestimates clinical severity, when symptoms are positional, or when surgical planning depends on understanding occult instability or motion-dependent contact.

Advanced Quantitative Imaging

Advanced quantitative MRI techniques offer biological resolution that conventional sequences cannot match. Diffusion tensor imaging (DTI) reflects axonal integrity and orientation, with reduced fractional anisotropy and increased radial diffusivity reported above and below sites of compression; recent systematic reviews and meta-analyses have confirmed its capacity to discriminate DCM from healthy controls and to track severity, although acquisition variability and the absence of harmonized thresholds continue to limit clinical adoption.[35,36] Magnetization transfer (MT) imaging probes macromolecular content, with MT ratio reductions tracking myelin loss; tract-specific MT measurements across dorsal, lateral, and ventral columns have recently been shown to provide insight into DCM severity beyond what is achievable with whole-cord measurement.[37] Myelin water imaging, which estimates the fraction of water trapped between myelin lamellae, provides a more specific index of myelination, although clinical translation remains in its early stages.[36] T2*-weighted sequences and gray-to-white matter signal ratio analyses provide complementary windows into compartment-specific injury.[38] Adoption of these techniques has been slowed by acquisition complexity, multivendor variability, and limited integration into routine workflows, although standardized acquisition protocols developed under international consortium efforts are beginning to address these barriers.[39]

Artificial Intelligence-driven Morphometrics and Radiomics

Morphometric features

A pragmatic and rapidly maturing alternative to advanced acquisition is the extraction of quantitative information from the T2-weighted images that are already obtained universally. Open-source pipelines, such as the Spinal Cord Toolbox, enable robust automated cord segmentation, vertebral level labeling, and measurement of geometric features at every level.[40] From these segmentations, morphometric features, cross-sectional area, antero-posterior and right-left diameters, eccentricity, solidity, and orientation, can be computed reproducibly. In our unpublished morphometric analysis of 350 patients with DCM drawn from the AO Spine North America and AO Spine International prospective cohorts,[41,42] severe myelopathy was associated with reductions in cross-sectional area, antero-posterior diameter, and right-left diameter at both compressed and noncompressed segments compared with mild and moderate disease, a finding consistent with the global cord involvement described earlier. Importantly, features extracted from outside the maximally compressed segment carried independent prognostic signal.

Radiomics

Radiomic feature extraction extends the morphometric approach by quantifying texture, shape, and first-order intensity descriptors that capture tissue heterogeneity invisible to the unaided eye. Standardized using the Image Biomarker Standardization Initiative (IBSI) framework and platforms such as PyRadiomics, radiomic features can be derived reproducibly from routine T2-weighted images and are well suited to multicenter aggregation.[43,44] In our complementary unpublished radiomics analysis of 204 patients drawn from the same multicenter prospective cohorts,[41,42] T2-weighted radiomic features extracted separately from compressed and noncompressed segments improved prediction of 1 year postoperative outcomes when added to clinical variables. Top-ranking features included gray-level co-occurrence matrix inverse variance, neighboring gray-tone difference matrix strength, root-mean-square intensity, elongation, and surface-to-volume ratio, which can be cautiously interpreted as imaging surrogates of tissue heterogeneity, demyelination, gliosis, edema, and remote degeneration.

Machine learning integration

When morphometric and radiomic features are integrated with clinical variables in supervised machine-learning models, modest but consistent gains in discrimination are observed across multiple outcomes. In our morphometric analysis, Extreme Gradient Boosting models combining clinical and morphometric features improved area under the curve (AUC) for the MCID in mJOA from approximately 0.70 to 0.76, and for SF-36 Physical Component Summary (PCS) improvement from approximately 0.75 to 0.77, compared with clinical-only models. In the parallel radiomics analysis, AUC for MCID in mJOA increased from 0.735 to 0.781 with combined clinical and all-radiomic features; AUC for 30% improvement in SF-36 PCS increased from 0.73 to 0.834 when compressed-segment radiomics were added (**Fig. 2**); and for a global composite outcome combining mJOA, SF-36 PCS, and NDI, regression performance improved from R^2 of 0.103 to 0.414 when noncompressed radiomic features were incorporated (see **Fig. 2**).

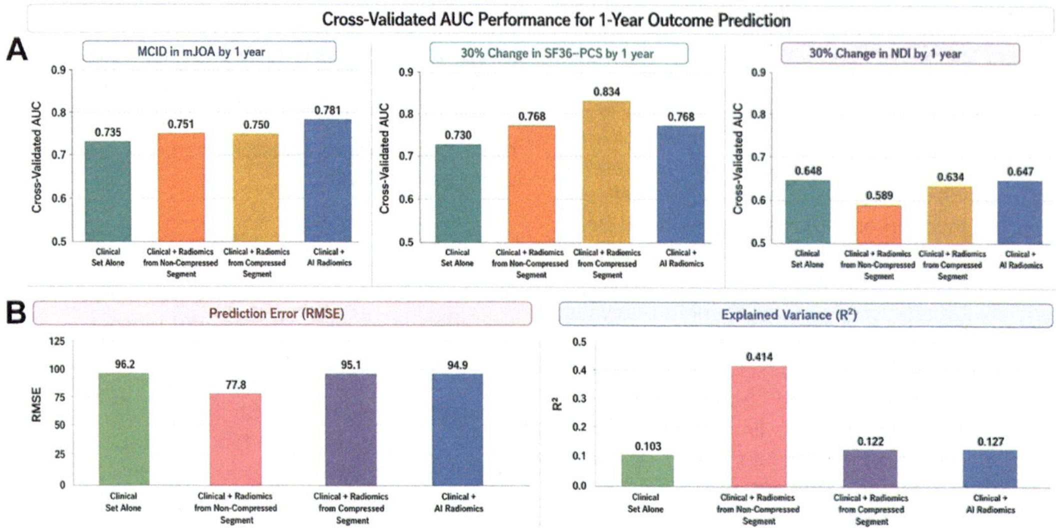

Fig. 2. Predictive performance of clinical and radiomic models for 1 year postoperative outcomes in degenerative cervical myelopathy. (*A*) Cross-validated area under the receiver operating characteristic curve (AUC) for models predicting achievement of minimum clinically important difference (MCID) in modified Japanese Orthopedic Association score (mJOA), 30% or greater improvement in SF-36 Physical Component Summary (SF36-PCS), and 30% or greater improvement in Neck Disability Index (NDI) at 1 year after surgery. Four predictor sets were compared: baseline clinical variables alone, clinical variables plus radiomics from the noncompressed spinal cord segment, clinical variables plus radiomics from the compressed segment, and clinical variables plus radiomics from both segments. (*B*) Prediction error and explained variance for the continuous global outcome score, summarized using root mean squared error (RMSE) and coefficient of determination (R^2). Higher AUC and R^2 values indicate better predictive performance, whereas lower RMSE indicates lower prediction error. Radiomic features were extracted from baseline T2-weighted MRI and added to routinely available clinical predictors to assess whether quantitative imaging biomarkers improved prognostication beyond clinical data alone.

Methodologically, however, machine-learning models can overfit small datasets, and reported performance can be inflated by information leakage, feature selection performed outside the training fold, or the absence of external validation; clinically useful models must demonstrate discrimination, calibration, decision-curve utility, fairness across demographic groups, robustness to scanner differences, and interpretability sufficient for shared decision-making.[45] **Table 2** summarizes recently identified quantitative imaging biomarkers for spinal cord compression and DCM.

PROGNOSTICATION: TOWARD PRECISION MEDICINE IN SPINAL CORD COMPRESSION

Traditional Prognostic Factors

Traditional prognostic factors in DCM include older age, longer symptom duration, higher baseline severity, presence and intensity of T2 hyperintensity, smoking, and selected comorbidities such as diabetes mellitus and psychiatric illness.[46,47] Tetreault and colleagues,[46,47] leveraging data from the AO Spine North America and AO Spine International prospective cohorts, derived clinical prediction models in which baseline mJOA, age, smoking status, and gait impairment ranked among the most important predictors of postoperative recovery; in those analyses, imaging variables did not enter the final model. T2 signal abnormalities, including focal hyperintensity and the ratio of T1 hypointensity to T2 hyperintensity, have been shown to correlate with severity and to portend poorer recovery, although the strength of this association varies across cohorts and outcome measures.[5,34]

Limitations of Linear Prognostic Models

These factors are modestly predictive at the group level but disappointing at the individual level. Linear and logistic models built upon these variables struggle with nonlinear interactions, missing data, and the inherent heterogeneity of DCM phenotypes, while their generalizability across populations and health care systems is uncertain.[46–48] As clinical prediction tools, they remain useful but inadequate for the granular, individualized counseling that contemporary practice demands. Indeed, the temporal evolution of compressive

Table 2
Emerging quantitative biomarkers in spinal cord compression and degenerative cervical myelopathy

Modality	Biological Signal Captured	Readiness for Clinical Use	Key Limitations
Dynamic MRI (flexion-extension)	Motion-dependent compression and instability	Available; selective use	Protocol heterogeneity; risk of overcalling clinically irrelevant findings
DTI	Axonal integrity and orientation; tract-specific microstructure	Research and selected clinical centers	Acquisition variability; lack of harmonized thresholds
MT	Macromolecular and myelin content	Research	Vendor variability; specialized acquisition
Myelin water imaging	Myelin fraction	Early research	Acquisition complexity; limited clinical translation
Automated morphometrics (Spinal Cord Toolbox)	CSA, AP/RL diameters, eccentricity, solidity at compressed and noncompressed segments	Translation-ready; pipeline available	Quality control across scanners; need for normalization
Radiomics (PyRadiomics, IBSI-compliant)	Texture, shape, and intensity heterogeneity reflecting tissue microstructure	Translation-ready in research workflows	Sensitivity to acquisition; risk of overfitting in small samples
Machine learning integration	Multimodal prediction of MCID in mJOA, NDI, SF-36, and surgical conversion	Research; awaiting prospective validation	External validation, calibration, fairness, and interpretability
Longitudinal trajectory biomarkers (eg, noncompressed CSA Δ/y)	Rate of remote cord atrophy as marker of progression	Emerging from prospective cohorts	Requires serial standardized imaging; longer follow-up

disease, with its propensity for stepwise progression and remote injury, is poorly captured by single-snapshot models that do not incorporate longitudinal change.[32]

Predictive Modeling and Machine Learning

Machine learning offers a more flexible analytical framework. Supervised models can integrate clinical, demographic, imaging, electrophysiological, and longitudinal data; capture nonlinear interactions between predictors; and tolerate the missingness that pervades real-world cohorts.[45,48] Recent research using gradient-boosted classifiers and unsupervised clustering approaches has identified clinically meaningful DCM phenotypes with distinct profiles and divergent long-term functional and neurologic outcomes, supporting the use of data-driven stratification in routine prognostic assessment.[49] The morphometric and radiomic models summarized earlier add an imaging biomarker layer to these efforts and demonstrate measurable gains in discrimination over clinical-only models for some, though not all, outcomes.

Unpublished Work Integration: Toward Trajectory-based Prediction

A complementary insight has emerged from longitudinal analyses in mild DCM. Whereas baseline T2-weighted morphometrics are largely indistinguishable between patients who will deteriorate and those who will remain stable, the rate of change of these metrics, particularly in the noncompressed cord, can be informative. In our exploratory support vector classifier trained on T2-weighted imaging features in 41 patients with mild DCM followed prospectively in the NH-DCM study, longitudinal features achieved an AUC of 0.762 for predicting surgical conversion, compared with 0.638 for a clinical-only model; this finding did not reach significance owing to the small sample size and event count. Cross-sectional comparison of conservatively managed NH-DCM patients with surgically managed mild patients from the AO Spine cohorts further demonstrated that surgical patients had approximately twice the MSCC ratio at the compression site and a greater number of compressed levels, while noncompressed cord measurements were structurally comparable, suggesting that compression-site burden, rather than global cord morphology at baseline, is the principal initial discriminator of management.

The implication of these data is that the future of prognostication in compressive disease is likely to depend less upon a single baseline snapshot and more upon the trajectory.[32] The prognostic shift from snapshot to trajectory aligns naturally with a precision-medicine framework in which individualized timing of intervention replaces fixed thresholds derived from population averages.[16]

EVOLVING TREATMENT PARADIGMS

Traditional Approach

Surgical decompression remains the standard of care for moderate and severe DCM, as well as for patients with progressive neurologic deterioration; large prospective multicenter studies have confirmed that decompression improves neurologic function, disability, and quality of life across the severity spectrum.[41,50] The 2017 AO Spine clinical practice guideline endorsed surgery for moderate and severe DCM and offered conditional recommendations for mild DCM and for nonmyelopathic patients with cord compression and corticospinal signs[33]; the 2025 AO Spine clinical practice recommendations have updated and refined these positions in light of accumulating evidence on natural history, surgical risk, and patient-reported outcomes.[51] In mild DCM, however, the optimal management strategy continues to be debated, with reasonable arguments on both sides supported by patients who deteriorate during observation and patients who remain stable for years.[52]

The phrase "time is spine," originally articulated in the context of acute traumatic spinal cord injury, where early decompression within 24 hours has been associated with improved AIS-grade conversion and shorter rehabilitation, has been increasingly extended to DCM.[53,54] Emerging evidence suggests that earlier intervention in DCM may protect against cumulative ischemic, inflammatory, and neurodegenerative injury, although the supporting evidence base remains less mature than in traumatic injury.[55]

Personalized Surgical Decision-making

If timing is biologically variable, then personalization is essential. The combination of imaging biomarkers, machine-learning predictions, and patient-specific clinical factors provides a route toward individualized risk stratification. Rapidly progressing patients can be identified for earlier intervention, whereas stable patients may be safely observed with structured surveillance.[16,49] Tools that integrate noncompressed CSA trajectory, radiomic phenotype, electrophysiological deterioration, and clinical risk factors are beginning to take shape, though prospective validation is still required. A practical precision-medicine workflow is necessarily sequential: confirmation of clinical myelopathy and exclusion of mimics; characterization of the anatomic compression as static, dynamic, focal, or multilevel; assessment of biological cord injury through signal change, atrophy, microstructural metrics, and radiomic features; longitudinal evaluation of stability versus progression; and integration with patient-specific goals, frailty, comorbidity, and surgical risk. A proposed workflow for the development and application of radiomics-derived prognostic biomarkers is shown in **Fig. 3**.

Emerging Therapeutic Concepts

Beyond decompression, the therapeutic landscape is expanding in directions that align with the multifactorial pathobiology of compression. Riluzole, a sodium-channel blocker with antiexcitotoxic properties, has been evaluated as a perioperative adjunct in the CSM-Protect randomized phase 3 trial; the primary analysis did not show significant improvement in functional recovery beyond decompressive surgery, but the trial established feasibility and provided important methodological lessons for the field.[56] In acute traumatic injury, the RISCIS trial offers a parallel example: riluzole has biological plausibility and signals in selected analyses, but definitive adoption requires careful interpretation of trial design, endpoints, and subgroups.[57] Pharmacologic adjuncts targeting BSCB integrity, neuroinflammation, microglial polarization, and excitotoxicity are under active investigation, and regenerative approaches including cell-based therapies, biomaterial scaffolds, and neuromodulation are being tested in carefully selected trauma and chronic compression cohorts; representing the long-term horizon of the field.[58,59] In each case, clinical success will depend on identifying the right patients at the right biological stage, and biomarker-enriched trials will likely be necessary to demonstrate benefit. A neuroprotective agent is unlikely to show effect if enrolled patients already harbor irreversible tissue loss, if the outcome measure is insensitive

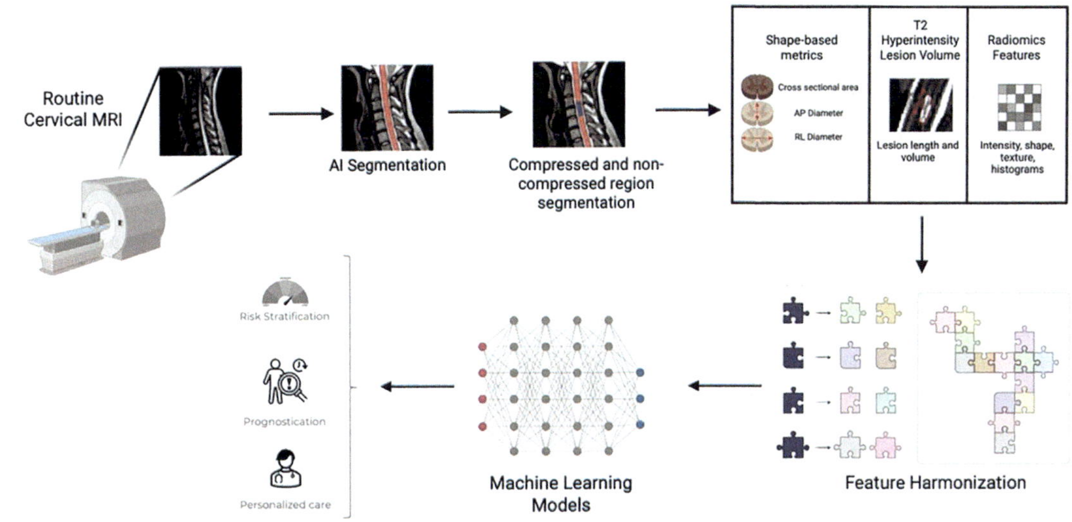

Fig. 3. Proposed AI-radiomics workflow for degenerative cervical myelopathy biomarker development. Routine clinical cervical MRI can be used as the input for automated or semiautomated spinal cord segmentation, allowing separation of compressed and noncompressed cord segments. Quantitative imaging biomarkers may then be extracted across complementary domains, including shape-based morphometric metrics such as cross-sectional area, antero-posterior diameter, and right–left diameter; T2-hyperintensity lesion metrics such as lesion length, lesion volume, and axial damage ratio; and high-dimensional radiomic features describing image intensity, shape, texture, and histogram-based characteristics. After feature harmonization to reduce scanner-related and acquisition-related variability, these imaging features can be integrated with clinical data in machine-learning models to support individualized prognostication, risk stratification, and selection of therapeutic pathways in degenerative cervical myelopathy. (*Created in* BioRender. Lab, F. (2026) https://BioRender.com/ob5af22.)

to subtle preservation, or if the biological target is not present in the study population.

FUTURE DIRECTIONS AND KNOWLEDGE GAPS

Realizing the promise of precision medicine in spinal cord compression will require coordinated progress on several fronts. Imaging acquisition protocols must be standardized across vendors and centers so that quantitative biomarkers are comparable across institutions; the spinal cord MRI generic protocol provides a foundation but has yet to achieve universal adoption.[39] Machine-learning models, including the morphometric and radiomic approaches described earlier, must be prospectively validated in independent multicenter datasets and tested for fairness across demographic subgroups before clinical deployment.[45] Implementation studies must address how AI-derived risk scores integrate with clinical decision-making, the user interface, the medicolegal framework, and the lived experience of patients and surgeons. Longitudinal datasets remain a particular priority. Cross-sectional associations can identify candidate biomarkers, but clinical decisions depend on prediction. Mild DCM, in particular, requires repeated clinical and imaging assessment to identify early deterioration, distinguish stable from progressive disease, and define clinically meaningful imaging change—a problem that the trajectory-based morphometric data described in this article are intended to inform. Fluid biomarkers, including cerebrospinal fluid and serum markers of inflammation, glial activation, axonal injury, and BSCB integrity, are likely to add additional biological dimensions; a recent systematic review and meta-analysis has summarized current evidence in DCM, although DCM-specific validation remains limited.[60]

Ethical and equity considerations are also important. Predictive models trained on cohorts from high-resource settings may not generalize to global populations and may inadvertently encode existing disparities in access to imaging and surgery. Bridging the gap between research-grade imaging analysis and bedside use will require investment in automation, quality control, regulatory pathways, and clinician training.

SUMMARY

Spinal cord compression has outgrown its origins as a static, mechanical concept. It is dynamic in time, multifactorial in mechanism, and systemic in distribution. Mechanical narrowing initiates a cascade that includes ischemia, BSCB disruption, neuroinflammation, demyelination, and remote degeneration; this cascade unfolds over years and extends well beyond the maximally compressed segment. Diagnostic tools are moving from qualitative MRI and ordinal clinical scales toward quantitative MRI, dynamic MRI, automated morphometrics, radiomics, and machine-learning models that capture this complexity. Prognostic thinking is shifting from group-level averages to individualized trajectories, and from snapshot assessment to longitudinal monitoring. Surgical decision-making is evolving from binary decompression-versus-observation toward precision risk management informed by biological readouts. The future of the field lies in precision, personalization, and prediction—in matching the right biological intervention to the right patient at the right biological moment in the natural history of disease.

CLINICS CARE POINTS

- Spinal cord compression should be conceptualized and discussed with patients as a dynamic biological process rather than as a fixed mechanical lesion; this framing supports more accurate counseling regarding heterogeneous progression and recovery trajectories.
- Conventional T2-weighted MRI is necessary but insufficient for prognostication; the absence of frank cord compression on a single imaging study does not exclude DCM, and the presence of severe compression does not mandate immediate surgery in the absence of clinical or biological deterioration.
- Dynamic MRI in flexion and extension should be considered when neutral imaging underestimates clinical severity, when symptoms are positional, or when surgical planning depends on identifying motion-dependent compression that is occult on standard sequences.
- In mild DCM, baseline imaging and clinical metrics alone are limited in their ability to identify patients at risk of deterioration; serial assessment with attention to noncompressed cord cross-sectional area and other quantitative features is increasingly informative and supports structured surveillance protocols.
- Quantitative morphometric and radiomic features extracted from routine T2-weighted MRI, when integrated with clinical variables in machine-learning models, can modestly but meaningfully improve prediction of postoperative outcomes; these tools should be regarded as decision-support adjuncts rather than replacements for clinical judgment.
- Surgical decompression remains the standard of care for moderate and severe disease and for progressive deterioration, but the optimal management of mild DCM requires individualized assessment that integrates anatomic, biological, and longitudinal information rather than relying on isolated mJOA thresholds.
- Emerging neuroprotective and regenerative adjuncts will require careful patient selection, biomarker-enriched trial designs, and outcome measures sensitive to the biological substrate that each therapy targets.

DECLARATION OF ARTIFICIAL INTELLIGENCE AND ARTIFICIAL INTELLIGENCE-ASSISTED TECHNOLOGIES IN THE WRITING PROCESS

During the preparation of this article, the authors used ChatGPT to enhance clarity of the text. After using this tool/service, the authors reviewed and edited the content as needed and take full responsibility for the content of the publication.

DISCLOSURE

M.G. Fehlings wishes to acknowledge support from the Robert Campeau Family Foundation/Dr C.H. Tator Chair in Brain and Spinal Cord Research at UHN.

REFERENCES

1. Nouri A, Tetreault L, Singh A, et al. Degenerative cervical myelopathy: epidemiology, genetics, and pathogenesis. Spine 2015;40(12):E675–93.
2. Tetreault L, Goldstein CL, Arnold P, et al. Degenerative cervical myelopathy: a spectrum of related disorders affecting the aging spine. Neurosurgery 2015;77(Suppl 4):S51–67.
3. Baptiste DC, Fehlings MG. Pathophysiology of cervical myelopathy. Spine J 2006;6(6 Suppl):190S–7S.
4. Karadimas SK, Erwin WM, Ely CG, et al. Pathophysiology and natural history of cervical spondylotic myelopathy. Spine 2013;38(22 Suppl 1):S21–36.
5. Nouri A, Martin AR, Kato S, et al. The relationship between MRI signal intensity changes, clinical presentation, and surgical outcome in degenerative cervical myelopathy: analysis of a global cohort. Spine 2017;42(24):1851–8.
6. Hilton B, Tempest-Mitchell J, Davies BM, et al. Cord compression defined by MRI is the driving factor behind the decision to operate in degenerative cervical myelopathy despite poor correlation

with disease severity. PLoS One 2019;14(12):e0226020.
7. Thompson K, Travers H, Ngan A, et al. Updates in current concepts in degenerative cervical myelopathy: a systematic review. J Spine Surg 2024;10(2):313–26.
8. Badhiwala JH, Ahuja CS, Akbar MA, et al. Degenerative cervical myelopathy - update and future directions. Nat Rev Neurol 2020;16(2):108–24.
9. Wilson JRF, Badhiwala JH, Moghaddamjou A, et al. Degenerative cervical myelopathy; A review of the latest advances and future directions in management. Neurospine 2019;16(3):494–505.
10. Smith SS, Stewart ME, Davies BM, et al. The prevalence of asymptomatic and symptomatic spinal cord compression on magnetic resonance imaging: a systematic review and meta-analysis. Glob Spine J 2021;11(4):597–607.
11. Tetreault L, Kopjar B, Nouri A, et al. The modified Japanese orthopaedic association scale: establishing criteria for mild, moderate and severe impairment in patients with degenerative cervical myelopathy. Eur Spine J 2017;26(1):78–84.
12. Kopjar B, Tetreault L, Kalsi-Ryan S, et al. Psychometric properties of the modified Japanese orthopaedic association scale in patients with cervical spondylotic myelopathy. Spine 2015;40(1):E23–8.
13. Treanor C, Gallagher C, Lenehan W, et al. Flipping the mJOA: clinical utility of the modified Japanese orthopaedic association score as a tool for detecting degenerative cervical myelopathy. Brain Spine 2024;4:102853.
14. Davies BM, Kwon BK, Fehlings MG, et al. AO spine RECODE-DCM: why prioritize research in degenerative cervical myelopathy? Glob Spine J 2022;12(1 Suppl):5S–7S.
15. Davies BM, Mowforth O, Wood H, et al. Improving awareness could transform outcomes in degenerative cervical myelopathy [AO spine RECODE-DCM research priority number 1]. Glob Spine J 2022;12(1_suppl):28S–38S.
16. Al-Shawwa A, Cadotte DW. Advancing precision medicine in degenerative cervical myelopathy. J Clin Med 2025;14(23):8344.
17. Fehlings MG, Rao SC, Tator CH, et al. The optimal radiologic method for assessing spinal canal compromise and cord compression in patients with cervical spinal cord injury. Part II: results of a multicenter study. Spine 1999;24(6):605–13.
18. Tator CH, Fehlings MG. Review of the secondary injury theory of acute spinal cord trauma with emphasis on vascular mechanisms. J Neurosurg 1991;75(1):15–26.
19. Akter F, Yu X, Qin X, et al. The pathophysiology of degenerative cervical myelopathy and the physiology of recovery following decompression. Front Neurosci 2020;14:138.
20. Dohle E, Beardall S, Chang A, et al. Human spinal cord tissue is an underutilised resource in degenerative cervical myelopathy: findings from a systematic review of human autopsies. Acta Neurochir 2023;165(5):1121–31.
21. Kim HW, Yong H, Shea GKH. Blood-spinal cord barrier disruption in degenerative cervical myelopathy. Fluids Barriers CNS 2023;20(1):68.
22. Schmidt TP, Jütten K, Bertram U, et al. Blood spinal cord barrier disruption recovers in patients with degenerative cervical myelopathy after surgical decompression: a prospective cohort study. Sci Rep 2023;13(1):7389.
23. Tu J, Vargas Castillo J, Das A, et al. Degenerative cervical myelopathy: insights into its pathobiology and molecular mechanisms. J Clin Med 2021;10(6):1214.
24. Yu WR, Liu T, Kiehl TR, et al. Human neuropathological and animal model evidence supporting a role for Fas-mediated apoptosis and inflammation in cervical spondylotic myelopathy. Brain 2011;134(Pt 5):1277–92.
25. Henderson FC, Geddes JF, Vaccaro AR, et al. Stretch-associated injury in cervical spondylotic myelopathy: new concept and review. Neurosurgery 2005;56(5):1101–13 [discussion: 1101–113].
26. Baram A, El Choueiri J, Brembilla C, et al. Dynamic MRI in degenerative cervical myelopathy: a systematic review of radiological markers, correlations, and outcomes. J Clin Med 2025;15(1):265.
27. Nigro L, Donnarumma P, Tarantino R, et al. Static and dynamic cervical MRI: two useful exams in cervical myelopathy. J Spine Surg 2017;3(2):212–6.
28. Hupp M, Pfender N, Vallotton K, et al. The restless spinal cord in degenerative cervical myelopathy. AJNR Am J Neuroradiol 2021;42(3):597–609.
29. Grabher P, Mohammadi S, Trachsler A, et al. Voxel-based analysis of grey and white matter degeneration in cervical spondylotic myelopathy. Sci Rep 2016;6(1):24636.
30. Vallotton K, David G, Hupp M, et al. Tracking white and gray matter degeneration along the spinal cord axis in degenerative cervical myelopathy. J Neurotrauma 2021;38(21):2978–87.
31. David G, Vallotton K, Hupp M, et al. Extent of cord pathology in the Lumbosacral enlargement in non-traumatic versus traumatic spinal cord injury. J Neurotrauma 2022;39(9–10):639–50.
32. Tetreault LA, Karadimas S, Wilson JR, et al. The natural history of degenerative cervical myelopathy and the rate of hospitalization following spinal cord injury: an updated systematic review. Glob Spine J 2017;7(3 Suppl):28S–34S.
33. Fehlings MG, Tetreault LA, Riew KD, et al. A clinical practice guideline for the management of degenerative cervical myelopathy: introduction, rationale, and scope. Glob Spine J 2017;7(3 Suppl):21S–7S.

34. Tetreault LA, Dettori JR, Wilson JR, et al. Systematic review of magnetic resonance imaging characteristics that affect treatment decision making and predict clinical outcome in patients with cervical spondylotic myelopathy. Spine 2013;38(22 Suppl 1):S89–110.
35. Mohammadi M, Roohollahi F, Farahbakhsh F, et al. Diffusion tensor imaging in diagnosing and evaluating degenerative cervical myelopathy: a systematic review and meta-analysis. Glob Spine J 2025; 15(1):267–83.
36. Martin AR, Aleksanderek I, Cohen-Adad J, et al. Translating state-of-the-art spinal cord MRI techniques to clinical use: a systematic review of clinical studies utilizing DTI, MT, MWF, MRS, and fMRI. Neuroimage, Clin 2016;10:192–238.
37. Haynes G, Muhammad F, Weber KA, et al. Tract-specific magnetization transfer ratio provides insights into the severity of degenerative cervical myelopathy. Spinal Cord 2024;62(12):700–7.
38. Martin AR, De Leener B, Cohen-Adad J, et al. Clinically feasible microstructural MRI to quantify cervical spinal cord tissue injury using DTI, MT, and T2*-Weighted imaging: assessment of normative data and reliability. AJNR Am J Neuroradiol 2017; 38(6):1257–65.
39. Cohen-Adad J, Alonso-Ortiz E, Abramovic M, et al. Generic acquisition protocol for quantitative MRI of the spinal cord. Nat Protoc 2021;16(10):4611–32.
40. De Leener B, Lévy S, Dupont SM, et al. SCT: spinal cord toolbox, an open-source software for processing spinal cord MRI data. Neuroimage 2017;145(Pt A):24–43.
41. Fehlings MG, Ibrahim A, Tetreault L, et al. A global perspective on the outcomes of surgical decompression in patients with cervical spondylotic myelopathy: results from the prospective multicenter AOSpine international study on 479 patients. Spine 2015;40(17):1322–8.
42. Fehlings MG, Barry S, Kopjar B, et al. Anterior versus posterior surgical approaches to treat cervical spondylotic myelopathy: outcomes of the prospective multicenter AOSpine North America CSM study in 264 patients. Spine 2013;38(26):2247–52.
43. Zwanenburg A, Vallières M, Abdalah MA, et al. The image biomarker standardization initiative: standardized quantitative radiomics for high-throughput image-based phenotyping. Radiology 2020;295(2): 328–38.
44. van Griethuysen JJM, Fedorov A, Parmar C, et al. Computational radiomics system to decode the radiographic phenotype. Cancer Res 2017;77(21): e104–7.
45. Lee S, Jung JY, Mahatthanatrakul A, et al. Artificial intelligence in spinal imaging and patient care: a review of recent advances. Neurospine 2024;21(2): 474–86.
46. Tetreault LA, Kopjar B, Vaccaro A, et al. A clinical prediction model to determine outcomes in patients with cervical spondylotic myelopathy undergoing surgical treatment: data from the prospective, multi-center AOSpine North America study. J Bone Joint Surg Am 2013;95(18):1659–66.
47. Tetreault LA, Côté P, Kopjar B, et al, AOSpine North America and International Clinical Trial Research Network. A clinical prediction model to assess surgical outcome in patients with cervical spondylotic myelopathy: internal and external validations using the prospective multicenter AOSpine north American and international datasets of 743 patients. Spine J 2015;15(3):388–97.
48. Merali ZG, Witiw CD, Badhiwala JH, et al. Using a machine learning approach to predict outcome after surgery for degenerative cervical myelopathy. PLoS One 2019;14(4):e0215133.
49. Pedro KM, Alvi MA, Hejrati N, et al. Machine learning-based cluster analysis identifies four unique phenotypes of patients with degenerative cervical myelopathy with distinct clinical profiles and long-term functional and neurological outcomes. EBioMedicine 2024;106:105226.
50. Fehlings MG, Wilson JR, Kopjar B, et al. Efficacy and safety of surgical decompression in patients with cervical spondylotic myelopathy: results of the AOSpine North America prospective multi-center study. J Bone Joint Surg Am 2013;95(18):1651–8.
51. Fehlings MG, Evaniew N, Ter Wengel PV, et al. AO spine clinical practice recommendations for diagnosis and management of degenerative cervical myelopathy: evidence based decision making - a review of cutting edge recent literature related to degenerative cervical myelopathy. Glob Spine J 2025;15(5):2585–93.
52. Rhee J, Tetreault LA, Chapman JR, et al. Nonoperative versus operative management for the treatment degenerative cervical myelopathy: an updated systematic review. Glob Spine J 2017;7(3 Suppl):35S–41S.
53. Badhiwala JH, Ahuja CS, Fehlings MG. Time is spine: a review of translational advances in spinal cord injury. J Neurosurg Spine 2019;30(1):1–18.
54. Fehlings MG, Vaccaro A, Wilson JR, et al. Early versus delayed decompression for traumatic cervical spinal cord injury: results of the surgical timing in acute spinal cord injury study (STASCIS). PLoS One 2012;7(2):e32037.
55. Fasinella MR, Benato A, Creatura D, et al. Degenerative cervical myelopathy: timing of surgery. EFORT Open Rev 2025;10(6):403–15.
56. Fehlings MG, Badhiwala JH, Ahn H, et al. Safety and efficacy of riluzole in patients undergoing decompressive surgery for degenerative cervical myelopathy (CSM-Protect): a multicentre, double-blind, placebo-controlled, randomised, phase 3 trial. Lancet Neurol 2021;20(2):98–106.

57. Fehlings MG, Moghaddamjou A, Harrop JS, et al. Safety and efficacy of riluzole in acute spinal cord injury study (RISCIS): a multi-center, randomized, placebo-controlled, double-blinded trial. J Neurotrauma 2023; 40(17–18):1878–88.
58. Fehlings MG, Honda S, Vajkoczy P, et al. Emerging advances in spinal cord injury: an introductory overview. Brain Spine 2025;5:104307.
59. Alvi MA, Pedro KM, Quddusi AI, et al. Advances and challenges in spinal cord injury treatments. J Clin Med 2024;13(14):4101.
60. Arora H, Darabi H, Wolsh CC, et al. Assessment of cerebrospinal fluid and blood-based biomarkers in degenerative cervical myelopathy: systematic review and meta-analysis. Glob Spine J 2026;16(3): 1619–32.

Epidemiology of Traumatic and Nontraumatic Spinal Cord Injury

Impact of Demographic Changes and Regional Differences

Narihito Nagoshi, MD, PhD

KEYWORDS

• Spinal cord injury • Epidemiology • Aging population • Nontraumatic SCI • Regional differences

KEY POINTS

- The epidemiology of spinal cord injury (SCI) is shifting globally, with a growing proportion of nontraumatic SCI (NTSCI) driven by population aging.
- Falls have become the leading cause of SCI in many high-income countries, replacing road traffic injuries.
- NTSCI is frequently underdiagnosed due to its insidious onset, highlighting the importance of early detection of degenerative and neoplastic conditions.
- Early surgical decompression within 24 hours is associated with improved neurologic outcomes in acute SCI.
- Region-specific prevention strategies and data-driven health care planning are essential to address the increasing global burden of SCI.

INTRODUCTION

Spinal cord injury (SCI) is broadly classified based on its cause into traumatic (TSCI) and nontraumatic (NTSCI). TSCI is defined as an acute injury to the spinal cord resulting from abrupt mechanical trauma, including traffic collisions, accidental falls, sports-related trauma, or violent incidents. In contrast, NTSCI denotes a condition in which the spinal cord is gradually damaged by nontraumatic pathologies, including spinal tumors, infections, and degenerative cervical myelopathy—such as cervical spondylotic myelopathy (CSM) or ossification of the posterior longitudinal ligament (OPLL)—as well as vascular disorders (**Fig. 1**). Both types result in permanent motor and sensory deficits and can lead to secondary complications like pressure ulcers, respiratory and cardiovascular issues, and psychological problems, causing life-long severe disability and high health care costs.[1] Thus, understanding the epidemiology of TSCI and NTSCI is essential for devising prevention strategies, planning health care resources and systems, and optimizing patient outcomes.

Epidemiologically, TSCI and NTSCI exhibit distinct characteristics, and their profiles have changed markedly in recent years.[2–7] Historically, prevention efforts have focused on the more visible causes of TSCI, such as road traffic injuries; however, with population aging and the increasing burden of chronic diseases, the relative importance of NTSCI has grown across many regions (**Table 1**). Accordingly, this review addresses global incidence trends, sex differences, regional variations, the rising prevalence of NTSCI in aging

Department of Orthopaedic Surgery, Keio University School of Medicine, 35 Shinanomachi, Shinjuku-ku, Tokyo 160-8582, Japan
E-mail address: nagoshi@keio.jp

Neurosurg Clin N Am 37 (2026) 469–478
https://doi.org/10.1016/j.nec.2026.05.001

Abbreviations

CSM	cervical spondylotic myelopathy
HICs	high-income countries
HIV	human immunodeficiency virus
LMICs	low-income and middle-income countries
NTSCI	nontraumatic SCI
OPLL	ossification of the posterior longitudinal ligament
SCI	spinal cord injury
TB	tuberculosis
TSCI	traumatic SCI

Table 1
Epidemiologic shift in spinal cord injury across aging societies

	Past	Present
Age group	Younger adults	Older adults
Etiology	High-energy trauma	Low-energy falls Degenerative conditions
Epidemiology	TSCI-dominant	Increasing NTSCI

societies, and the increasing contribution of falls among older adults. Finally, we discuss the public health and clinical implications of these shifts, ranging from prevention to early diagnosis and personalized rehabilitation. An integrated summary of the epidemiologic and clinical characteristics of SCI is presented in **Table 2**.

INCIDENCE

The global incidence of SCI remains substantial. A 2024 meta-analysis estimated the pooled worldwide incidence at approximately 23.8 cases per million population per year.[8] Based on available data, the pooled incidence of TSCI was 26.5 cases per million, whereas the pooled incidence of NTSCI was 17.9 cases per million.

Since 2000, the annual incidence of TSCI has remained consistently high but relatively stable, generally ranging between 20 and 45 cases per million population per year.[8] In contrast, year-based analyses in the same meta-analysis suggested that NTSCI incidence increased after 2007 and subsequently stabilized at approximately 25 to 35 cases per million population per year in many regions.[8] This epidemiologic shift reflects the growing contribution of nontraumatic etiologies to the overall burden of SCI.

POPULATION DEMOGRAPHICS

One prominent trend since 2000 has been the aging of the SCI patient population. Several countries have reported that the average age at the time of injury has increased by over 10 years in the past few decades.[9–12] For example, in the United States, the mean age at injury for TSCI rose from about 41 years in the 1990s to about 51 years in the early 2010s,[9] and in Europe, recent cohorts have shown median ages at injury in the 50s to 60s.[10–12] The proportion of new SCI cases occurring in older adults (65 years and above) has also increased, with the United States seeing the share of SCI in seniors more than double from the late 1990s to the early 2010s.[9] A study in Ontario, Canada, found that SCI incidence among older women increased at an average rate of 4.3% per year,[7] suggesting an increasing vulnerability in the elderly. Many of these injuries in older individuals are caused by falls and often result in incomplete cervical cord injuries.[13]

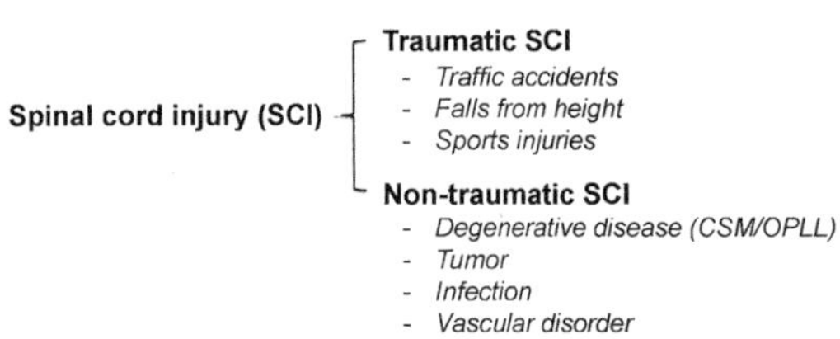

Fig. 1. Classification of traumatic and nontraumatic spinal cord injury.

Older patients with SCI experience substantially worse early and long-term survival compared with younger individuals. Specifically, patients aged 65 years or older have an approximately 6 fold higher risk of death following injury than younger adults, and more than double the mortality risk compared with age-matched, sex-matched, and comorbidity-matched noninjured controls.[7] In addition, older individuals with SCI have higher rates of hospital readmission and greater health care utilization. These demographic shifts highlight the need for prevention strategies specifically focused on older adults—especially fall prevention—as well as for medical management approaches adapted to the unique needs of the aging SCI population.

TSCI has traditionally been more common in male individuals, with the incidence of SCI consistently higher in men than in women worldwide.[3] Young men have long been the highest risk group due to greater exposure to high-energy trauma (vehicle operation, contact sports, and military service). However, with the rise in SCI among older adults, the sex disparity is narrowing in the higher age brackets. NTSCI shows an even smaller gender gap, with a male-to-female ratio on the order of 1.3 to 1.5:1.[14,15] This trend suggests that the

Table 2
Integrated framework of epidemiology and management in spinal cord injury

Domain	TSCI	NTSCI	Clinical Implications
Typical population	Younger individuals	Older individuals	Aging shifts burden toward NTSCI
Main causes	Traffic accidents and high-energy trauma	Degenerative disease, tumor, and infection	Etiology-specific prevention required
Temporal trend	Relatively stable incidence	Increasing proportion globally	Changing health care demand
Onset	Sudden	Gradual, often delayed diagnosis	Need for early detection systems
Acute management	Emergency stabilization and early decompression	Urgent imaging and etiology-specific treatment	Early diagnosis and timely intervention are critical
Prevention	Road safety and occupational safety	Early diagnosis and infection control	Region-specific strategies essential
Long-term care	Rehabilitation and complication prevention	Chronic disease management	Integrated care models required

increasing contribution of causes with less pronounced sex differences (ie, NTSCI) is gradually attenuating the overall gender gap in SCI. Nevertheless, male individuals remain at higher risk in nearly every age group, and prevention efforts should continue to focus on risk behaviors that are more common in men.[3]

REGIONAL DIFFERENCES

The epidemiology of SCI varies greatly by region and socioeconomic context. According to a 2024 systematic review, reported SCI incidence rates range widely from about 7 to 152 cases per million population per year in different regions.[8] In general, low-income and middle-income countries (LMICs) tend to have higher reported TSCI incidence than high-income countries (HICs).[16,17] Regions where multiple risk factors coincide—such as high rates of traffic accidents, widespread occupational work at height, and insufficient safety infrastructure—experience extremely high TSCI rates. Indeed, a recent systematic review reported that national SCI incidence estimates vary widely, with some countries reporting rates exceeding 50 cases per million population.[3] A review of provincial data in China found that SCI incidence ranged from approximately 14.6 to 60.6 per million across regions, with higher rates observed in more industrialized areas with heavy traffic.[18] By contrast, many HICs report relatively lower SCI incidence rates than low-income and middle-income regions, although this difference may partly reflect variations in data availability and reporting quality.[3] North America represents an exception among developed regions, with reported traumatic SCI (TSCI) incidence rates of approximately 30 to 40 cases per million population, substantially higher than those in Western Europe and Australia.[19] This difference may partly reflect more comprehensive case ascertainment through established national trauma and SCI registries.

Notably, the currently available epidemiologic data are skewed toward North America, Europe, and Oceania, and reliable data remain lacking for large portions of Asia, Africa, and Latin America.[3] In many LMICs, surveillance systems are weak, and hospital-based studies may fail to capture patients who die before reaching medical care or those treated outside of formal health care facilities. As a result, SCI incidence in developing regions is likely underestimated, and the true burden may be higher than reported.

The causes of TSCI also differ markedly by region. A recent global estimate reported that approximately 47% of new SCIs were due to falls, surpassing the roughly 25% caused by road traffic accidents.[3] However, road traffic accidents remain the leading cause of SCI in many LMICs. In nations across Africa, Asia, and the Middle East, motor vehicle collisions are reported to account for about 40% to 60% of TSCI cases.[20] Falls are also a globally important cause, but the nature of falls leading to SCI varies by region. In HICs, low-level falls on the same plane (trips or falls from standing height) among the elderly have been increasing yearly and are becoming a leading cause of SCI.[13] In developing countries, a substantial proportion of TSCI results from falls from height, particularly among young, economically active individuals engaged in high-risk occupations such as farming and construction work.[20] SCI due to violence (eg, gunshot or stab wounds) can also comprise a significant share in certain regions. In the United States, gunshot injuries have historically caused around 10% to 20% of SCIs, and in some parts of Africa, conflict and social unrest have led to an increase in war-related spinal injuries.[6,21] Sports and recreational trauma account for less than 10% of SCIs globally, but they are not negligible in specific subpopulations—for instance, cervical SCI from diving accidents, contact-sport injuries, or winter sports injuries in mountainous areas occur at noteworthy rates.[22] Overall, LMICs see many cases of SCI in young male individuals resulting from high-energy trauma (traffic crashes or falls from height), whereas HICs are witnessing an increase in SCI due to low-energy falls in the elderly.[6,23] This difference suggests that prevention strategies must be tailored to regional risk patterns. In LMICs, establishing and enforcing road traffic safety laws and workplace fall-prevention measures are of paramount importance, while in HICs, preventing falls in the home environment and managing osteoporosis are critical priorities.

The profile of NTSCI etiologies also varies by region. In high-income areas (eg, North America and Western Europe), degenerative spinal diseases and neoplastic lesions are the major causes of NTSCI.[24] Degenerative conditions such as CSM or OPLL, and spinal tumors (including intramedullary neoplasms and metastatic lesions to the spine), account for a large share of NTSCI cases. A systematic global review reported that degenerative conditions typically account for 18% to 33% of NTSCI cases, while spinal tumors contribute to approximately 20% to 44%.[24] In contrast, infectious diseases contribute a greater proportion of NTSCI in developing countries. Spinal tuberculosis (Pott's disease) is a classic cause of nontraumatic paraplegia in South Asia and sub-Saharan Africa, and some reports attribute 15% to 30% of NTSCI cases to tuberculosis (TB).[25] Human immunodeficiency virus (HIV)-associated myelopathy and parasitic infections (such as schistosomiasis in endemic regions) are also observed as causes of NTSCI in these areas.[25] With increasing life expectancy, however, degenerative and neoplastic NTSCI etiologies are expected to become more common in LMICs in the future.

Overall, NTSCI in developed countries is predominantly associated with diseases of older age (degenerative and neoplastic causes), whereas in lower income regions a relatively larger share of NTSCI stems from untreated infections or congenital abnormalities, and the average age at onset tends to be younger. In all regions, patients with NTSCI are older on average than patients with TSCI, although in places where infections are a main cause, NTSCI can occur in midadulthood. Furthermore, because NTSCI arises without an obvious traumatic trigger, it is often diagnosed late; consequently, improving health care providers' awareness and recognition of NTSCI remains a challenge in both high-income and low-income settings.[26]

PREVENTION AND TREATMENT

Traumatic Injury Prevention Strategies

Road traffic and occupational safety

Road traffic collisions remain the largest cause of neurotrauma (including TSCI) worldwide, especially in LMICs.[6] Interventions such as motorcycle helmet laws, seatbelt enforcement, anti–drunk-driving campaigns, and workplace fall-prevention programs are recommended to reduce these injuries. For example, a global analysis emphasizes that improved road safety regulations and occupational safety measures can significantly lower TSCI incidence in these regions.[6]

Falls in the elderly

In high-income and aging societies, falls have become a leading cause of SCI among older adults.[5] Community-based fall-prevention programs (balance and strength training, home hazard modifications, medication review, osteoporosis treatment, and so forth) are broadly advocated to curb fall-related SCIs.[6]

Sports and recreation injuries

Sports-related activities account for a significant subset of TSCIs in youth, calling for targeted preventive efforts. Rule changes in sports have proven effective—for instance, banning head-first tackling in American football (enacted in 1976) led to a dramatic drop in catastrophic cervical spine injuries.[22] Similarly, safer rugby scrum techniques and stricter enforcement of no-diving zones in shallow water have reduced spinal injuries. A systematic review noted that diving is a leading sport cause of SCI in many countries, and it recommended public education (eg, warning signage and lifeguards at swimming areas) to prevent devastating diving injuries.[22] Continued improvements in protective sports gear and coaching of proper techniques remain necessary to further lessen these tragic injuries.

Nontraumatic Spinal Cord Injury Prevention

Early detection of degenerative myelopathy

Many NTSCIs are due to chronic degenerative conditions. Clinical vigilance for early signs of cervical myelopathy (eg, gait imbalance or hand clumsiness) is crucial, because timely surgical decompression can halt progression before irreversible damage occurs.[27,28] Indeed, previous studies conclude that early surgical intervention for degenerative cervical myelopathy is essential to minimizing long-term disability and maximizing quality of life.[29,30]

Metastatic spinal cord compression

In oncology, preventing SCI means early identification and treatment of spinal metastases. Clinical guidelines (eg, NICE 2023) stress prompt MRI evaluation and intervention at the first sign of cord compression, rather than waiting for profound neurologic deficits.[31] Early radiotherapy or surgical stabilization for patients with vertebral metastases can avert paralysis and improve outcomes. In practice, establishing clear pathways for urgent referral and treatment of metastatic spinal cord compression has been shown to prevent neurologic injury and improve prognosis.[31]

Infections (tuberculosis and human immunodeficiency virus)

Proper management of infections can greatly reduce NTSCI. In regions where TB is endemic, early diagnosis and full treatment of spinal TB (Pott's disease) are vital. Delayed diagnosis leads to worse outcomes, whereas treating spinal TB in its early stages achieves disease cure in approximately 95% of patients and prevents permanent paraplegia.[32] Likewise, HIV-associated myelopathy has become far less frequent since the advent of antiretroviral therapy—now less than 10% of patients with acquired immunodeficiency syndrome develop HIV-related myelopathy—highlighting how controlling infections can avert spinal cord damage.[33,34] Overall, strengthening infectious disease control is an integral part of NTSCI prevention.

Acute Phase Care

Rapid imaging and diagnosis

Efficient emergency protocols are equally important for both TSCI and NTSCI (**Fig. 2**). Prehospital responders are trained to suspect SCI even in low-mechanism injuries if neurologic signs are present and to immobilize the spine.[35] Upon hospital arrival, prompt MRI is indicated for any acute myelopathic symptoms without obvious trauma. For example, in a cancer patient with new limb weakness, urgent MRI can confirm spinal cord compression so that treatment is not delayed.[31] Guidelines for metastatic spinal cord compression (SCC) recommend obtaining MRI immediately when cord compression is suspected, to facilitate treatment within 24 hours.[31] In clinical practice, expedited MRI or computed tomography imaging in the emergency department facilitates the differentiation of traumatic fractures, epidural hematomas, spinal abscesses, and neoplastic lesions, enabling timely surgical or medical intervention to minimize spinal cord damage.[36,37]

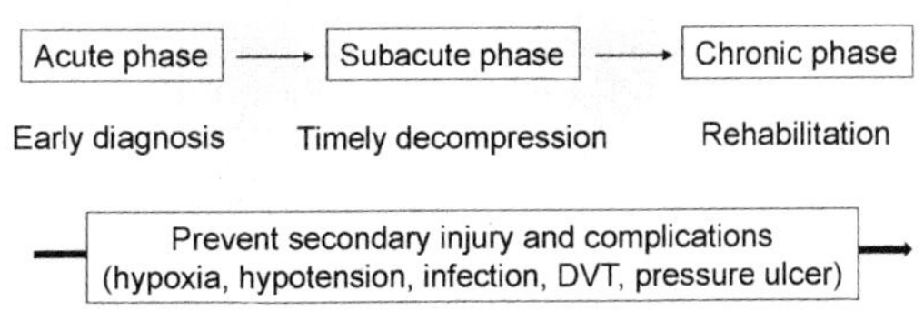

Fig. 2. Clinical continuum of spinal cord injury from acute to chronic phases.

Urgent decompression

Modern acute SCI management adopts the mantra "Time is Spine," reflecting that the timing of intervention is critical. Growing evidence shows that early surgical decompression (ideally within 24 hours of injury) leads to significantly better neurologic outcomes in acute SCI.[38,39] A 2021 pooled analysis of 1548 patients found that those who underwent surgery less than 24 hours after injury had superior 1 year motor and sensory recovery and higher rates of improvement in the American Spinal Injury Association Impairment Scale grade, compared to those decompressed later.[40] Moreover, motor recovery declined steeply as surgical delay increased during the first 24 to 36 hours after injury, after which recovery plateaued.[40] These findings have prompted calls to make less than 24 hour surgical intervention a standard goal in trauma systems. Clinical guidelines are being updated to reflect that, whenever feasible, patients with acute SCI should be transferred to a spine center and decompressed as soon as possible, since early surgery is safe and offers clear benefits in neurologic recovery.[39]

Special considerations in older patients

Acute SCI in elderly patients poses additional challenges. Older individuals often have medical comorbidities that must be managed alongside the spinal injury.[41] Early surgery might be medically complex if the patient is on blood thinners or has unstable vital signs. Intensive care for older patients with SCI focuses on avoiding secondary complications: strict pulmonary hygiene to prevent pneumonia, vigilant infection control to prevent sepsis, deep vein thrombosis prophylaxis, and early gentle mobilization to avert pressure ulcers and deconditioning.[42–44] Studies show that elderly patients with SCI have substantially higher rates of acute complications like pneumonia, urinary tract infection, and sepsis than younger cohorts, contributing to higher early mortality.[45] For example, a recent Italian registry noted that as the proportion of elderly SCI cases increased, the case-fatality rate during initial hospitalization more than tripled (from ~17% in 2009 to 57% in 2020).[46] This stark statistic underlines the importance of meticulous supportive care in the acute phase. In summary, organizing regionalized trauma systems with specialized spine centers, ensuring rapid imaging, early surgical decompression, and providing tailored critical care are all key to optimizing acute SCI outcomes.

Rehabilitation and Long-term Care

Geriatric rehabilitation

SCI in older adults often involves nontraumatic causes and multiple chronic conditions (eg, arthritis, cardiac issues, and cognitive decline). Rehabilitation for this group must prioritize basic mobility and self-care independence over athletic goals. Studies confirm that older patients with SCI recover function more slowly and are more prone to complications during rehab and after discharge.[47,48] They may require longer inpatient stays and specialized, multidisciplinary rehab teams to manage complex medical needs. Incorporating bone health (osteoporosis treatment to prevent fractures) and fall-prevention strategies into rehabilitation is also recommended, given the high risk of osteoporosis and falls in this population.[49] Thorough discharge planning is critical, as many older patients return to homes ill-suited for wheelchairs and face a high risk of falls postdischarge.

Home and community support

Effective long-term management of SCI extends beyond the hospital. Continuous care via community health services can reduce complications and prevent rehospitalization.[50] Older patients with SCI often rely on aging spouses or live alone, making in-home support essential. Early coordination with home health nursing, personal care aides, outpatient therapy, and family education is strongly advised.[50] In rapidly aging regions (eg, East Asia), health systems are moving to integrate medical follow-up with social support (home modifications, transportation, and meal services) to support older SCI survivors in the community.[51] Such integrated care models not only improve safety and independence but also help contain long-term health care costs by preventing avoidable complications. When living at home becomes unsafe despite support, timely transition to assisted living or skilled nursing facilities should be arranged to ensure the patient's well-being.

Managing "invisible" disabilities in incomplete spinal cord injury

Many patients with nontraumatic or incomplete SCI regain the ability to walk, yet suffer "hidden" deficits such as severe spasticity, neuropathic pain, and impaired hand function.[50,52,53] These issues can drastically reduce quality of life if left unaddressed. Long-term care plans must include proactive spasticity management (medications like baclofen or Botox injections and physical therapy techniques) and neuropathic pain management (appropriate medications and counseling), as well as occupational therapy to improve fine motor skills for daily tasks.[54–56] Regular follow-up in specialized SCI clinics is ideal to monitor and treat secondary complications (pressure ulcers, neurogenic bladder/bowel dysfunction, shoulder overuse injuries, and so forth) that may emerge over time.[26] Research on patients with incomplete SCI emphasizes the need for ongoing outpatient therapy and periodic re-evaluations to maintain functional gains and catch late-onset issues.[57] These follow-up strategies are particularly important for managing residual or "invisible" impairments—such as subtle motor dysfunction, pain, or spasticity—that may not be fully captured during the acute or inpatient phase.

ECONOMIC IMPACT

SCI imposes a substantial lifelong economic burden on individuals, health care systems, and society. In HICs, the estimated lifetime direct medical cost per patient ranges from approximately USD 1.5 million to 3 million, depending on injury severity.[58] A large proportion of these costs is incurred during the first year after injury, driven by acute hospitalization, surgical treatment, and inpatient rehabilitation, while long-term expenses continue to accumulate due to chronic complications and ongoing medical care.[6] In addition to direct health care costs, SCI results in considerable indirect costs, including loss of employment, reduced productivity, decreased tax revenue, and increased reliance on disability benefits and caregiving services.

Globally, the overall burden of SCI is increasing as a result of population growth and aging, even in regions where age-adjusted incidence rates have stabilized. Data from the Global Burden of Disease studies demonstrate a marked increase in the number of individuals living with SCI, a trend that is expected to continue.[6] In aging societies, particularly in East Asia, the growing incidence of fall-related and osteoporosis-associated SCI among older adults is expected to further increase long-term health care and social care expenditures. Consequently, the global economic costs associated with SCI are projected to escalate in the coming decades.

Given the extraordinarily high lifetime costs per case, prevention is widely regarded as one of the most cost-effective strategies to reduce the economic impact of SCI.[59] Many causes of SCI are preventable through relatively low-cost interventions, such as road safety enforcement and fall-prevention programs for older adults. These measures can avert injuries that would otherwise result in substantial long-term medical and social costs, making prevention a high-value public health investment.[60]

At the same time, changing patient demographics require health care systems to optimize resource allocation. Greater investment in postacute and long-term services, including outpatient rehabilitation, home-based care, and caregiver support, may reduce secondary complications, prevent hospital readmissions, and lower overall costs.[61] In addition, promoting independence and social participation among people with SCI has important economic benefits.[62] Improved access to rehabilitation, assistive technologies, and employment support can increase workforce participation, reduce dependence on public assistance, and enhance overall productivity.

Finally, robust epidemiologic data and national or international SCI registries are essential for evidence-based policy and efficient resource planning.[62] Accurate data enable policymakers to identify emerging trends, evaluate cost–benefit relationships, and prioritize interventions with the greatest economic and societal return. Together, strengthened prevention efforts, optimized care delivery, and data-driven policy planning offer viable pathways to mitigate the growing global economic burden of SCI.

SUMMARY

- Global SCI incidence is stable overall, but the proportion of NTSCI is rising, particularly in aging populations.
- Falls are now the leading cause of SCI in many HICs, overtaking road traffic injuries.
- NTSCI often results from degenerative, neoplastic, or infectious conditions and may be diagnosed late due to gradual onset.
- Early surgical decompression (within 24 hours) significantly improves outcomes in acute SCI.
- Older patients with SCI have higher complication and mortality rates, requiring specialized rehabilitation and long-term care strategies.
- Integrated care models, including home health support and community-based services, are vital for aging SCI populations.
- Robust epidemiologic surveillance and SCI registries are essential for shaping cost-effective, data-driven policy responses.
- Prevention (falls, trauma, and infections) remains the most economically efficient strategy to reduce long-term SCI burden.

CLINICS CARE POINTS

- Consider degenerative cervical myelopathy in older adults presenting with gait disturbance, hand clumsiness, or recurrent falls, even in the absence of trauma.
- Obtain urgent MRI in patients with cancer who develop new limb weakness, sensory changes, or sphincter dysfunction to exclude metastatic spinal cord compression.
- Transfer patients with acute SCI to specialized spine centers whenever possible, aiming for decompression within 24 hours.
- Low-energy falls in older adults can cause significant cervical SCI despite the absence of fracture; maintain a high index of suspicion.
- Screen for respiratory complications, urinary tract infection, pressure injuries, and venous thromboembolism early in elderly SCI patients.
- Persistent neuropathic pain, spasticity, and hand dysfunction should be actively assessed during long-term follow-up, even in ambulatory patients.

DECLARATION OF ARTIFICIAL INTELLIGENCE AND ARTIFICIAL INTELLIGENCE-ASSISTED TECHNOLOGIES IN THE WRITING PROCESS

During the preparation of this article, the author used ChatGPT (OpenAI) in order to refine grammar and correcting typographical errors. The tool/service was applied exclusively to improve clarity and readability and did not influence the scientific content, data interpretation, or conclusions. After using this tool/service, the author reviewed and edited the content as needed and takes full responsibility for the content of the publication.

DISCLOSURE

The authors declare no conflicts of interest.

REFERENCES

1. Diop M, Epstein D. A systematic review of the impact of spinal cord injury on costs and health-related quality of life. PharmacoEcon Open 2024;8: 793–808.

2. Choi Y, Leigh JH, Jeon J, et al. Trends in the incidence and etiology of non-traumatic spinal cord injury in Korea: a nationwide population-based study from 2007 to 2020. J Korean Med Sci 2023;38:e158.
3. Collaborators GBDSCI. Global, regional, and national burden of spinal cord injury, 1990-2019: a systematic analysis for the global burden of disease study 2019. Lancet Neurol 2023;22:1026–47.
4. Ge L, Arul K, Ikpeze T, et al. Traumatic and nontraumatic spinal cord injuries. World Neurosurg 2018;111:e142–8.
5. Kim HS, Lim KB, Kim J, et al. Epidemiology of spinal cord injury: changes to its cause amid aging population, a single center study. Ann Rehabil Med 2021;45:7–15.
6. Kim M, Jeong W, Jang S, et al. Spinal cord injury epidemiology and causes: a worldwide analysis with 2050 projections. Healthcare (Basel) 2025;13(20):2552.
7. Wilson JR, Cronin S, Fehlings MG, et al. Epidemiology and impact of spinal cord injury in the elderly: results of a fifteen-year population-based cohort study. J Neurotrauma 2020;37:1740–51.
8. Lu Y, Shang Z, Zhang W, et al. Global incidence and characteristics of spinal cord injury since 2000-2021: a systematic review and meta-analysis. BMC Med 2024;22:285.
9. Jain NB, Ayers GD, Peterson EN, et al. Traumatic spinal cord injury in the United States, 1993-2012. JAMA 2015;313:2236–43.
10. Niemeyer MJS, Lokerman RD, Sadiqi S, et al. Epidemiology of traumatic spinal cord injury in the Netherlands: emergency medical service, hospital, and functional outcomes. Top Spinal Cord Inj Rehabil 2020;26:243–52.
11. Josefson C, Rekand T, Lundgren-Nilsson A, et al. Epidemiology of spinal cord injury in adults in Sweden, 2016-2020: a retrospective registry-based study. Neuroepidemiology 2025;59:334–42.
12. Barbiellini Amidei C, Salmaso L, Bellio S, et al. Epidemiology of traumatic spinal cord injury: a large population-based study. Spinal Cord 2022;60:812–9.
13. Miyakoshi N, Suda K, Kudo D, et al. A nationwide survey on the incidence and characteristics of traumatic spinal cord injury in Japan in 2018. Spinal Cord 2021;59:626–34.
14. Khadour FA, Khadour YA, Meng L, et al. Epidemiology features of traumatic and non-traumatic spinal cord injury in China, wuhan. Sci Rep 2024;14:1640.
15. Mackiewicz-Milewska M, Cisowska-Adamiak M, Glowacka-Mrotek I, et al. Traumatic vs. non-traumatic spinal cord injury-epidemiology, complications, and neurological status during rehabilitation. J Clin Med 2025;14(15):5209.
16. Chiu WT, Lin HC, Lam C, et al. Review paper: epidemiology of traumatic spinal cord injury: comparisons between developed and developing countries. Asia Pac J Public Health 2010;22:9–18.
17. van den Berg ME, Castellote JM, Mahillo-Fernandez I, et al. Incidence of spinal cord injury worldwide: a systematic review. Neuroepidemiology 2010;34:184–92 [discussion: 92].
18. Chen C, Qiao X, Liu W, et al. Epidemiology of spinal cord injury in China: a systematic review of the Chinese and English literature. Spinal Cord 2022;60:1050–61.
19. Cripps RA, Lee BB, Wing P, et al. A global map for traumatic spinal cord injury epidemiology: towards a living data repository for injury prevention. Spinal Cord 2011;49:493–501.
20. Golestani A, Shobeiri P, Sadeghi-Naini M, et al. Epidemiology of traumatic spinal cord injury in developing countries from 2009 to 2020: a systematic review and meta-analysis. Neuroepidemiology 2022;56:219–39.
21. Sidhu GS, Ghag A, Prokuski V, et al. Civilian gunshot injuries of the spinal cord: a systematic review of the current literature. Clin Orthop Relat Res 2013;471:3945–55.
22. Chan CW, Eng JJ, Tator CH, et al. Epidemiology of sport-related spinal cord injuries: a systematic review. J Spinal Cord Med 2016;39:255–64.
23. Chen Y, Tang Y, Allen V, et al. Aging and spinal cord injury: external causes of injury and implications for prevention. Top Spinal Cord Inj Rehabil 2015;21:218–26.
24. New PW, Cripps RA, Bonne Lee B. Global maps of non-traumatic spinal cord injury epidemiology: towards a living data repository. Spinal Cord 2014;52:97–109.
25. Musubire AK, Meya DB, Bohjanen PR, et al. A systematic review of non-traumatic spinal cord injuries in Sub-Saharan Africa and a proposed diagnostic algorithm for resource-limited settings. Front Neurol 2017;8:618.
26. Molinares DM, Gater DR, Daniel S, et al. Nontraumatic spinal cord injury: epidemiology, etiology and management. J Personalized Med 2022;12(11):1872.
27. Nouri A, Tetreault L, Singh A, et al. Degenerative cervical myelopathy: epidemiology, genetics, and pathogenesis. Spine (Phila Pa 1976) 2015;40:E675–93.
28. Fehlings MG, Tetreault LA, Riew KD, et al. A clinical practice guideline for the management of patients with degenerative cervical myelopathy: recommendations for patients with mild, moderate, and severe disease and nonmyelopathic patients with evidence of cord compression. Glob Spine J 2017;7:70S–83S.
29. Nagoshi N, Yamane J, Okubo T, et al. Impact of symptom duration on surgical outcomes and functional recovery in degenerative cervical myelopathy: insights

from a prospective multicenter study. Spine (Phila Pa 1976) 2025.
30. Matsukura Y, Egawa S, Inose H, et al. Preoperative symptom duration influences neurological recovery and patient-reported outcome measures after surgical treatment of cervical ossification of the posterior longitudinal ligament. Spine (Phila Pa 1976) 2023; 48:1259–65.
31. Spinal metastases and metastatic spinal cord compression, NICE Clinical Guidelines, No. 234. London: National Institute for Health and Care Excellence (NICE); 2023. Available at: https://www.ncbi.nlm.nih.gov/books/NBK595817/.
32. Glassman I, Nguyen KH, Giess J, et al. Pathogenesis, diagnostic challenges, and risk factors of Pott's disease. Clin Pract 2023;13:155–65.
33. Rezaie A, Parmar R, Rendon C, et al. HIV-associated vacuolar myelopathy: a rare initial presentation of HIV. SAGE Open Med Case Rep 2020;8:2050313X20945562.
34. Di Rocco A, Simpson DM. AIDS-associated vacuolar myelopathy. AIDS Patient Care STDS 1998;12:457–61.
35. Feller R, Furin M, Alloush A, et al. EMS immobilization techniques, . StatPearls [Internet]. Treasure Island (FL): StatPearls Publishing; 2026.
36. Kuah T, Vellayappan BA, Makmur A, et al. State-of-the-Art imaging techniques in metastatic spinal cord compression. Cancers (Basel) 2022;14.
37. Laur O, Nandu H, Titelbaum DS, et al. Nontraumatic spinal cord compression: MRI primer for emergency department radiologists. Radiographics 2019;39: 1862–80.
38. Ramakonar H, Fehlings MG. 'Time is spine': new evidence supports decompression within 24 h for acute spinal cord injury. Spinal Cord 2021;59: 933–4.
39. Fehlings MG, Tetreault LA, Wilson JR, et al. A clinical practice guideline for the management of patients with acute spinal cord injury and central cord syndrome: recommendations on the timing (</=24 hours versus >24 hours) of decompressive surgery. Glob Spine J 2017;7:195S–202S.
40. Badhiwala JH, Wilson JR, Witiw CD, et al. The influence of timing of surgical decompression for acute spinal cord injury: a pooled analysis of individual patient data. Lancet Neurol 2021;20:117–26.
41. Krassioukov AV, Furlan JC, Fehlings MG. Medical co-morbidities, secondary complications, and mortality in elderly with acute spinal cord injury. J Neurotrauma 2003;20:391–9.
42. Raab AM, Brinkhof MWG, Berlowitz DJ, et al. Respiratory function and respiratory complications in spinal cord injury: protocol for a prospective, multicentre cohort study in high-income countries. BMJ Open 2020;10:e038204.
43. Reyes MRL, Elmo MJ, Menachem B, et al. A primary care provider's guide to managing respiratory health in subacute and chronic spinal cord injury. Top Spinal Cord Inj Rehabil 2020;26:116–22.
44. Prevention of venous thromboembolism in individuals with spinal cord injury: Clinical practice guidelines for health care providers, 3rd edition; consortium for spinal cord medicine. Top Spinal Cord Inj Rehabil 2016;22:209–40.
45. Mirzaeva L, Lobzin S, Tcinzerling N, et al. Complications and mortality after acute traumatic spinal cord injury in Saint Petersburg, Russia. Spinal Cord 2020; 58:970–9.
46. Conti A, Campagna S, Gianino MM, et al. Incidence and mortality of spinal cord injury from 2008 to 2020: a retrospective population-based cohort study in the Piedmont region, Italy. Spinal Cord 2023;61:99–105.
47. Scivoletto G, Morganti B, Ditunno P, et al. Effects on age on spinal cord lesion patients' rehabilitation. Spinal Cord 2003;41:457–64.
48. Stenimahitis V, Gharios M, Fletcher-Sandersjoo A, et al. Long-term outcome and predictors of neurological recovery in cervical spinal cord injury: a population-based cohort study. Sci Rep 2024;14: 20945.
49. Seijas V, Schrepfer L, Posada AM, et al. Evidence-based recommendations for the rehabilitation and management of the ageing population with spinal cord injury: a systematic review of clinical practice guidelines. Eur J Phys Rehabil Med 2024;60: 433–44.
50. Paker N, Soy D, Kesiktas N, et al. Reasons for rehospitalization in patients with spinal cord injury: 5 years' experience. Int J Rehabil Res 2006;29:71–6.
51. He AJ, Tang VFY. Integration of health services for the elderly in Asia: a scoping review of Hong Kong, Singapore, Malaysia, Indonesia. Health Policy 2021;125:351–62.
52. Nagoshi N, Yamane J, Okubo T, et al. Prevalence and surgical outcomes of neuropathic pain in degenerative cervical myelopathy: a multicenter prospective cohort study. Spine (Phila Pa 1976) 2026;51:9–15.
53. Nagoshi N, Yamane J, Okubo T, et al. Clinical indicators of surgical outcomes in degenerative cervical myelopathy assessed using the JOACMEQ: a prospective multicenter study. Spine (Phila Pa 1976) 2025;50:1319–26.
54. Billington ZJ, Henke AM, Gater DR Jr. Spasticity management after spinal cord injury: the here and now. J Personalized Med 2022;12(5):808.
55. Hagen EM, Rekand T. Management of neuropathic pain associated with spinal cord injury. Pain Ther 2015;4:51–65.
56. Ciardi G, Lamberti G, Avanzi M. Using "functional hand" protocol to improve hand function following a spinal cord injury: an explorative study. Acta Biomed 2023;94:e2023255.

57. Yilmaz F, Sahin F, Aktug S, et al. Long-term follow-up of patients with spinal cord injury. Neurorehabil Neural Repair 2005;19:332–7.
58. Merritt CH, Taylor MA, Yelton CJ, et al. Economic impact of traumatic spinal cord injuries in the United States. Neuroimmunol Neuroinflamm 2019;6:9.
59. Bellon K, Kolakowsky-Hayner SA, Chen D, et al. Evidence-based practice in primary prevention of spinal cord injury. Top Spinal Cord Inj Rehabil 2013;19:25–30.
60. Tyroch AH, Davis JW, Kaups KL, et al. Spinal cord injury. A preventable public burden. Arch Surg 1997;132:778–81.
61. Hesari M, Alizadeh SD, Malekzadeh H, et al. 30- and 90-Day readmission rates following traumatic spinal cord injury: a systematic review and meta-analyses. Glob Spine J 2025;15:2480–9.
62. McDaid D, Park AL, Gall A, et al. Understanding and modelling the economic impact of spinal cord injuries in the United Kingdom. Spinal Cord 2019;57:778–88.

Pathobiology of Spinal Cord Compression

Nicole Ossandón-Pino, MSc[a,b], Pia M. Vidal, PhD[a,b,*]

KEYWORDS

• Neuroinflammation • Gut dysbiosis • Ischemia • Biomarkers

KEY POINTS

- Degenerative cervical myelopathy (DCM) is associated with a systemic activation of the immune system, reflected by increased circulating immune cells and elevated serum biomarkers such as of cytokines.
- DCM causes spinal cord hypoxia, inflammation and remodeling of microvasculature.
- Peripheral immune response and gut dysbiosis in DCM is sex-dependent.

INTRODUCTION

Spinal cord injuries (SCIs) are the leading cause of disability across both young and elderly populations. These injuries are classified into traumatic and non-traumatic injuries, which differ mainly in their etiology and pathophysiological progression. Traumatic injuries most commonly results from external mechanical forces, such as traffic accidents and falls, whereas non-traumatic injuries are mainly caused by degenerative changes of the spinal column, aging-related process, and neoplastic conditions.[1] These distinct etiologies lead to different patterns of injury evolution. Traumatic SCI is initiated by primary mechanical damage, characterized by vascular disruption, focal hemorrhage, ischemia, and neuroglial necrosis. This primary insult may mainly result from laceration or transection, and is often exacerbated by persistent post-traumatic compression.[2]

Within minutes of injury, innate immune responses are rapidly activated, including astrocyte and microglia activation with an inflammatory phenotype (eg, IL-1α, IL-6, and TNF-α expression)[3]; infiltration of peripheral immune cells facilitated by hemorrhage and blood-spinal cord barrier disruption, and upregulation of endothelial adhesion molecules (ICAM-1, VCAM-1), which promote leukocyte recruitment and amplify inflammation.[4] The secondary phase involves a prolonged cascade of biochemical and structural damage that may persist for months, including ionic imbalance and excitotoxicity (eg, glutamate accumulation, calcium overload, and mitochondrial dysfunction), oxidative stress with lipid peroxidation, and progressive tissue degeneration. These processes converge with Wallerian degeneration, edema, microvascular thrombosis, and expansion of the ischemic area, further exacerbating the initial injury.[5] Later on, a glial scar progressively forma, consisting of reactive astrocytes, oligodendrocytes, meningeal cells, activated microglia, and infiltrating fibroblasts, along with increased extracellular matrix proteoglycans (eg, neurocan, versican) that inhibit axonal growth.[6–8] This structure acts as both a physical and biochemical barrier to regeneration while also restricting lesion spread.[4] This phase lead to remodeling of lesion microenvironment, with peripheral retraction of reactive astrocytes, accumulation of phagocytic macrophages in necrotic areas, and clearance of cellular debris. Microglia localize to the lesion border,

[a] Neuroimmunology and Regeneration of the Central Nervous System Unit, Biomedical Science Research Laboratory, Department of Basic Sciences, Faculty of Medicine, Universidad Católica de La Santísima Concepción, Concepción, Chile; [b] Neuromet Group, Universidad Católica de La Santisima Concepción, Concepción, Chile
* Corresponding author. Neuroimmunology and Regeneration of the Central Nervous System Unit, Biomedical Science Research Laboratory, Department of Basic Sciences, Faculty of Medicine, Universidad Católica de La Santísima Concepción, Concepción, 4090541, Chile.
E-mail address: pvidal@ucsc.cl

Neurosurg Clin N Am 37 (2026) 479–487
https://doi.org/10.1016/j.nec.2026.05.002

Abbreviations

DCM	degenerative cervical myelopathy
GALT	gut-associated lymphoid tissue
HIF-1	hypoxia-inducible factor
IL	Interlukin
Nfl	neurofilament light chain
OPLL	ossification of the posterior longitudinal ligament
SCI	spinal cord injury
TNF	tumor necrosis factor

where along to astrocytes contribute to the regulation of inflammation and tissue repair.[7] In contrast, non-traumatic SCI typically involves a slow and progressive compression of the spinal cord, with a temporarily diffuse inflammatory response leading to chronic and sustained inflammation, ischemia, vascular compromise and remodeling, as well as demyelination.[9–11] Rather than an abrupt mechanical insult, these types of injuries involve sustained microenvironment stress, progressive vascular compromise. Although similar cellular players are involved (eg, astrocytes, microglia, and infiltrating immune cells) their activation profiles tend to be more heterogeneous and prolonged. Consequently, tissue damage evolves over longer timeframes, with a greater contribution of chronic inflammation, maladaptive repair, and progressive neurodegeneration.[11–14] Additional differences have been described between both types of injuries, including the development of a post-traumatic cyst in traumatic SCI,[9] sex-related incidence ratio,[15] development of respiratory complications,[16] and the presence of immediate vascular disruption following traumatic SCI.[10] Despite these differences, both types of injuries share key pathophysiological features. For example, axonal degeneration and demyelination extending rostrally and caudally from the injury site,[9] highlighting potentially convergent mechanisms of neurodegeneration.

Degenerative cervical myelopathy (DCM) is the most common form of non-traumatic SCI. It comprises a heterogeneous group of pathologies characterized by degenerative deterioration of the spinal cord in adults.[17] There are 2 main causes contributing to the development of DCM, the static and dynamic factors.[11] These include conditions such as cervical spondylosis, ossification of the ligamentum flavum, ossification of the posterior longitudinal ligament, and degenerative disc disease,[18] all of which ultimately lead to chronic spinal cord compression. The clinical presentation of DCM is highly variable, ranging from asymptomatic individuals to patients with neurologic impairment (**Fig. 1**A–C). The symptomatic patients may present with a wide spectrum of manifestations, from mild sensory and motor symptoms to severe complications such as neurogenic bladder dysfunction and, in severe cases, tetraplegia.[19,20] There is a poor or even absent direct correlation between the degree of spinal cord compression and clinical symptom severity.[18] Instead, accumulating evidence suggest that functional plasticity, both in response to chronic compression and following surgical decompression, plays a key role in determining clinical outcomes.[21,22]

NEUROINFLAMMATION

Several signaling pathways have been implicated in the processes of neuroinflammation and neurodegeneration. At the systemic level, a preclinical mouse of DCM shows an increased frequency of circulating T lymphocytes.[23] In patients with DCM, elevated serum levels of inflammatory and neuroaxonal markers (eg, Interlukin (IL)-6, neurofilament light chain (Nfl) have been reported).[24] A recent prospective study has suggested presurgical serum levels of Nfl, IL-6, and brain-derived neurotophic factor as potential biomarkers to distinguish control versus DCM patients.[24] Furthermore, at the systemic level, increased IL-6 serum levels have been correlated with symptom severity in DCM patients.[25]

During DCM the recruitment of immune cells from the periphery is thought to contribute to the neuroinflammatory response observed at the spinal cord level.[14] This process is mainly characterized by the mobilization and activation of macrophages and/or microglial cells at the site of compression,[13,14,26] that have been shown to contribute to the development of DCM symptomatology[27] in a sex-dependent manner. In the twy/twy preclinical mouse model, overexpression of the complement protein C1q in microglia has been reported. C1q is well known for its role in synapse elimination and neuronal death.[28] Additionally, activation of the Cyr61 pathway has been observed. Cyr61 is an extracellular matrix protein expressed at sites of inflammation and plays a critical role in the recruitment of inflammatory macrophages.[29] Furthermore, strong neuronal Fas immunoreactivity has been described,[26] along with increased expression of cleaved caspase-3 and TUNEL-positive cells in both gray and white matter.[30] This signaling pathway has been implicated in the progressive apoptosis of neurons and oligodendrocytes.[26] In the context of neuroinflammation, astrocytes undergo a phenotypic shift toward a reactive, inflammatory state, commonly referred to as the A1 phenotype.[31] This transition is driven by an inflammatory microenvironment

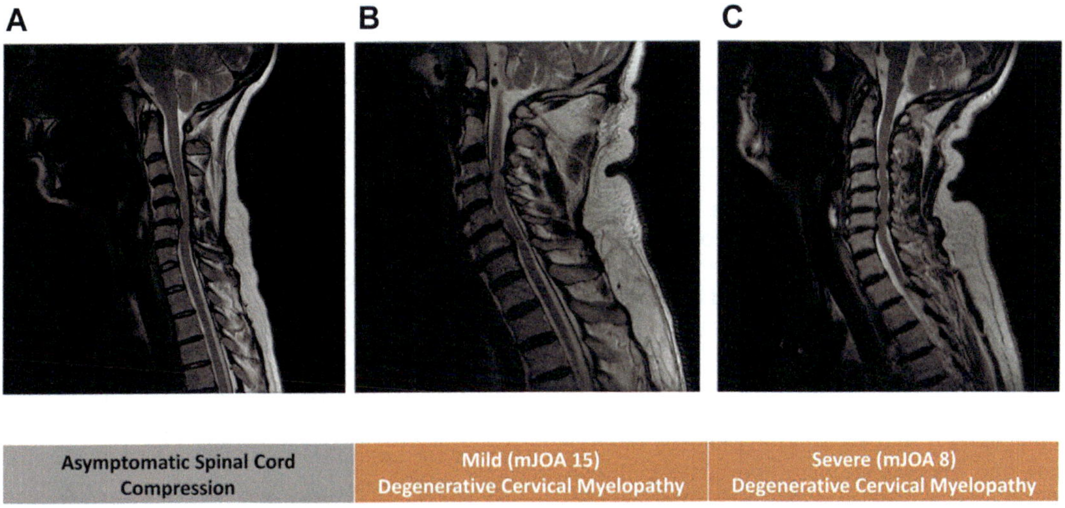

Fig. 1. Cord compression does not represent DCM. Series of T2 weight sagittal cervical spine MRI. Cord compression is commonly incidental (*A*), even with hyperintensity signal change, and the amount of compression weakly correlates to the disease severity (A vs B vs C). (*B*) represents a T2 MRI of a mild DCM patient, whereas (*C*) shows a severe DCM patient. DCM, degenerative cervical myelopathy. (Davies BM, Mowforth O, Gharooni A-A, et al. A New Framework for Investigating the Biological Basis of Degenerative Cervical Myelopathy [AO Spine RECODE-DCM Research Priority Number 5]: Mechanical Stress, Vulnerability and Time. Global Spine Journal. 2022;12(1_suppl):78S-96S. https://doi.org/10.1177/21925682211057546.)

enriched in inflammatory cytokines, such as tumor necrosis factor (TNF)-α and IL-1β, mainly released by activated microglia.[32] Activation of the NF-κB signaling pathway in reactive astrocytes promotes the expression of complement-related genes, contributing to synaptic dysfunction and neuronal injury.[33] Additionally, these activated astrocytes release chemoattractant signals (eg, CXCL10, CINC-1, and CINC-2) that facilitate the recruitment of peripheral immune cells, including T lymphocytes and neutrophils. Thus, contributing to amplify local inflammation and tissue damage at the site of injury.[34]

METABOLIC AND BIOENERGETIC FAILURE IN THE COMPRESSED SPINAL CORD

During the progression of compression, the microvascular network gradually becomes compromised, leading to reduced blood flow and, consequently, decreased oxygen and nutrient supply, thereby establishing a state of persistent hypoxia and ischemia.[35] The anterior spinal artery supplies a large proportion of the spinal cord's internal blood flow. Occlusion of the anterior spinal artery and radicular arteries disrupts blood supply to the pial plexus surrounding the spinal cord, resulting in ischemia, inflammation, hypoxia, and cell apoptosis.[36] The presence of compression-associated oxidative stress mediators, such as reactive oxygen species and superoxide dismutase, is linked to lipid peroxidation of cell membranes, precipitating spinal cord degeneration.[37] Under hypoxic conditions, angiogenesis is promoted by the induction of Hypoxia-inducible factor (HIF-1) α, vascular endothelial growth factor, and angiopoietin-2, as a compensatory response aimed at counteracting vessel damage and restoring oxygen delivery via newly formed vascular pathways.[38] Furthermore, increased HIF-1α expression upregulates matrix metalloproteinase-9 expression, which contributes to proteolytic damage of tight junctions and the basement membrane, leading to disruption of the blood-brain barrier following spinal cord compression. This disruption facilitates immune cell infiltration and exacerbates neuroinflammation.[39]

Concurrently, ischemia reduces ATP levels, impairing Na^+/K^+-ATPase function and promoting mitochondrial dysfunction. In this context, stabilization of HIF-1α reprograms cellular metabolism by inducing genes involved in erythropoiesis, glucose uptake (GLUT1/3), and anaerobic glycolysis, in an attempt to sustain energy production.[40] However, this adaptive response is insufficient in over time. Chronic hypoxia is particularly toxic to oligodendrocytes, and their loss results in axonal demyelination.[41] Moreover, mitochondrial damage disrupts the Krebs cycle and oxidative phosphorylation, leading to a sustained bioenergetic deficit.[42] Cells subsequently undergo severe metabolic impairment, with an approximately 25% reduction in the metabolome, promoting neuronal deterioration driven by glutamate-mediated excitotoxicity.[43]

ISCHEMIA–REPERFUSION INJURY IN DEGENERATIVE CERVICAL MYELOPATHY

Surgical decompression is a common and effective treatment for the majority of DCM[44] patients.[45] Delayed decompression has been linked with ischemia-reperfusion injury, which exacerbates neuroinflammation.[46] This process is characterized by the release of inflammatory cytokines, activation of astrocytes and an monocytic response, and has been associated to suboptimal neurologic recovery in approximately 9.3% of patients undergoing surgery.[47] Ischemia-reperfusion injury further activates the immune system by promoting immune cell infiltration into the spinal cord parenchyma,[48] and inducing the release of cytokines and chemoattractants (eg, TNF-α, CCL-2, CCL-3, CCL-5, CXCL1, IL-1β, IL-6). Thereby sustaining inflammation and impairing neurologic recovery in s subset of DCM patients.[47]

PERIPHERAL IMMUNITY AND THE GUT–SPINAL CORD AXIS

SCI leads to systemic immune dysregulation due to loss of descending inhibitory control from the brain over preganglionic sympathetic neurons that innervate different organs below the level of injury. This disruption results in a loss of regulatory feedback from the sympathetic nervous system, ultimately contributing to systemic immune and metabolic dysfunction.[49,50] It has been reported that following traumatic SCI, increased cytokine production and changes in the leukocyte populations within the gut-associated lymphoid tissue (GALT), correlate with shifts gut bacteria abundance.[51,52] However, considerably less is known about these processes in non-traumatic SCI.

It has been reported that 16% of patients with DCM present with gastrointestinal comorbidities, which may influence both disease progression and recovery after surgical decompression.[53,54] Studies in both human patients and animal models of traumatic SCI and non-traumatic SCI (eg, disc herniation, disc degeneration, and DCM) have demonstrate significant changes in gut microbiota composition following injury, as well as significant effects on functional recovery following microbiota modulation.[55–60] Changes in the gut microbiota, known as gut dysbiosis, have been identified as key contributors to increased lesion size and exacerbated neuroinflammation within the spinal cord.[52] In addition to taxonomic shifts, SCI is associated with functional alterations in the gut microbiota, including changes in the production of gut-derived metabolites, such as short chain fatty acids. These changes have been shown to correlate with injury severity and duration.[57] Distinct microbial profiles have been reported according to lesion completeness, and clinical factors such as antibiotic exposure further exacerbate gut dysbiosis by favoring opportunistic taxa over beneficial commensals.[56] Two Mendelian randomization studies have identified specific bacterial taxa and associated metabolic pathways linked to intervertebral disc degeneration[58] and cervical spondylosis.[61] The implicated pathways include mixed acid fermentation, glycolysis and related degradation pathways, as well as D-galactose degradation V, with notable associations involving *Parabacteroides johnsonii* and *Alistipes senegalensis*. However, these analyses did not account for potential confounding factors such as sex, which may influence both gut microbiota composition and disease susceptibility. At the preclinical level, a mouse model of DCM has shown that gut dysbiosis is more pronounced in males than in females,[59] and that gut microbiota influences the recruitment of different immune cell populations within the spinal cord.[27] Given that DCM is more prevalent in men,[62] these findings suggest that sex-dependent alterations in the gut microbiota may contribute to disease progression and the development of comorbidities through activation of the immune system.[27] Collectively, these findings support the hypothesis that impaired gastrointestinal function arises from altered sympathetic input to the gut, leading to gut inflammation, immune dysfunction within the GALT, and the development of gut dysbiosis. Future research should focus on experimental models to clarify the mechanistic links between gut microbiota and SCI, with the ultimate goal of translating these findings to clinical settings.

A recent preclinical study using a thoracic spinal cord contusion model has highlighted the importance of temporal dynamics in the immune response, as well as the role of the spinal cord meninges in supporting post-injury vascular repair.[63] In this study, aging was shown to impair myeloid and T cell recruitment through altered cytokine production. This immune cell recruitment is key to promote tissue repair, as it contributes to the clearance of cellular debris and the regulation of post-injury remodeling processes after injury (eg, glial scar formation in traumatic SCI models).[64,65]

CLINICAL IMPLICATIONS AND FUTURE THERAPEUTIC DIRECTIONS

Advances in the understanding of the pathobiology of spinal cord compression are key for the development of early biomarkers, optimization of

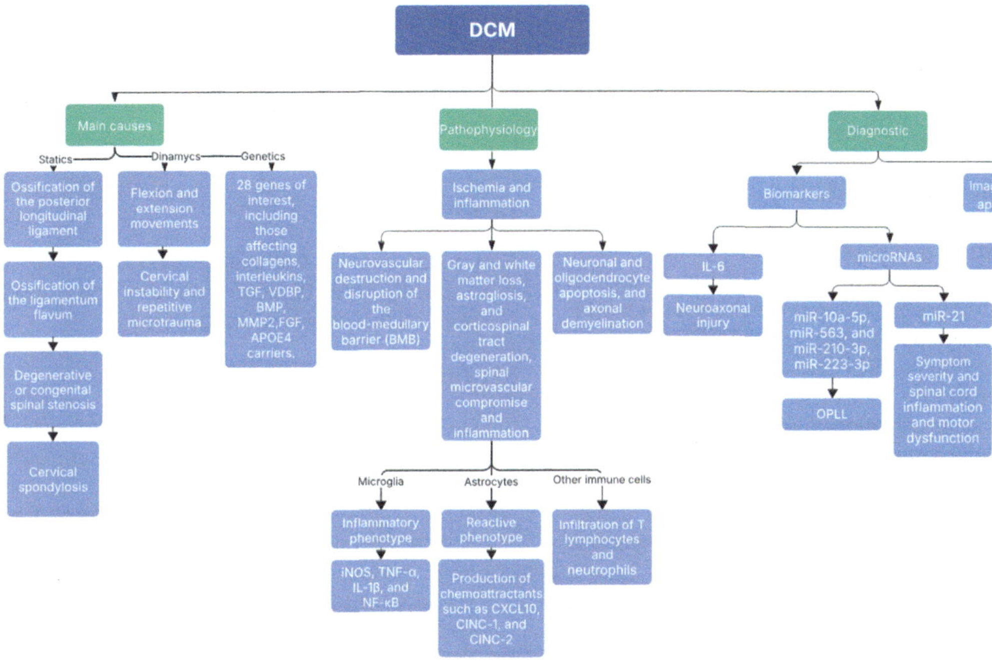

Fig. 2. Integrated pathophysiological mechanisms and biomarker landscape of DCM. This schematic summarizes the multifactorial pathophysiology of DCM. Static and dynamic mechanical factors interplay with genetic susceptibility to drive chronic spinal cord compression. Subsequent ischemia and neuroinflammation lead to blood-spinal cord barrier disruption, microvascular dysfunction, glial activation, immune cell infiltration, and progressive gray and white matter degeneration with axonal injury and demyelination. Emerging biomarkers associated with DCM include inflammatory mediators (eg, IL-6) as markers of neuroaxonal injury and dysregulated microRNAs linked to disease severity, spinal cord inflammation, motor dysfunction, and ossification-related phenotypes. DCM, degenerative cervical myelopathy.

therapeutic strategies, and refinement of intervention timing (**Fig. 2**). Although surgical decompression remains the gold standard treatment for DCM patients, accumulating evidence indicates that, while decompression effectively halts cord compression, it does not result in neurological improvement in all patients.[46,66,67]

One of the most promising clinical applications of these mechanistic insights lies in the identification of reliable biomarkers for disease stratification and prognosis. Elevated serum levels of IL-6, as well as markers of neuroaxonal injury, including Nfl, have been reported in patients with DCM.[24] These biomarkers may reflect ongoing neuroinflammatory and neurodegenerative processes that are not fully captured by conventional imaging. Another emerging biomarker, are microRNAs. Several microRNAs are differentially expressed in ossification of the posterior longitudinal ligament (OPLL) patients compared with non-OPLL and degenerative disc disease, as well DCM versus healthy controls (eg, miR-10a-5p, miR-563, and miR-210-3p, miR-223-3p).[68–70] Among these candidates, miR-21 has consistently emerged as a promising prognostic biomarker in DCM. Increased miR-21 expression has been reported in patient cohorts and correlates with symptom severity, findings that have been validated in a preclinical DCM model.[71] Experimental studies further indicate that miR-21 contributes to spinal cord inflammation and motor dysfunction,[71] supporting its role not only as a biomarker but also as a potential modulator of disease pathobiology. In the future, circulating biomarkers could support earlier diagnosis, help identify patients at higher risk of progression, and assist in predicting functional recovery following surgical decompression. However, their clinical utility will depend on validation in large, longitudinal cohorts and on integration with clinical and radiological parameters. An emerging area of interest is the contribution of gut–spinal cord axis to disease progression. Alterations in gut microbiota composition and increased intestinal permeability may promote systemic inflammation, influencing immune cell recruitment to the injured spinal cord.[27,52,59] Modulation of peripheral immune responses through dietary interventions, probiotics, or targeted immunotherapies represents a novel and potentially low-risk approach to attenuate chronic inflammation.

For example, nutritional supplementation with bioactive compounds, such as docosahexaenoic acid and curcumin, as well as selected herbal formulations, have been associated with improved motor function, reduced pain-related behavior, and modulation of neurotrophic and oxidative stress pathways in preclinical models.[72,73] Along these lines, the clinical trial NCT04659408 was designated to generate preliminary data to inform a future randomized controlled trial at evaluating the effects of prebiotic and probiotic supplementation on gut dysbiosis and gastrointestinal dysfunction in traumatic SCI patients. An initial pilot study focused on assessing the safety and feasibility of this intervention in elite athletes with SCI as the study population.[74] While this field remains in its early stages, it highlights the importance of considering spinal cord compression as a systemic disorder rather than a purely local mechanical problem.

The timing of surgical intervention represents another critical area in which biological insights may inform clinical decision-making. The well-recognized discrepancy between the degree of spinal cord compression and clinical severity[18] suggests that dynamic processes such as neuroinflammation, metabolic dysfunction, and neural plasticity play a major role in determining neurological outcomes.[21,22] These processes likely evolve over time, creating biological windows during which intervention may prevent irreversible neuronal damage. Earlier surgical decompression, guided not only by structural findings but also by biological markers of active injury, may therefore improve long-term outcomes.[47]

These insights support a shift toward a more integrated and personalized management of spinal cord compression. Future therapeutic strategies are likely to combine timely surgical decompression with biomarker-guided risk stratification and targeted adjunct therapies aimed at modulating inflammation, metabolism, and systemic immune responses. Such a multimodal approach has the potential to improve neurological outcomes and quality of life for patients with DCM, while also opening new avenues for translational research.

CLINICS CARE POINTS

- Systemic immune alterations and gut dysbiosis are emerging factors that may influence DCM development and recovery after spinal cord surgical decompression.
- Neurological decline in DCM may continue despite stable radiographic findings; clinical examination remains essential for treatment decisions.
- Functional impairment in DCM reflects not only structural spinal cord compression but also adaptive and maladaptive plastic changes accross brain and spinal cord networks.

DISCLOSURE

P.M. Vidal received financial support of the FAA II/2025 and DI-FMEI 02/2025 from the Universidad Católica de la Santísima Concepción.

REFERENCES

1. Ge L, Arul K, Ikpeze T, et al. Traumatic and nontraumatic spinal cord injuries. World Neurosurg 2018;111:e142–8.
2. Alizadeh A, Dyck SM, Karimi-Abdolrezaee S. Traumatic spinal cord injury: an overview of pathophysiology, models and acute injury mechanisms. Front Neurol 2019;10. https://doi.org/10.3389/fneur.2019.00282.
3. Hellenbrand DJ, Quinn CM, Piper ZJ, et al. Inflammation after spinal cord injury: a review of the critical timeline of signaling cues and cellular infiltration. J Neuroinflammation 2021;18(1):284.
4. Ng SY, Lee AYW. Traumatic brain injuries: pathophysiology and potential therapeutic targets. Front Cell Neurosci 2019;13. https://doi.org/10.3389/fncel.2019.00528.
5. Lascu CF, Hozan CT, Vindis K, et al. Spinal cord injury physiopathology and its causative models: a review study. J Biochem Technol 2023;14(4–2023):19–24.
6. Okada S, Hara M, Kobayakawa K, et al. Astrocyte reactivity and astrogliosis after spinal cord injury. Neurosci Res 2018;126:39–43.
7. Bellver-Landete V, Bretheau F, Mailhot B, et al. Microglia are an essential component of the neuroprotective scar that forms after spinal cord injury. Nat Commun 2019;10(1):518.
8. Asher RA, Morgenstern DA, Shearer MC, et al. Versican is upregulated in CNS injury and is a product of oligodendrocyte lineage cells. J Neurosci 2002;22(6):2225–36.
9. David G, Mohammadi S, Martin AR, et al. Traumatic and nontraumatic spinal cord injury: pathological insights from neuroimaging. Nat Rev Neurol 2019;15(12):718–31.
10. Ahuja CS, Wilson JR, Nori S, et al. Traumatic spinal cord injury. Nat Rev Dis Primers 2017;3(1):17018.
11. Badhiwala JH, Ahuja CS, Akbar MA, et al. Degenerative cervical myelopathy — update and future directions. Nat Rev Neurol 2020;16(2):108–24.
12. Witiw CD, Fehlings MG. Degenerative cervical myelopathy. CMAJ (Can Med Assoc J) 2017;189(3):E116.

13. Hirai T, Uchida K, Nakajima H, et al. The prevalence and phenotype of activated microglia/macrophages within the spinal cord of the hyperostotic mouse (twy/twy) changes in response to chronic progressive spinal cord compression: implications for human cervical compressive myelopathy. In: Block ML, editor. PLoS One 2013;8(5):e64528.
14. Yu WR, Karadimas SK, Hong J, et al. An examination of the role of CX3CR1 in the pathobiology of degenerative cervical myelopathy: evidence from human and mouse tissue. J Clin Med 2025; 15(1):82.
15. Mackiewicz-Milewska M, Cisowska-Adamiak M, Głowacka-Mrotek I, et al. Traumatic vs. non-traumatic spinal cord injury—epidemiology, complications, and neurological status during rehabilitation. JCM 2025;14(15):5209.
16. Spinal cord injury and degenerative cervical myelopathy. Handb Clin Neurol 2022;189:241–57. https://doi.org/10.1016/B978-0-323-91532-8.00006-9. Elsevier.
17. Nouri A, Tetreault L, Singh A, et al. Degenerative cervical myelopathy: epidemiology, genetics, and pathogenesis. Spine (Phila Pa 1976) 2015;40(12):E675–93.
18. Smith SS, Stewart ME, Davies BM, et al. The prevalence of asymptomatic and symptomatic spinal cord compression on magnetic resonance imaging: a systematic review and meta-analysis. Glob Spine J 2021;11(4):597–607.
19. Oh T, Lafage R, Lafage V, et al. Comparing quality of life in cervical spondylotic myelopathy with other chronic debilitating diseases using the short form survey 36-Health survey. World Neurosurg 2017; 106:699–706.
20. Scheuren PS, Hupp M, Pfender N, et al. Contact heat evoked potentials reveal distinct patterns of spinal cord impairment in degenerative cervical myelopathy beyond MRI lesions. Eur J Neurol 2025;32(1):e70001.
21. Xie B, Ni H, Yao J, et al. Functional and structural brain remodeling in patients with degenerative cervical myelopathy following cervical decompression surgery. Commun Med 2025;5(1):191.
22. Sweetman H, Rahman M, Vedantam A, et al. Subclinical respiratory dysfunction and impaired ventilatory adaptation in degenerative cervical myelopathy. Exp Neurol 2024;371:114600.
23. Ulndreaj A, Ávila A, Hong J, et al. Acute systemic white blood cell changes following degenerative cervical myelopathy (DCM) in a mouse model. IJMS 2022;23(19):11496.
24. Vedantam A, Rahman M, Salam S, et al. Serum protein biomarkers for degenerative cervical myelopathy: a prospective study. J Neurosurg Spine 2025;42(6): 718–26.
25. Du S, Sun Y, Zhao B. Interleukin-6 serum levels are elevated in individuals with degenerative cervical myelopathy and are correlated with symptom severity. Med Sci Monit 2018;24:7405–13.
26. Yu WR, Liu T, Kiehl TR, et al. Human neuropathological and animal model evidence supporting a role for Fas-mediated apoptosis and inflammation in cervical spondylotic myelopathy. Brain 2011;134(5): 1277–92.
27. Ossandón-Pino N, Musleh-Vega S, Pacheco JM, et al. Antibiotic administration decreases microglia and macrophage recruitment in a sex-dependent manner following degenerative cervical myelopathy. Mol Neurobiol 2025;63(1):1.
28. Yousefpour N, Tansley SN, Locke S, et al. Targeting C1q prevents microglia-mediated synaptic removal in neuropathic pain. Nat Commun 2025;16(1):4590.
29. Takano M, Kawabata S, Komaki Y, et al. Inflammatory cascades mediate synapse elimination in spinal cord compression. J Neuroinflammation 2014; 11(1):40.
30. He Z, Tang T, Zhu Z, et al. Development of a mouse model of chronic ventral spinal cord compression: Neurobehavioral, radiological, and pathological changes. JOR SPINE 2024;7(3):e1350.
31. Lawrence JM, Schardien K, Wigdahl B, et al. Roles of neuropathology-associated reactive astrocytes: a systematic review. Acta Neuropathol Commun 2023;11(1):42.
32. Liu LR, Chen LJ, Shuang BJ, et al. Interaction of microglia and astrocytes in the neurovascular unit. Front Immunol 2020;11. https://doi.org/10.3389/fimmu.2020.01024.
33. Xu X, Zhang A, Zhu Y, et al. MFG-E8 reverses microglial-induced neurotoxic astrocyte (A1) via NF-κB and PI3K-Akt pathways. J Cell Physiol 2019; 234(1):904–14.
34. Kim S, Son Y. Astrocytes stimulate microglial proliferation and M2 polarization in vitro through crosstalk between astrocytes and microglia. Int J Mol Sci 2021;22(16):8800.
35. Akter F, Yu X, Qin X, et al. The pathophysiology of degenerative cervical myelopathy and the physiology of recovery following decompression. Front Neurosci 2020;14. Available at: https://www.frontiersin.org/articles/10.3389/fnins.2020.00138. Accessed May 27, 2023.
36. Ren ZX, Xu JH, Cheng X, et al. Pathophysiological mechanisms of chronic compressive spinal cord injury due to vascular events. Neural Regen Res 2023;18(4):790.
37. Yao M, Li G, Pu P-M, et al. Neuroinflammation and apoptosis after surgery for a rat model of double-level cervical cord compression. Neurochem Int 2022;157:105340.
38. Lee P, Chandel NS, Simon MC. Cellular adaptation to hypoxia through hypoxia inducible factors and beyond. Nat Rev Mol Cell Biol 2020;21(5): 268–83.

39. Cheng X, Long H, Chen W, et al. The correlation between hypoxia-inducible factor-1α, matrix metalloproteinase-9 and functional recovery following chronic spinal cord compression. Brain Res 2019;1718:75–82.
40. Long HQ, Li GS, Cheng X, et al. Role of hypoxia-induced VEGF in blood-spinal cord barrier disruption in chronic spinal cord injury. Chinese Journal of Traumatology 2015;18(5):293–5.
41. Hernandez-Gerez E, Fleming IN, Parson SH. A role for spinal cord hypoxia in neurodegeneration. Cell Death Dis 2019;10(11):861.
42. Wu L, Niu Z, Hu X, et al. Regional cerebral metabolic levels and turnover in awake rats after acute or chronic spinal cord injury. FASEB J 2020;34(8):10547–59.
43. Dolci S, Mannino L, Bottani E, et al. Therapeutic induction of energy metabolism reduces neural tissue damage and increases microglia activation in severe spinal cord injury. Pharmacol Res 2022;178:106149.
44. Fehlings MG, Ibrahim A, Tetreault L, et al. A global perspective on the outcomes of surgical decompression in patients with cervical spondylotic myelopathy: results from the prospective multicenter AOSpine international study on 479 patients. Spine 2015;40(17):1322.
45. Algahtani AY, Bamsallm M, Alghamdi KT, et al. Cervical spinal cord ischemic reperfusion injury: a comprehensive narrative review of the literature and case presentation. Cureus 2022;14. https://doi.org/10.7759/cureus.28715.
46. Karadimas SK, Laliberte AM, Tetreault L, et al. Riluzole blocks perioperative ischemia-reperfusion injury and enhances postdecompression outcomes in cervical spondylotic myelopathy. Sci Transl Med 2015;7(316):316ra194.
47. Vidal PM, Karadimas SK, Ulndreaj A, et al. Delayed decompression exacerbates ischemia-reperfusion injury in cervical compressive myelopathy. JCI Insight 2017;2(11). https://doi.org/10.1172/jci.insight.92512.
48. Smith PD, Puskas F, Meng X, et al. The evolution of chemokine release supports a bimodal mechanism of spinal cord ischemia and reperfusion injury. Circulation 2012;126(11_suppl_1):S110–7.
49. Wulf MJ, Tom VJ. Consequences of spinal cord injury on the sympathetic nervous system. Front Cell Neurosci 2023;17. https://doi.org/10.3389/fncel.2023.999253.
50. Carpenter RS, Marbourg JM, Brennan FH, et al. Spinal cord injury causes chronic bone marrow failure. Nat Commun 2020;11(1):3702.
51. O'Connor G, Jeffrey E, Madorma D, et al. Investigation of microbiota alterations and intestinal inflammation post-spinal cord injury in rat model. J Neurotrauma 2018;35(18):2159–66.
52. Kigerl KA, Hall JCE, Wang L, et al. Gut dysbiosis impairs recovery after spinal cord injury. J Exp Med 2016;213(12):2603–20.
53. Davies BM, Munro C, Khan DZ, et al. Outcomes of degenerative cervical myelopathy from the perspective of persons living with the condition: findings of a semistructured interview process with partnered internet survey. Glob Spine J 2022;12(3):432–40.
54. Nouri A, Badhiwala JH, Kato S, et al. The relationship between gastrointestinal comorbidities, clinical presentation and surgical outcome in patients with DCM: analysis of a global cohort. J Clin Med 2020;9(3):624.
55. Gungor B, Adiguzel E, Gursel I, et al. Intestinal microbiota in patients with spinal cord injury. PLoS One 2016;11(1):e0145878.
56. Bazzocchi G, Turroni S, Bulzamini MC, et al. Changes in gut microbiota in the acute phase after spinal cord injury correlate with severity of the lesion. Sci Rep 2021;11(1):12743.
57. Jing Y, Yang D, Bai F, et al. Spinal cord injury-induced gut dysbiosis influences neurological recovery partly through short-chain fatty acids. npj Biofilms Microbiomes 2023;9(1):1–15.
58. Fang M, Liu W, Wang Z, et al. Causal associations between gut microbiota with intervertebral disk degeneration, low back pain, and sciatica: a Mendelian randomization study. Eur Spine J 2024;33(4):1424–39.
59. Farkas C, Retamal-Fredes E, Ávila A, et al. Degenerative cervical myelopathy induces sex-specific dysbiosis in mice. Front Microbiol 2023;14. https://doi.org/10.3389/fmicb.2023.1229783.
60. Rajasekaran S, Soundararajan DCR, Tangavel C, et al. Human intervertebral discs harbour a unique microbiome and dysbiosis determines health and disease. Eur Spine J 2020;29(7):1621–40.
61. Zhang J, Wang B, Du P, et al. Gut-disc axis: a Mendelian randomization study on the relationship between gut microbiota and cervical spondylosis. Medicine 2025;104(7):e41536.
62. Nouri A, Tessitore E, Molliqaj G, et al. Degenerative cervical myelopathy: development and natural history [AO spine RECODE-DCM research priority number 2]. Glob Spine J 2022;12(1 Suppl):39S–54S.
63. Salvador AFM, Dykstra T, Rustenhoven J, et al. Age-dependent immune and lymphatic responses after spinal cord injury. Neuron 2023;111(14):2155–69.e9.
64. Anderson MA, Burda JE, Ren Y, et al. Astrocyte scar formation aids central nervous system axon regeneration. Nature 2016;532(7598):195–200.
65. Brennan FH, Li Y, Wang C, et al. Microglia coordinate cellular interactions during spinal cord repair in mice. Nat Commun 2022;13(1):4096.
66. Future perspectives after the guidelines of degenerative cervical myelopathy: a narrative review. J Clin Orthop Trauma 2025;68:103104.
67. Evaniew N, Burger LD, Dea N, et al. Deterioration after surgery for degenerative cervical myelopathy: an observational study from the Canadian

spine outcomes and research network. Spine 2023;48(5):310.

68. Divi SN, Markova DZ, D'Antonio ND, et al. Circulating microRNAs may be predictive of degenerative cervical myelopathy. Spine 2024;49(20):1393.

69. Vansteenkiste DP, Fenger JM, Fadda P, et al. MicroRNA expression in the cerebrospinal fluid of dogs with and without cervical spondylomyelopathy. J Vet Intern Med 2019;33(6):2685–92.

70. MicroRNA-10a, -210, and -563 as circulating biomarkers for ossification of the posterior longitudinal ligament. Spine J 2019;19(4):735–43. https://doi.org/10.1016/j.spinee.2018.10.008.

71. Laliberte AM, Karadimas SK, Vidal PM, et al. Mir21 modulates inflammation and sensorimotor deficits in cervical myelopathy: data from humans and animal models. Brain Commun 2021;3(1):fcaa234.

72. Yan R, Chen R, Wang J, et al. Jingshu Keli and its components notoginsenoside R1 and ginsenoside Rb1 alleviate the symptoms of cervical myelopathy through Kir3.1 mediated mechanisms. CNS Neurol Disord: Drug Targets 2019;18(8):631–42.

73. Holly LT, Blaskiewicz D, Wu A, et al. Dietary therapy to promote neuroprotection in chronic spinal cord injury. J Neurosurg Spine 2012;17(2):134–40.

74. Hertig-Godeschalk A, Glisic M, Ruettimann B, et al. The feasibility of a randomized controlled cross-over trial to assess the effect of probiotic and prebiotic supplementation on the health of elite wheelchair athletes. Pilot Feasibility Stud 2023; 9(1):99.

Pathophysiology and Repair Potential in Degenerative Cervical Myelopathy

Sebastian A. Lares, BSc[a], Nader Hejrati, MD[b,c],
James D. Guest, MD, PhD, FAANS[a,d,*]

KEYWORDS

• Spinal cord injury • Degenerative cervical myelopathy • Neuroplasticity and recovery
• Demyelination • Apoptosis • Ischemia

KEY POINTS

- Degenerative cervical myelopathy (DCM) represents a chronic, progressive injury state characterized by sustained mechanical compression, ischemia, apoptosis, inflammation, and demyelination, distinct from acute traumatic SCI.
- Pathology extends beyond the compression site, involving distributed degeneration and network-level changes across the spinal cord and brain.
- Functional impairment reflects a balance between axonal dysfunction (potentially reversible) and irreversible structural loss, highlighting a critical window for intervention.
- Surgical decompression halts ongoing injury and may enable recovery through relief of distortion, remyelination, restored perfusion, and neuroplasticity, though outcomes are limited by chronicity and age.
- Emerging therapies—including neuromodulation and pharmacologic agents—aim to enhance recovery by targeting residual circuitry and repair mechanisms.

INTRODUCTION

In the aging population of the 21st century, compression of the spinal cord due to age-associated degenerative spinal changes is increasingly important as a source of neurologic disability. When the compression is severe and causes impairment of function, the treatment is surgical decompression, which can be followed by variable recovery due to *endogenous mechanisms*. It is of great interest to determine if advanced recovery technologies that have been applied to *traumatic spinal cord injury* (tSCI) are also helpful in compressive myelopathy, which has recently been unified under the term degenerative cervical myelopathy (DCM).[1]

The development of treatment approaches must be grounded in a thorough understanding of pathophysiology. In this article, we review the relevant pathophysiology to anticipate which treatments investigated for tSCI may be relevant to DCM. While we have learned much about the spinal cord's responses to injury in the tSCI field, there are important differences because myelopathy is

[a] The Miami Project to Cure Paralysis, Miller School of Medicine, Miami, FL, USA; [b] Department of Neurosurgery and Spine Center, HOCH Health Ostschweiz, St. Gallen, Switzerland; [c] Faculty of Medicine, University of Basel, Basel, Switzerland; [d] Department of Neurological Surgery, University of Miami Miller School of Medicine, Miami, FL, USA
* Corresponding author. Neurological Surgery, and Christine E. Lynn Rehabilitation Center, Miller School of Medicine, 1095 NW 14th Terrace, Miami, FL 33136.
E-mail address: Jguest@med.miami.edu

Neurosurg Clin N Am 37 (2026) 489–504
https://doi.org/10.1016/j.nec.2026.05.012

Abbreviations	
BSCB	blood-spinal cord barrier
CST	corticospinal tract
DCM	degenerative cervical myelopathy
MS	multiple sclerosis
MTR	magnetization transfer ratio
MWF	myelin water fraction
MWI	myelin water imaging
OPC	oligodendrocyte progenitor cell
PWI	perfusion-weighted MRI
rTMS	repetitive transcranial magnetic stimulation
SCBF	spinal cord blood flow
tSCI	traumatic spinal cord injury
tSCS	transcutaneous spinal cord stimulation

a gradual process that typically affects older individuals. It is thus important to understand the effects of advancing age on recovery processes,[2] which require both tissue repair and circuit neuroplasticity.[3] Advancing age is consistently associated with lower postoperative DCM recovery potential, even though older patients can still improve clinically.[4]

While the neurologic improvement following surgical decompression must be largely due to improved axonal and neuronal function, we have relatively limited insight into the specific recovery processes. Mechanistically, chronic compression produces ischemia, axonal loss, demyelination, inflammation, and network reorganization. Decompression may lead to a period of tissue repair and plasticity in residual circuitry, but the extent of "reversible" substrate may be reduced and compounded by longer symptom duration and more advanced cord injury at presentation.[5] Consistent with this, there may be a *ceiling* of functional recovery after surgery.[6]

The Compressed Spinal Cord as a Distinct Biological State

Although DCM and acute tSCI may ultimately produce overlapping clinical manifestations of motor, sensory, and autonomic dysfunction, their biological mechanisms differ in important respects. tSCI results from a sudden mechanical insult that causes immediate axonal disruption, hemorrhage, rapidly expanding edema, and necrosis.[7,8] Secondary injury mechanisms, including excitotoxic stress, inflammation, vascular compromise, apoptosis, and demyelination, evolve rapidly after this discrete primary event and contribute to progressive tissue loss before stabilization of the focal lesion occurs, which is characterized by deposition of a glial scar.[7,9] The single tSCI injury is followed by extensive neuroplastic adaptations throughout the nervous system, depending on its severity.

In contrast, DCM develops gradually as a consequence of progressive degenerative changes of the cervical spine, leading to canal narrowing, spinal tissue compression, and abnormal strains. Changes include disc bulging and osteophyte formation, ligamentum flavum hypertrophy or invagination, and dynamic tethering during neck movement.[7] The temporal profile of neural injury in DCM is prolonged, often evolving over months to years before clinical presentation.[10] There is usually no single inciting event that demarcates a primary from secondary injury; instead, ongoing compression sustains a biological environment characterized by continued mechanical deformation and metabolic stress (**Fig. 1** and **Table 1**). Thus, the secondary injury processes that are generally time-limited after tSCI may persist indefinitely in myelopathy.

Although DCM and tSCI share downstream processes such as axonal degeneration, demyelination, inflammatory signaling, vascular alterations, and apoptotic cell death,[7,10] the manner in which these processes unfold differs substantially. In DCM, mechanical deformation is chronic and repetitive. Experimental compression models demonstrate oligodendrocyte apoptosis, resulting in segmental demyelination, impaired axonal conduction, reactive astrogliosis, and neuronal loss.5 Mechanical stress, hypoperfusion,[11] and inflammatory activation[12] act in concert under sustained compression to generate a persistent, progressive injury environment. Also, it is extremely rare for DCM to become as severe as a complete SCI, and autonomic disturbances more prominently affect the bladder than blood pressure.[13] Profound dysautonomia, such as autonomic dysreflexia, is rare in DCM.14

Degenerative Cervical Myelopathy Is Associated with Distributed Pathology Within the Neural Axis

Established DCM produces axonal injury at the site of compression. As in tSCI, loss of axons at the epicenter is expected to result in anterograde and retrograde Wallerian degeneration along long tracts, particularly the corticospinal tracts (CSTs) and dorsal columns.[15,16] In Wallerian degeneration, the associated myelin of degenerating axons is removed by macrophages, leaving behind depleted tissue primarily composed of astrocytes and microglia. Quantitative MRI studies have demonstrated microstructural abnormalities above and below the DCM stenotic level, with reduced fractional anisotropy and altered diffusivity within

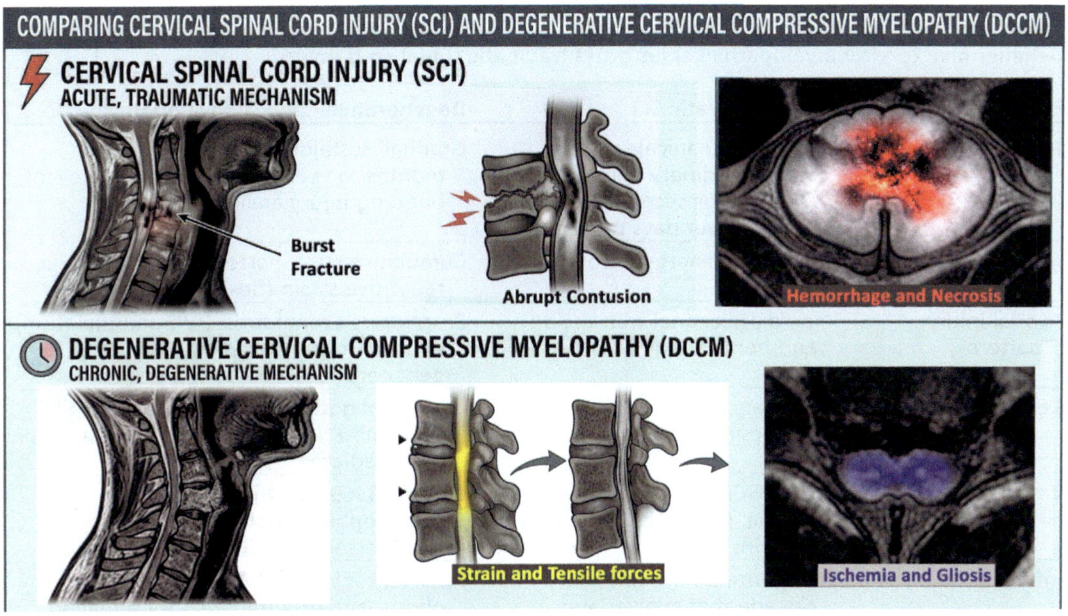

Fig. 1. The distinctions between acute traumatic spinal cord injury and chronic compressive myelopathy are indicated. These include the abrupt contusive event that initiates SCI and the extent of hemorrhage and necrosis (not seen in compressive myelopathy). Also, the compressive and motion-related tensile forces associated with myelopathy are indicated as a gradient (yellow, lower middle panel). Unlike acute SCI, DCM is associated with chronic ischemia (blue, lower-right panel).

the CST and posterior columns at rostral cervical levels (eg, C2/C3) that align anatomically with known tract trajectories.[10,17,18] This component of remote degeneration in DCM may be explained as tract-specific Wallerian degeneration secondary to focal axonal injury.

However, recent quantitative MRI investigations, including multiparametric structural imaging, diffusion tensor imaging (DTI), magnetization transfer imaging, and perfusion-sensitive techniques, have reported additional changes that extend beyond classical tract-restricted Wallerian patterns. Grabher and colleagues (2017) reported ventral horn gray matter alterations in DCM, suggesting neuronal compartment involvement in addition to white matter tract changes.[19] Studies have demonstrated gray and white matter atrophy at rostral cervical levels and, in some reports, at caudal segments distant from the compression site.[10,18] Furthermore, perfusion-sensitive imaging has suggested impaired microvascular parameters above the stenosis,[20] raising the possibility of hemodynamic contributions to tissue injury beyond the maximal stenosis. Multicenter quantitative MRI studies have found supraspinal structural changes, including thalamic and corticospinal pathway alterations, in DCM patients,21 findings interpreted as evidence of network-level or trans-synaptic degeneration.

Structural and diffusion imaging above the level of compression demonstrate microstructural alterations within the ventral horns without measurable atrophy, whereas the dorsal horns exhibit volumetric reduction without corresponding diffusivity changes.[19] Ventral horn diffusivity alterations correlate with CST abnormalities, suggesting early involvement of motor neuronal pools, while dorsal horn atrophy relates more closely to sensory dysfunction.[19] Quantitative MRI further demonstrates infralesional microstructural abnormalities and tissue loss extending into the lumbar enlargement, indicating that the effects of chronic compression involve distributed network changes.[10,22,23] DCM may thus exhibit more widespread, active, region-specific pathology than post-tSCI Wallerian degeneration.

Mechanisms of Injury in Chronic Spinal Cord Compression

Cumulative mechanical loading and tissue strain

Dynamic imaging and patient-specific modeling studies support the idea that DCM is driven not only by "static" stenosis but also by repetitive, motion-dependent, spatially nonuniform tissue deformation (**Table 2**). Using 3D registration of flexion/extension MRI, Stoner and colleagues

Table 1
Degenerative cervical myelopathy versus acute traumatic spinal cord injury

Feature	Acute Traumatic SCI	Degenerative Cervical Myelopathy
Temporal profile	Sudden mechanical insult; discrete primary injury followed by secondary cascade over days to weeks	Gradual, sustained compression over months to years; no single inciting event; ongoing injury environment
Mechanical loading	Single high-energy deformation	Cumulative static narrowing and dynamic repetitive strain (flexion/extension)
Axonal injury pattern	Immediate axonal transection and hemorrhage at impact site	Progressive axonal stress (APP accumulation) with preserved continuity; Wallerian degeneration in advanced stages
Demyelination	Secondary demyelination in peri-lesional zones	Primary oligodendrocyte apoptosis with segmental demyelination; potential intermediate recoverable state
Vascular response	Acute BSCB breach with rapid edema; permeability to large proteins resolves within ~2 wk	Chronic BSCB dysfunction without catastrophic breach; sustained ischemia from vessel distortion and hyalinization
Inflammation	Rapid, intense inflammatory cascade that evolves and partially resolves	Persistent microglial activation, reactive gliosis, and proinflammatory signaling under ongoing compression
Spatial distribution	Focal epicenter with rostro-caudal secondary degeneration; more severe tract-specific disruption	Spatially heterogeneous; region-specific gray matter changes (ventral horn diffusivity vs dorsal horn atrophy); remote degeneration to lumbar enlargement
Neuroplasticity	Abrupt deafferentation triggers rapid cortical map reorganization	Gradual deafferentation drives progressive, severity-dependent redistribution within established sensorimotor circuits
Recovery substrate	Abrupt loss limits residual substrate; rapid stabilization of lesion	Partially preserved axonal continuity and distributed redundant circuitry; recovery potential shaped by duration of compression

Comparison of key biological features distinguishing DCM from acute traumatic SCI.

showed that in healthy subjects principal strain during physiologic motion is relatively evenly distributed along the cervical cord, whereas in cervical myelopathy the cord displaces less and exhibits higher principal strain concentrated at mid-cervical levels, consistent with segmental "tethering" and strain amplification at/near compressive levels during everyday neck motion.[24] Extending this concept, Rahman and colleagues used patient-specific FE models and reported that intramedullary stress and strain at the level of maximum compression during neck flexion correlate with preoperative neurologic dysfunction, including sensorimotor hand impairment and overall disease severity, linking abnormal, repetitive flexion-associated loading to clinically meaningful deficits.[25]

Finite element analyses indicate that repetitive strain in DCM follows distinct intramedullary distribution patterns shaped by compression morphology and dynamic "pincer" mechanics. In the 3D FE analysis by Nishida and colleagues, simulated ligamentum flavum invagination during extension produced stress concentrations that differed by the pattern of anterior cord deformation. With central-type anterior compression, stress localized to the posterior horn and portions of posterior/lateral funiculi (beneath the posterior invagination), whereas lateral-type compression produced stress in gray matter and lateral funiculus on the compression side with additional stress in posterior structures contralaterally under ligamentum flavum indentation; diffuse-type deformation yielded a wider stress field spanning gray matter plus lateral and posterior funiculi.[26]

Thus, tissue injury in DCM arises from the interaction among spinal canal and recess degenerative patterns, mechanical stress, intrinsic tissue vulnerability, and exposure duration.[27]

Vascular dysfunction and chronic ischemia

A central question in DCM is the extent to which chronic ischemia contributes to tissue injury. Early

Table 2
Pathophysiology of degenerative cervical myelopathy

Mechanism	Key Features in DCM	Clinical Significance
Cumulative mechanical loading	Static canal narrowing + dynamic flexion–extension strain; cumulative burden over time (AO Spine RECODE framework)	Injury severity depends on magnitude × duration × tissue vulnerability, not single-timepoint canal diameter
Axonal injury	APP accumulation reflecting impaired axonal transport; GAP-43 upregulation and sprouting after decompression	Axons may be dysfunctional but structurally intact, retaining potential for physiologic recovery
Oligodendrocyte apoptosis and demyelination	Caspase-dependent apoptosis of myelinating cells; segmental demyelination with preserved axonal profiles	Conduction failure can exceed structural axonal loss; demyelination may mark a recoverable intermediate state
Vascular dysfunction	Vessel wall thickening, hyalinization; reduced spinal cord blood flow; HIF-1α/VEGF upregulation	Medial gray matter and terminal-branch territories are earliest affected; decompression partially restores perfusion
BSCB impairment	Chronic tight-junction disruption; elevated CSF:serum protein ratios; abnormal contrast enhancement	Permits inflammatory infiltration and serum-derived factors; sustains ischemia–inflammation cycle
Inflammatory activation	Microglial activation; reactive astrogliosis; proinflammatory microenvironment	Drives both demyelination (oligodendrocyte loss) and neuronal apoptosis; M2 phenotype required for repair
Neuronal and gray matter loss	Anterior horn motor neuron apoptosis; ventral horn diffusivity changes preceding clinical deficits; dorsal horn volumetric atrophy	Region-specific vulnerability; motor deficits correlate with ventral horn/CST changes; sensory deficits with dorsal horn atrophy
Wallerian degeneration	Disruption of descending motor tracts in advanced/prolonged compression	Marks transition from potentially recoverable dysfunction to irreversible structural loss

Principal injury mechanisms in chronic spinal cord compression and their clinical significance.

perfusion-weighted MRI perfusion-imaging imaging (PWI) studies demonstrated reduced perfusion indices at the level of maximal compression, with partial normalization after decompression, suggesting that spinal cord blood flow (SCBF) is dynamically constrained rather than irreversibly lost.[28] More recent dynamic susceptibility contrast MRI investigations have shown abnormal hemodynamic parameters consistent with impaired microvascular perfusion and oxygen delivery at compressed segments, with perfusion metrics correlating with clinical severity and neurologic impairment.[29]

Diffusion-based techniques further refine this picture. Intravoxel incoherent motion MRI, which provides a noncontrast surrogate of microvascular perfusion, demonstrates reduced perfusion fractions at and even rostral to the site of maximal stenosis, indicating that vascular compromise may extend longitudinally beyond the focal compressive level.[20] Complementing imaging data, intraoperative power Doppler ultrasonography has directly demonstrated reduced regional SCBFs in patients with cervical spondylotic myelopathy, with measurable increases following decompression.[30,31] Across modalities, studies indicate that the chronically compressed cord is in a state of persistent hypoperfusion with impaired vascular reserve.

Histopathologic findings from human autopsy series align with these observations. Classic clinicopathologic studies of CSM describe selective gray matter involvement, cavitation, and necrosis within the anterior horns and central cord, often disproportionate to purely white matter tract compression.[32] The relative vulnerability of metabolically active gray matter neurons, particularly anterior horn cells, is consistent with chronic hypoxic stress. Additional reports describe microvascular changes, including hyalinization and narrowing of intramedullary arterioles, as well as gliosis and myelin loss in a watershed-like distribution.

Taken together, human imaging, intraoperative hemodynamic measurements, and histopathology converge on a model in which DCM represents a state of mechanical deformation compounded by chronic microvascular insufficiency. The pathology appears to involve subthreshold, repetitive ischemic stress where baseline perfusion is reduced, and vascular reserve is limited, rendering the cord susceptible to episodic hypoperfusion during neck motion, systemic hypotension, or dynamic "pincer" compression. Decompression may therefore confer benefit not only by relieving structural distortion but also by restoring perfusion reserve and mitigating ongoing ischemic injury.

Loss of blood–brain barrier function and inflammation

An intact spinal cord microvascular endothelium is essential for maintaining blood–spinal cord barrier integrity, thereby limiting the entry of circulating inflammatory mediators/cells and reducing vasogenic edema within spinal cord tissue.[33] Differences in vascular response further underscore this contrast. In acute tSCI, primary trauma disrupts the blood-spinal cord barrier (BSCB), leading to rapid edema and leakage of serum macromolecules; permeability to large proteins typically diminishes over subsequent weeks, although alterations in smaller molecules may persist.[34] In DCM, by contrast, BSCB dysfunction occurs in a sustained progressive manner. Elevated cerebrospinal fluid-to-serum protein ratios, abnormal MRI contrast enhancement, and histologic evidence of tight junction disruption under sustained compression indicate chronic barrier impairment.[34] Rather than resolving after an acute event, vascular dysfunction in DCM persists under ongoing mechanical stress, contributing to a prolonged state of ischemia and inflammatory activation.[34] However, after surgical treatment, there is evidence from human studies that barrier function can be restored.[35]

Inflammatory cascades and apoptosis

tSCI is characterized by an immediate influx of neutrophils through the BSCB, leading to lipid peroxidation and necrosis.[36] This severe inflammatory event does not occur in DCM; rather, there is long-term microglial activation, influx of CD11/CD45 macrophages, transitions between M1 and M2 macrophage states, and influx of CD4 helper T cells.[37] In DCM, mechanical stress and hypoxia converge with inflammatory signaling pathways to promote cellular injury. Microglial activation and reactive gliosis further sustain a proinflammatory microenvironment.[5] Tumor necrosis factor-α (TNFα)-dependent signaling has also been implicated in oligodendrocyte death in chronic compression models, further linking inflammation to white matter injury in myelopathy.

In models of cervical compressive myelopathy, oligodendrocyte apoptosis and demyelination are described as early features of injury and may precede or amplify later axonal degeneration, helping explain how chronic compression can produce substantial conduction failure before complete axonal loss is established. Chronic compression models demonstrate activation of caspase-dependent pathways in both oligodendroglia and neurons,[38] and shifts in pro-apoptotic signaling.[5,39] Oligodendrocyte apoptosis contributes directly to demyelination, whereas neuronal apoptosis within anterior horn regions correlates with progressive motor deficits.[31,39] These processes exist along a continuum: early inflammatory activation may impair conduction and synaptic function, whereas sustained apoptotic signaling culminates in structural cell loss. Oligodendrocytes appear especially vulnerable because they sit at the intersection of several injurious processes: ischemia from microvascular compromise, glutamate-mediated excitotoxicity, oxidative stress, and inflammatory signaling.[40] Relative to many other neural cell types, oligodendroglia have high metabolic demands to maintain their extensive myelin, comparatively limited antioxidant defenses, and marked sensitivity to AMPA/kainate receptor activation,[41] all of which make them prone to apoptosis when tissue perfusion and homeostasis are disturbed.[42]

Axonal dysfunction versus irreversible loss

Clinical studies have indicated that conduction slowing of neurophysiologic potentials correlates with compression severity,[43] and, in some cases, conduction improvement can be demonstrated at the time of decompression[44] or at follow-up.[45] A potentially critical distinction in DCM lies between axonal dysfunction and irreversible axonal loss. An important question is whether axons whose function has been compromised, such as by myelin distortion, local demyelination, or impaired axonal transport, can recover useful function. In chronic human tSCI, neurofilament-positive axons lacking myelin have been identified in pericavity regions, indicating that axonal continuity can persist despite loss of surrounding myelin.[46] In experimental models of chronic cervical compression, intra-axonal accumulation of amyloid precursor protein has been observed, consistent with impaired axonal transport under sustained focal mechanical stress.[6] Following decompression, increased GAP-43 expression and evidence of axonal sprouting have been reported, indicating structural remodeling when axonal continuity is preserved.[6] In contrast, prolonged compression is associated with Wallerian degeneration and disruption of descending motor tracts in advanced stages.[39] Once axonal transection and substantial neuronal loss occur, the intrinsic capacity for recovery is markedly reduced. Our understanding of whether such axons that remain structurally intact but are functionally compromised can undergo physiologic recovery after relief of compression is incomplete. In conditions such as amyotrophic lateral sclerosis (ALS), compensatory collateral innervation of muscle fibers occurs when motor neurons are lost. Whether this form of compensation is present in DCM is uncertain.[47,48]

Demyelination and Its Potential Repair

Detecting demyelination in vivo

Across several CNS diseases, the question of myelin repair is important, with multiple sclerosis (MS) being the most notable example, as well as tSCI.[49,50] Demyelination may mark a window of recoverable dysfunction in the compressed spinal cord. In DCM, myelin disruption cannot be reliably inferred from conventional MRI alone, as standard structural MRI lacks specificity for microstructural alterations such as demyelination.[51] However, myelin water imaging (MWI) studies in patients with DCM demonstrate reductions in myelin water fraction that correlate with abnormal somatosensory evoked potentials, providing in vivo evidence of decreased myelin content associated with impaired spinal cord conduction.[52] Conventional MRI metrics, such as the degree of compression, show limited correlation with functional deficits, whereas MWI provides complementary, more myelin-specific information.[52] Within the pathophysiological framework of DCM, demyelination is a biologically meaningful component of white matter injury.

Consequences beyond conduction slowing

Myelin supports both saltatory impulse conduction and axonal viability through trophic mechanisms, and its disruption has consequences that extend beyond slowed signaling. White matter injury in chronic compression reflects the high vulnerability of myelinating cells to excitotoxic perturbation.[53] Redistribution of sodium and potassium channels along demyelinated segments and impaired axonal transport can produce conduction block even when axonal continuity is preserved.[54] Sustained demyelination increases susceptibility to secondary axonal degeneration.[54] If remyelination occurs before irreversible degeneration, physiologic recovery remains possible; if not, progressive axonal loss may ensue.

The microenvironment for remyelination

Whether demyelination in chronic compression is reversible depends in part on the surrounding cellular and inflammatory microenvironment. Spontaneous remyelination is well documented in experimental toxin-based systems, but its efficiency requires coordinated immune and glial responses. Macrophage depletion impairs oligodendrocyte remyelination following toxin-induced demyelination, indicating that inflammatory cells are necessary for effective repair.[55] Moreover, a shift toward an M2 microglial and macrophage phenotype promotes oligodendrocyte progenitor cell (OPC) differentiation and remyelination, mediated in part by prodifferentiation factors such as activin-A.[56] These findings indicate that the inflammatory response, as shaped by macrophage and microglial phenotype, is not uniformly detrimental; rather, its *specific* cellular and molecular profile determines whether it supports or impedes remyelination. In DCM, where chronic mechanical deformation is accompanied by sustained ischemia and glial activation, the microenvironment may progressively lose its capacity to support effective OPC maturation.

Evidence of remyelination in multiple sclerosis

In MS, some spontaneous remyelination has been documented in human neuropathology, demonstrating that endogenous repair occurs in the adult CNS.[57] In vivo MRI studies further support remyelination dynamics using myelin-sensitive quantitative metrics. Myelin water fraction (MWF) imaging shows that newly forming MS lesions often exhibit early MWF reduction consistent with demyelination, followed in some lesions by MWF increases over time, consistent with partial remyelination or "myelin recovery" during lesion evolution.[58,59] Similarly, longitudinal magnetization transfer ratio (MTR) studies identify lesion subregions with dynamic decreases in MTR followed by subsequent MTR recovery, changes widely interpreted as reflecting demyelination followed by remyelination.

Taken together, available evidence suggests that demyelination in chronic spinal cord compression occupies a dynamic position along a continuum of injury. Early in the disease course, myelin disruption may reflect a potentially recoverable state in which axons remain structurally intact and capable of functional restoration. Over time, however, sustained mechanical stress, ischemia, and maladaptive inflammatory signaling may reduce the microenvironment's permissiveness for remyelination and increase the likelihood of *secondary axonal degeneration*. The question of reversibility is therefore inseparable from the timing of intervention and the biological context in which repair must occur.

Neuroplastic Responses to Gradual Injury

Supraspinal reorganization

The biological consequences of chronic compression are not confined to the spinal cord itself (**Table 3**). If DCM represents a distinct and progressively evolving pathologic state at the level of the cord, it must likewise involve progressive alterations within supraspinal networks. Neuroplasticity in DCM should therefore be understood as a continuous, adaptive process that unfolds in parallel with ongoing mechanical deformation, ischemia, demyelination, and axonal stress.

Neuroimaging studies support this network-level perspective. A systematic review of brain MRI in DCM demonstrates structural and functional alterations within the sensorimotor network, thalamus, cerebellum, and associative cortical regions.60 Gray matter reductions within primary sensorimotor cortices and cerebellar regions have been reported, accompanied by altered functional connectivity and task-related activation within motor and sensory networks.[60] Task-based functional MRI (fMRI) further shows that supraspinal recruitment scales with compression severity: greater spinal cord compression volume correlates with increased blood-oxygen-level-dependent (BOLD) signal and expanded activation in primary motor and somatosensory cortices, as well as in subcortical motor regions, including the cerebellum, thalamus, putamen, and caudate.[61] Together, these findings indicate that progressive impairment of ascending and descending pathways is associated with graded, distributed supraspinal reorganization.

Deafferentation as a driver of plasticity

A central driver of supraspinal reorganization in DCM is chronic and partial deafferentation. Progressive compression of the dorsal columns and CSTs degrades ascending sensory input and descending motor outputs. This deafferentation arises not from immediate axonal transection,

Table 3
Neuroplastic responses in degenerative cervical myelopathy

Response	Mechanism/Evidence	Functional Implication
Supraspinal cortical reorganization	Expanded BOLD activation in M1, S1, cerebellum, thalamus, putamen, caudate; scales with compression severity	Compensatory recruitment of parallel motor circuits to maintain output despite impaired spinal transmission
Altered functional connectivity	Modified sensorimotor, frontal, and cerebellar network connectivity on resting-state and task-based fMRI	Distributed network-level adaptation rather than purely focal spinal cord dysfunction
Chronic partial deafferentation	Degraded (not lost) ascending/ descending conduction from demyelination and microstructural disruption within preserved tracts	Cortex recalibrates to degraded input; structurally preserved pathways retain potential for functional recovery
Propriospinal relay formation	Spared corticospinal and brainstem fibers sprout onto propriospinal neurons, rerouting commands around focal disruption	Intrinsic spinal circuit reorganization provides substrate for compensation when axonal continuity is partially preserved
Descending pathway redundancy	Parallel reticulospinal, rubrospinal, and propriospinal systems converge on shared motoneuronal pools	Partial compromise of one tract does not equate to complete motor loss; distributed circuitry supports preserved function
Limits of plasticity	Longer symptom duration associated with poorer postoperative recovery; expanding cortical recruitment may reflect diminishing efficiency	Cumulative neuronal loss and gray matter atrophy progressively constrain adaptive capacity; plasticity delays but does not indefinitely prevent decline

Adaptive neural responses to chronic compression and their functional implications.
Abbreviations: BOLD, blood-oxygen-level-dependent; fMRI, functional magnetic resonance imaging.

but from microstructural changes that impair conduction within anatomically preserved pathways. As discussed earlier, histopathological and DTI studies demonstrate segmental demyelination, axonal injury, and reduced fractional anisotropy within these tracts, changes consistent with impaired conduction and microstructural disruption rather than complete axonal loss.[6,10,23,39] Neurophysiological studies further support this interpretation. Delayed central motor conduction time has been attributed to slowed conduction in demyelinated corticospinal fibers, and electrophysiological abnormalities may be detected even in presymptomatic stages of disease.[62] In contrast to the abrupt and often complete deafferentation observed in traumatic SCI, which induces rapid cortical map reorganization and synaptic remodeling,[63] DCM appears to drive a more gradual recalibration of sensorimotor networks. The cortex is not adapting to abrupt loss of input, but to degraded input. This distinction is biologically significant because plastic reorganization in DCM represents a response to gradually degrading yet structurally preserved pathways that may retain the potential for functional recovery.

Compensatory cortical recruitment and its limits

The functional consequences of such reorganization appear compensatory. Patients with more severe structural compression demonstrate greater activation within contralateral primary motor cortex and associated subcortical regions during simple motor tasks.[61] Network-level analyses further reveal altered connectivity within sensorimotor circuits and related frontal and cerebellar regions.[60] Such findings suggest redistribution of activity across parallel motor circuits. In practical terms, increased cortical engagement may allow preservation of function despite impaired spinal transmission.[64]

However, plasticity in DCM is limited. Clinical outcome studies demonstrate that longer preoperative symptom duration is associated with poorer postoperative functional recovery and quality-of-life outcomes, suggesting that prolonged compression may exceed the adaptive capacity of neural networks.[65] Consistent with this concept, greater compression severity is associated with greater cortical recruitment during motor tasks,61 yet this increased activation does not necessarily translate into preserved or fully recoverable function. Instead, expanding recruitment may indicate diminishing efficiency, in which larger neural populations are required to achieve equivalent motor output. Over time, cumulative neuronal loss and gray matter atrophy may constrain further adaptive remodeling. Plasticity may therefore delay functional decline, but it may not indefinitely prevent it under conditions of persistent mechanical and metabolic stress and may transition toward physiologic/network constraints consistent with a limited "reserve capacity".[66]

Functional Preservation Despite Axonal Loss

Redundancy in descending motor systems

Substantial neurologic function may persist in the presence of measurable axonal injury within the compressed spinal cord. This apparent paradox reflects the distributed, redundant organization of the descending, ascending, and propriospinal systems. Voluntary motor control is not mediated exclusively by the CST, but by parallel descending pathways, including reticulospinal projections, that converge upon shared interneuronal and motoneuronal pools.[67] The existence of multiple descending systems provides anatomic redundancy, such that partial compromise of one tract does not equate to complete loss of motor output.

Propriospinal relay pathways

Experimental studies further demonstrate that the spinal cord possesses an intrinsic capacity for circuit reorganization when long tracts are interrupted. Following incomplete injury in experimental animal studies, spared CST and brainstem fibers can sprout and form synaptic contacts onto propriospinal neurons, which in turn project to denervated segments below the lesion.[68] Such propriospinal detour pathways may transfer descending signals around areas of focal tract disruption. Subsequent work has confirmed that structural and functional reorganization of propriospinal connections promotes meaningful recovery, with short-distance fiber growth and synaptic rewiring serving as a substrate for compensation.[69] Although these studies arise primarily from traumatic models, the principles may be relevant to DCM, where axonal continuity is often partially preserved rather than abruptly transected.

Dissociation between structure and function

Clinical and imaging data in DCM further underscore that structural compromise does not directly correlate with functional impairment. Microstructural degeneration can be detected both at and remote from the site of compression, yet tract-specific injury in DCM is generally less severe than in traumatic injury.[10] Moreover, quantitative MRI metrics may demonstrate progression of tissue abnormality even when clinical status remains relatively stable.[23] Conversely, the degree of static cord compression on conventional MRI correlates poorly with symptom severity and functional disability, despite often influencing surgical decision-making.[70]

These observations suggest that a critical mass of structurally intact and functionally recruitable pathways may suffice to preserve meaningful neurologic function despite measurable axonal loss. Functional preservation despite axonal loss, therefore, represents not merely a compensatory phenomenon, but a biological opportunity: the chronically compressed spinal cord retains distributed circuitry that may be amenable to targeted modulation and repair.

Evidence from Surgical Decompression

Surgery as a biological stressor

The treatment of DCM is usually surgical decompression, which removes the major driver of pathology. However, the extent to which surgery is itself a stressor with systemic and local consequences is often underappreciated.[71] These arise from the consequences of anesthesia, local surgical bed inflammation and healing, and potential injury to the spinal cord, dura mater, and nerve roots during surgery.

Interpreting postoperative imaging

For the post-decompression context, this distinction has practical implications. If remote abnormalities predominantly represent secondary Wallerian degeneration, decompression may halt progression but cannot restore axons already lost; recovery would depend on spared fibers and adaptive plasticity. Conversely, if some remote changes reflect potentially reversible pathology—such as demyelination without axonal loss, metabolic dysfunction, or perfusion deficits—there may be a window for partial structural and functional recovery following surgical relief of compression. Determining which quantitative MRI signatures represent irreversible axonal degeneration versus modifiable tissue injury remains a central challenge in contemporary DCM research and is critical for interpreting postoperative imaging and guiding adjunctive neuroprotective or neuromodulatory strategies.

The postoperative repair window

Experimental decompression studies further underscore the importance of timing in shaping the repair environment. In a mouse model of DCM, delayed decompression is associated with exacerbated ischemia-reperfusion injury, prolonged cytokine elevation, persistent microglial activation, and poorer neurologic recovery compared with earlier intervention.[72] These observations suggest that prolonged hypoperfusion and persistent inflammatory activation could create a microenvironment less permissive for myelin repair. Complementary work in rat models of CSM demonstrates structural remodeling and recovery-associated plasticity following decompression, indicating that relief of mechanical stress can reactivate intrinsic repair programs when sufficient viable substrate remains.[6] Together, these data imply that remyelination capacity in chronic compression is time-sensitive and contingent upon the evolving vascular and inflammatory milieu.

Rehabilitation and Neuromodulation

Rehabilitation may be needed after surgical decompression to improve recovery from myelopathic deficits.[73] Neuromodulation to enhance recovery after DCM has not been extensively explored, but approaches such as transcutaneous spinal cord stimulation (tSCS), which is being implemented for chronic SCI,[74] represent biologically plausible strategies. However, these approaches may carry risk while compression remains ongoing, as increased neural excitation could, in theory, potentiate injury. A combination of intensive task practice with vagal nerve stimulation has shown recovery benefits after stroke and chronic SCI,[1] and could be tested in DCM.

Cortical and peripheral stimulation

As a postoperative adjunct, neuromodulation is premised on the principle that recovery after decompression depends not only on removal of mechanical and ischemic stress but also on the capacity of residual spinal and supraspinal networks to reorganize. Noninvasive cortical stimulation with repetitive transcranial magnetic stimulation (rTMS) has been explored in DCM to modulate corticospinal excitability, with systematic review data suggesting feasibility and preliminary signals of benefit for motor function and neuropathic pain, albeit in small and heterogeneous cohorts.[75] Peripheral and task-specific stimulation strategies have shown promise for hand recovery. Functional electrical stimulation paired with structured upper-limb training has been associated with improvements in reaching and grasping in DCM populations, supporting the concept that stimulation-augmented, use-dependent plasticity may enhance dexterity after decompression.[76,77] More recently, spinal neuromodulation approaches have been considered to directly modulate segmental excitability. While traditional cervical spinal cord stimulation has primarily targeted pain relief and lacks robust data on motor restoration in DCM, emerging noninvasive tSCS paradigms are being investigated as postoperative rehabilitation adjuncts, including protocols that pair tSCS with balance and gait training to enhance axial and lower-extremity control. Reviews of emerging therapies in DCM emphasize that such approaches are biologically plausible and increasingly studied, but remain investigational, and require adequately powered randomized trials to determine whether neuromodulation meaningfully augments hand dexterity, balance, and overall functional recovery beyond decompression and conventional rehabilitation alone.

Table 4
Potential therapeutic strategies for degenerative cervical myelopathy

Category	Agent/Approach	Mechanism	Evidence Status in DCM
Surgical	Decompression	Removes mechanical and ischemic stress; may trigger postoperative repair window with axonal sprouting and perfusion recovery	Standard of care; timing critical—delayed decompression associated with ischemia-reperfusion injury and poorer recovery
Neuromodulation	Repetitive TMS (rTMS)	Modulates corticospinal excitability	Feasibility demonstrated; preliminary signals for motor function and neuropathic pain in small DCM cohorts
Neuromodulation	Transcutaneous spinal cord stimulation (tSCS)	Modulates segmental spinal excitability; paired with balance/gait training	Established in chronic tSCI for upper-limb function; investigational in DCM as postoperative rehabilitation adjunct
Neuromodulation	Vagus nerve stimulation + task practice	Closed-loop stimulation promotes use-dependent plasticity	Recovery benefits demonstrated in stroke and chronic SCI; proposed for DCM but not yet tested
Neuromodulation	Functional electrical stimulation therapy	Stimulation-augmented, task-specific upper-limb training	Improvements in reaching/grasping reported in CSM; supports use-dependent plasticity for hand dexterity
Remyelination	Clemastine	Antimuscarinic promoting OPC differentiation via ERK1/2 signaling; increased myelin-associated transcription factor expression	Proof of principle in experimental SCI; not yet evaluated in DCM
Neuroprotection	Riluzole	Sodium channel blockade; reduces excitotoxicity	CSM-Protect phase 3 trial: safe but did not meet primary efficacy endpoint; no drug yet standard-of-care
Microvascular	Limaprost alfadex	Oral PGE1 analog; improves spinal cord microcirculation	Clinical studies in CSM populations report symptom improvement
Neuroprotection/ glial modulation	Ibudilast (MN-166)	Glial/immune modulation; putative neuroprotective effects	Randomized placebo-controlled trial as adjunct to surgery (NCT04631471)
Plasticity priming	Intermittent hypoxia	Neuroplasticity-priming rehabilitation strategy	Strong evidence in SCI paradigms; proposed for DCM but direct clinical evidence limited

Current and emerging interventions beyond surgical decompression, with evidence status.

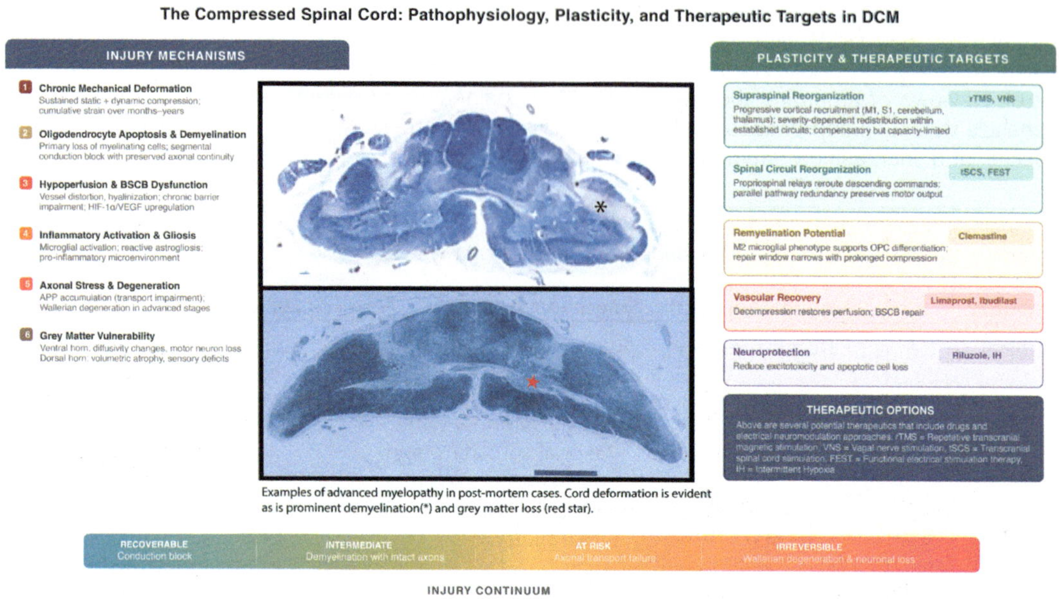

Fig. 2. Pathophysiology, plasticity, and therapeutic targets in DCM. In the central panel postmortem luxol-fast blue sections from individuals with chronic cervical compression myelopathy. In the upper central panel, a region of pallor associated with probable demyelination ± axonal loss is shown. In the lower central panel, there is marked gray matter loss, indicated with the red star.

Emerging Restorative Therapies

The spinal cord is capable of some endogenous repair; however the extent of this capacity in humans, particularly in older individuals and those with relevant comorbidities is unknown (**Table 4**). The morphology of lesions, which are often malacic and gliotic, is not favorable for intraparenchymal transplantation.

Remyelination agents

Drug-induced promotion of OPC differentiation provides additional evidence that demyelination may be biologically reversible under appropriate conditions. Clemastine, an antimuscarinic agent, promotes OPC differentiation and enhances the expression of myelin-associated transcription factors through activation of ERK1/2 signaling in experimental SCI.[78] Clinical evidence for clemastine as a remyelination-promoting therapy was shown in the optic pathway of MS, where a randomized cross-over trial demonstrated modest improvement in visual evoked potential (VEP) latency, consistent with enhanced myelin-dependent conduction, and supportive MRI myelin biomarker analyses. However, cell-type specificity (OPC differentiation) has not been demonstrated clinically, and a progressive-MS platform trial arm was halted due to accelerated disability progression, suggesting potential context-dependent risk.[79]

Neuroprotective, microvascular, and plasticity-priming strategies

A range of drug adjuncts aimed at neuroprotection, microvascular support, or plasticity priming have been explored in DCM as complements to decompression (**Fig. 2**). The CSM-Protect trial evaluated perioperative riluzole as a neuroprotective adjunct to decompressive surgery.[80] Limaprost alfadex (an oral prostaglandin E1 analog) has been studied in DCM-spectrum cohorts to improve microcirculation in the nerve roots and spinal cord.[81,82] Limaprost gained attention for vasculitic diseases and lumbar spinal stenosis in Japanese and Korean studies.[83] No conclusive studies have been conducted on DCM.

Ibudilast, a brain-penetrant phosphodiesterase and macrophage migration inhibition factor (MIF) inhibitor, enhances cyclic adenosine monophospahte response element-binding protein-(CREB) signaling while attenuating microglial-mediated TNF and interleukin 1β (IL-1β) production,[84] thereby shifting the injured spinal cord microenvironment toward a state permissive for activity-dependent synaptic remodeling and oligodendroglial repair. Ibudilast was shown to reduce whole-brain atrophy in MS[85] and gray matter atrophy.[86] It has progressed to formal evaluation as an adjunct to decompressive surgery in DCM through a randomized, placebo-controlled clinical trial pathway (ClinicalTrials.gov NCT04631471).

SUMMARY

Compressed spinal cord tissue is subject to several pathologic changes that are difficult to mitigate without decompression. DCM is associated with compensatory supraspinal reorganization; however, as disease severity/chronicity increases, these adaptations may become less effective and/or transition to maladaptive network states, potentially reducing the capacity for postoperative functional gains. Thus, it is essential to intervene with decompressive surgery before losses are unrecoverable. Both neuromodulatory and drug interventions are being explored to potentiate DCM recovery.

CLINICS CARE POINTS

- In DCM, progressive compression sustains ongoing spinal cord injury; timely decompression is essential before reversible substrate and neuroplastic reserve are exhausted.
- Decompression removes the major driver of injury, but postoperative improvement depends on preserved circuitry, remyelination potential, and rehabilitation-driven plasticity.
- Conventional MRI compression severity alone should not determine clinical judgment, because structural narrowing correlates imperfectly with disability and recovery potential.
- Postoperative rehabilitation should be considered integral to care.
- Neuromodulation may become a useful postoperative adjunct, but it remains investigational and may be inappropriate while substantial compression persists.

DISCLOSURE

The authors have nothing to disclose.

REFERENCES

1. Kilgard MP, Epperson JD, Adehunoluwa EA, et al. Closed-loop vagus nerve stimulation aids recovery from spinal cord injury. Nature 2025;643(8073):1030–6.
2. Freitas C, Perez J, Knobel M, et al. Changes in cortical plasticity across the lifespan. Front Aging Neurosci 2011;3:5.
3. Wilson JRF, Badhiwala JH, Jiang F, et al. The impact of older age on functional recovery and quality of life outcomes after surgical decompression for degenerative cervical myelopathy: results from an ambispective, propensity-matched analysis from the CSM-NA and CSM-I international, multi-center studies. J Clin Med 2019;8(10):1708.
4. Nakashima H, Tetreault LA, Nagoshi N, et al. Does age affect surgical outcomes in patients with degenerative cervical myelopathy? Results from the prospective multicenter AOSpine International study on 479 patients. J Neurol Neurosurg Psychiatr 2016;87(7):734–40.
5. Akter F, Yu X, Qin X, et al. The pathophysiology of degenerative cervical myelopathy and the physiology of recovery following decompression. Front Neurosci 2020;14:2020.
6. Dhillon RS, Parker J, Syed YA, et al. Axonal plasticity underpins the functional recovery following surgical decompression in a rat model of cervical spondylotic myelopathy. Acta Neuropathol Commun 2016; 4(1):89.
7. David G, Mohammadi S, Martin AR, et al. Traumatic and nontraumatic spinal cord injury: pathological insights from neuroimaging. Nat Rev Neurol 2019;15-(12):718–31.
8. Aarabi B, Sansur CA, Ibrahimi DM, et al. *Intramedullary lesion length on postoperative magnetic resonance imaging is a strong predictor of ASIA impairment scale grade conversion following decompressive surgery in cervical spinal cord injury. Neurosurgery 2017;80(4):610–20.
9. Tator CH, Fehlings MG. Review of the secondary injury theory of acute spinal cord trauma with emphasis on vascular mechanisms. J Neurosurg 1991;75(1):15–26.
10. Seif M, David G, Huber E, et al. Cervical cord neurodegeneration in traumatic and non-traumatic spinal cord injury. J Neurotrauma 2020;37(6):860–7.
11. Yamamoto S, Kurokawa R, Kim P. *Postdecompressive spinal cord blood flow increments in a cervical chronic myelopathy model in rats. J Neurosurg Spine 2021;35(2):202–10.
12. Takano M, Kawabata S, Komaki Y, et al. Inflammatory cascades mediate synapse elimination in spinal cord compression. J Neuroinflammation 2014;11:40.
13. Misawa T, Kamimura M, Kinoshita T, et al. Neurogenic bladder in patients with cervical compressive myelopathy. J Spinal Disord Tech 2005;18(4): 315–20.
14. Khanna K, Theologis AA, Tay B. Autonomic dysreflexia caused by cervical stenosis. Spinal Cord Ser Cases 2017;3:17102.
15. Becerra JL, Puckett WR, Hiester ED, et al. MR-pathologic comparisons of wallerian degeneration in spinal cord injury. AJNR Am J Neuroradiol 1995;16(1): 125–33.
16. Fischer T, Stern C, Freund P, et al. Wallerian degeneration in cervical spinal cord tracts is commonly seen in routine T2-weighted MRI after traumatic spinal cord injury and is associated with impairment in a retrospective study. Eur Radiol 2021;31(5):2923–32.
17. Grabher P, Mohammadi S, Trachsler A, et al. Voxel-based analysis of grey and white matter

degeneration in cervical spondylotic myelopathy. Sci Rep 2016;6(1):24636.
18. Vallotton K, David G, Hupp M, et al. Tracking white and gray matter degeneration along the spinal cord axis in degenerative cervical myelopathy. J Neurotrauma 2021;38(21):2978–87.
19. Grabher P, Mohammadi S, David G, et al. Neurodegeneration in the spinal ventral horn prior to motor impairment in cervical spondylotic myelopathy. J Neurotrauma 2017;34(15):2329–34.
20. Lebret A, Lévy S, Pfender N, et al. Investigation of perfusion impairment in degenerative cervical myelopathy beyond the site of cord compression. Sci Rep 2023;13(1):22660.
21. Freund P, Boller V, Emmenegger TM, et al. Quantifying neurodegeneration of the cervical cord and brain in degenerative cervical myelopathy: a multicentre study using quantitative magnetic resonance imaging. Eur J Neurol 2024;31(7):e16297.
22. David G, Seif M, Huber E, et al. In vivo evidence of remote neural degeneration in the lumbar enlargement after cervical injury. Neurology 2019;92(12): e1367–77.
23. Martin AR, De Leener B, Cohen-Adad J, et al. Monitoring for myelopathic progression with multiparametric quantitative MRI. PLoS One 2018;13(4): e0195733.
24. Stoner KE, Abode-Iyamah KO, Magnotta VA, et al. Measurement of in vivo spinal cord displacement and strain fields of healthy and myelopathic cervical spinal cord. J Neurosurg: Spine SPI 2019;31(1): 53–9.
25. Rahman M, Palmer P, Harinathan B, et al. Using finite element models to assess spinal cord biomechanics after cervical laminoplasty for degenerative cervical myelopathy. Diagnostics (Basel) 2024;14-(14):1497.
26. Nishida N, Kato Y, Imajo Y, et al. Biomechanical analysis of cervical spondylotic myelopathy: the influence of dynamic factors and morphometry of the spinal cord. J Spinal Cord Med 2012;35(4):256–61.
27. Davies BM, Mowforth O, Gharooni AA, et al. A new framework for investigating the biological basis of degenerative cervical myelopathy [AO spine RECODE-DCM research priority number 5]: mechanical stress, vulnerability and time. Glob Spine J 2022;12(1_suppl):78s–96s.
28. Uemura K, Matsumura A, Isobe T, et al. Perfusion-weighted magnetic resonance imaging of the spinal cord in cervical spondylotic myelopathy. Neurol Med Chir (Tokyo) 2006;46(12):581–8.
29. Ellingson BM, Woodworth DC, Leu K, et al. Spinal cord perfusion MR imaging implicates both ischemia and hypoxia in the pathogenesis of cervical spondylosis. World Neurosurg 2019;128:e773–81.
30. Tsuji T, Matsuyama Y, Sato K, et al. Evaluation of spinal cord blood flow during prostaglandin E1-induced hypotension with power doppler ultrasonography. Spinal Cord 2001;39(1):31–6.
31. Yamamoto S, Kurokawa R, Kim P. Postdecompressive spinal cord blood flow increments in a cervical chronic myelopathy model in rats. J Neurosurg Spine 2021;35(2):202–10.
32. Ito T, Oyanagi K, Takahashi H, et al. Cervical spondylotic myelopathy. Clinicopathologic study on the progression pattern and thin myelinated fibers of the lesions of seven patients examined during complete autopsy. Spine (Phila Pa 1976) 1996;21(7): 827–33.
33. Jin LY, Li J, Wang KF, et al. Blood-spinal cord barrier in spinal cord injury: a review. J Neurotrauma 2021; 38(9):1203–24.
34. Kim HW, Yong H, Shea GKH. Blood-spinal cord barrier disruption in degenerative cervical myelopathy. Fluids Barriers CNS 2023;20(1):68.
35. Schmidt TP, Jütten K, Bertram U, et al. Blood spinal cord barrier disruption recovers in patients with degenerative cervical myelopathy after surgical decompression: a prospective cohort study. Sci Rep 2023;13(1):7389.
36. Fleming JC, Norenberg MD, Ramsay DA, et al. The cellular inflammatory response in human spinal cords after injury. Brain 2006;129(Pt 12): 3249–69.
37. Hirai T, Uchida K, Nakajima H, et al. The prevalence and phenotype of activated microglia/macrophages within the spinal cord of the hyperostotic mouse (twy/twy) changes in response to chronic progressive spinal cord compression: implications for human cervical compressive myelopathy. PLoS One 2013;8(5):e64528.
38. Liu XZ, Xu XM, Hu R, et al. Neuronal and glial apoptosis after traumatic spinal cord injury. J Neurosci 1997;17-(14):5395–406.
39. Karadimas SK, Moon ES, Yu WR, et al. A novel experimental model of cervical spondylotic myelopathy (CSM) to facilitate translational research. Neurobiol Dis 2013;54:43–58.
40. Inukai T, Uchida K, Nakajima H, et al. Tumor necrosis factor-alpha and its receptors contribute to apoptosis of oligodendrocytes in the spinal cord of spinal hyperostotic mouse (twy/twy) sustaining chronic mechanical compression. Spine (Phila Pa 1976) 2009;34(26):2848–57.
41. McDonald JW, Althomsons SP, Hyrc KL, et al. Oligodendrocytes from forebrain are highly vulnerable to AMPA/kainate receptor-mediated excitotoxicity. Nat Med 1998;4(3):291–7.
42. Dewar D, Underhill SM, Goldberg MP. Oligodendrocytes and ischemic brain injury. J Cereb Blood Flow Metab 2003;23(3):263–74.
43. Rikita T, Tanaka N, Nakanishi K, et al. The relationship between central motor conduction time and spinal cord compression in patients with cervical

spondylotic myelopathy. Spinal Cord 2017;55(4): 419–26.
44. Bouchard JA, Bohlman HH, Biro C. Intraoperative improvements of somatosensory evoked potentials: correlation to clinical outcome in surgery for cervical spondylitic myelopathy. Spine (Phila Pa 1976) 1996; 21(5):589–94.
45. De Mattei M, Paschero B, Cocito D, et al. Motor evoked potentials in the post-surgical follow-up of cervical spondylotic myelopathy. Ital J Neurol Sci 1995;16(4):239–48.
46. Guest JD, Hiester ED, Bunge RP. Demyelination and schwann cell responses adjacent to injury epicenter cavities following chronic human spinal cord injury. Exp Neurol 2005;192(2):384–93.
47. Hattori S, Kawai K, Mabuchi Y, et al. The relationship between magnetic resonance imaging and quantitative electromyography findings in patients with compressive cervical myelopathy. Spine (Phila Pa 1976) 2010;35(8):E290–4.
48. Ojeda J, Vergara M, Ávila A, et al. Impaired communication at the neuromotor axis during Degenerative Cervical Myelopathy. Front Cell Neurosci 2024;17: 2023.
49. Crowe MJ, Bresnahan JC, Shuman SL, et al. Apoptosis and delayed degeneration after spinal cord injury in rats and monkeys. Nat Med 1997;3(1):73–6.
50. Totoiu MO, Keirstead HS. Spinal cord injury is accompanied by chronic progressive demyelination. J Comp Neurol 2005;486(4):373–83.
51. Nouri A, Martin AR, Mikulis D, et al. Magnetic resonance imaging assessment of degenerative cervical myelopathy: a review of structural changes and measurement techniques. Neurosurg Focus 2016; 40(6):E5.
52. Liu H, MacMillan EL, Jutzeler CR, et al. Assessing structure and function of myelin in cervical spondylotic myelopathy: evidence of demyelination. Neurology 2017;89(6):602–10.
53. Sánchez-Gómez MV, Alberdi E, Ibarretxe G, et al. Caspase-Dependent and caspase-independent oligodendrocyte death mediated by AMPA and kainate receptors. J Neurosci 2003;23(29):9519–28.
54. Plemel JR, Keough MB, Duncan GJ, et al. Remyelination after spinal cord injury: is it a target for repair? Prog Neurobiol 2014;117:54–72.
55. Kotter MR, Setzu A, Sim FJ, et al. Macrophage depletion impairs oligodendrocyte remyelination following lysolecithin-induced demyelination. Glia 2001;35(3):204–12.
56. Miron VE, Boyd A, Zhao JW, et al. M2 microglia and macrophages drive oligodendrocyte differentiation during CNS remyelination. Nat Neurosci 2013; 16(9):1211–8.
57. Patrikios P, Stadelmann C, Kutzelnigg A, et al. Remyelination is extensive in a subset of multiple sclerosis patients. Brain 2006;129(Pt 12):3165–72.
58. Laule C, Moore GRW. Myelin water imaging to detect demyelination and remyelination and its validation in pathology. Brain Pathol 2018;28(5):750–64.
59. Brown RA, Narayanan S, Arnold DL. Segmentation of magnetization transfer ratio lesions for longitudinal analysis of demyelination and remyelination in multiple sclerosis. Neuroimage 2013;66:103–9.
60. Rafati Fard A, Mowforth OD, Yuan M, et al. Brain MRI changes in degenerative cervical myelopathy: a systematic review. EBioMedicine 2024;99:104915.
61. Cronin AE, Detombe SA, Duggal CA, et al. Spinal cord compression is associated with brain plasticity in degenerative cervical myelopathy. Brain Commun 2021;3(3):fcab131.
62. Yu Z, Pan W, Chen J, et al. Application of electrophysiological measures in degenerative cervical myelopathy. Front Cell Dev Biol 2022;10:834668.
63. Mohammed H, Hollis ER 2nd. Cortical reorganization of sensorimotor systems and the role of intracortical circuits after spinal cord injury. Neurotherapeutics 2018;15(3):588–603.
64. Holly LT, Dong Y, Albistegui-DuBois R, et al. Cortical reorganization in patients with cervical spondylotic myelopathy. J Neurosurg Spine 2007; 6(6):544–51.
65. Tetreault L, Wilson JR, Kotter MRN, et al. Is preoperative duration of symptoms a significant predictor of functional outcomes in patients undergoing surgery for the treatment of degenerative cervical myelopathy? Neurosurgery 2019;85(5):642–7.
66. Rafati Fard A, Mowforth OD, Yuan M, et al. Brain MRI changes in degenerative cervical myelopathy: a systematic review. EBioMedicine 2024;99:104915.
67. Lemon RN. Descending pathways in motor control. Annu Rev Neurosci 2008;31:195–218.
68. Bareyre FM, Kerschensteiner M, Raineteau O, et al. The injured spinal cord spontaneously forms a new intraspinal circuit in adult rats. Nat Neurosci 2004; 7(3):269–77.
69. Filli L, Schwab ME. Structural and functional reorganization of propriospinal connections promotes functional recovery after spinal cord injury. Neural Regen Res 2015;10(4):509–13.
70. Hilton B, Tempest-Mitchell J, Davies BM, et al. Cord compression defined by MRI is the driving factor behind the decision to operate in Degenerative Cervical Myelopathy despite poor correlation with disease severity. PLoS One 2019;14(12):e0226020.
71. Ivascu R, Torsin LI, Hostiuc L, et al. The surgical stress response and Anesthesia: a narrative review. J Clin Med 2024;13(10):3017.
72. Vidal PM, Karadimas SK, Ulndreaj A, et al. Delayed decompression exacerbates ischemia-reperfusion injury in cervical compressive myelopathy. JCI Insight 2017;2(11):e92512.
73. Rahman M, Banerjee A, Yang Y, et al. Impact of postsurgical rehabilitation on outcomes for

degenerative cervical myelopathy. J Neurosurg Spine 2024;41(2):167–73.
74. Moritz C, Field-Fote EC, Tefertiller C, et al. Non-invasive spinal cord electrical stimulation for arm and hand function in chronic tetraplegia: a safety and efficacy trial. Nat Med 2024;30(5):1276–83.
75. Gharooni AA, Khan M, Yang X, et al. Therapeutic repetitive Transcranial Magnetic stimulation (rTMS) for neurological dysfunction in Degenerative cervical Myelopathy: an unexplored opportunity? Findings from a systematic review. J Clin Neurosci 2021;90: 76–81.
76. Popovic MR, Zivanovic V, Valiante TA. Restoration of upper limb function in an individual with cervical spondylotic myelopathy using functional electrical stimulation therapy: a case study. Front Neurol 2016;7:81.
77. Pastor D. Use of electrical stimulation and exercise to increase muscle strength in a patient after surgery for cervical spondylotic myelopathy. Physiother Theory Pract 2010;26(2):134–42.
78. Tong LY, Deng YB, Du WH, et al. Clemastine promotes differentiation of oligodendrocyte progenitor cells through the activation of ERK1/2 via muscarinic receptors after Spinal Cord injury. Front Pharmacol 2022;13:914153.
79. Green AJ, Gelfand JM, Cree BA, et al. Clemastine fumarate as a remyelinating therapy for multiple sclerosis (ReBUILD): a randomised, controlled, double-blind, crossover trial. Lancet 2017;390-(10111):2481–9.
80. Fehlings MG, Badhiwala JH, Ahn H, et al. Safety and efficacy of riluzole in patients undergoing decompressive surgery for degenerative cervical myelopathy (CSM-Protect): a multicentre, double-blind, placebo-controlled, randomised, phase 3 trial. Lancet Neurol 2021;20(2):98–106.
81. Sugawara T, Hirano Y, Higashiyama N, et al. Limaprost alfadex improves myelopathy symptoms in patients with cervical spinal canal stenosis. Spine (Phila Pa 1976) 2009;34(6):551–5.
82. Onda A, Kimura M. Comparisons between the efficacy of limaprost alfadex and pregabalin in cervical spondylotic radiculopathy : design of a randomized controlled trial. Fukushima J Med Sci 2018;64(2): 73–81.
83. Matsudaira K, Seichi A, Kunogi J, et al. The efficacy of prostaglandin E1 derivative in patients with lumbar spinal stenosis. Spine (Phila Pa 1976) 2009; 34(2):115–20.
84. Schwenkgrub J, Zaremba M, Joniec-Maciejak I, et al. The phosphodiesterase inhibitor, ibudilast, attenuates neuroinflammation in the MPTP model of Parkinson's disease. PLoS One 2017;12(7):e0182019.
85. Fox RJ, Coffey CS, Conwit R, et al. Phase 2 trial of ibudilast in progressive multiple sclerosis. N Engl J Med 2018;379(9):846–55.
86. Naismith RT, Bermel RA, Coffey CS, et al. Effects of Ibudilast on MRI Measures in the Phase 2 SPRINT-MS Study. Neurology 2021;96(4):e491–500.

Novel Outcome Measures for Traumatic and Nontraumatic Spinal Cord Injury

Muhammad Sulman, BS[a], Carl M. Zipser, MD, MA[b,*],
Allan R. Martin, MD, PhD, FRCSC[c]

KEYWORDS

- Spinal cord injury • Degenerative cervical myelopathy • Outcome measures
- Patient-reported outcomes • Clinician-reported outcomes • Psychometrics

KEY POINTS

- Current spinal cord injury (SCI)/degenerative cervical myelopathy (DCM) outcome measures often miss important domains (autonomic, bowel/bladder/sexual, and dorsal column function) and may lack responsiveness across severities.
- Patient-reported outcome measures and clinician-reported outcome measures provide complementary information; multidimensional batteries or hybrid outcome measures (eg, DCM-subjective and outcome severity) are required for comprehensive assessment.
- SCI-specific functional tools (eg, spinal cord independence measure) and focal measures (eg, graded redefined assessment of strength, sensibility, and prehension) can be more sensitive than generic scales.
- Technology-enabled measures (wearables, imaging/neurophysiology biomarkers) may improve precision and real-world monitoring.
- Consensus frameworks (eg, AO Spine RECODE-DCM) support standardization to improve trial comparability and evidence synthesis.

INTRODUCTION

Spinal cord injury (SCI) represents a major cause of neurologic disability worldwide, encompassing traumatic and nontraumatic etiologies. Nontraumatic dysfunction is typically associated with chronic compression of the spinal cord due to age-related degenerative changes, resulting in neurologic impairment, known as degenerative cervical myelopathy (DCM).[1,2] DCM is the leading cause of spinal cord dysfunction in adults in developed countries, with an estimated prevalence of 1% to 5%,[3–5] and rising surgical intervention rates.[6–8]

Clinical presentation differs markedly between traumatic and nontraumatic dysfunction, particularly in the disease onset, course, and symptom profile. Traumatic spinal cord injury (tSCI) can affect both younger and elderly individuals with acute neurologic deficits, oftentimes with severe autonomic nervous system dysfunction, whereas DCM primarily occurs in older adults (peak

[a] School of Medicine, University of California, Davis, 4610 X Street, Sacramento, CA 95817, USA; [b] Spinal Cord Injury Center, Balgrist University Hospital, University of Zurich, Forchstrasse 340, 8008 Zurich, Switzerland; [c] Department of Neurological Surgery, University of California, Davis, 4610 X Street, Sacramento, CA 95817, USA
* Corresponding author.
E-mail address: carl.zipser@balgrist.ch

Neurosurg Clin N Am 37 (2026) 505–521
https://doi.org/10.1016/j.nec.2026.05.013
1042-3680/26/

Abbreviations

6MWT	6-min walk test
10MWT	10-m walk test
CAT	computer adaptive testing
CPG	clinical practice guideline
CROMs	clinician-reported outcome measures
CSM	cervical spondylotic myelopathy
DCM	degenerative cervical myelopathy
DCM-SOS	Degenerative cervical myelopathy subjective and outcome severity score
EQ-5D	EuroQol-5 Dimension
FIM	Functional Independence Measure
GRASSP	Graded Redefined Assessment of Strength, Sensibility, and Prehension
GRASSP-M	GRASSP-myelopathy
GTE	global treatment effect
ICC	intraclass correlation coefficient
ISNCSCI	International Standards for Neurologic Classification of spinal cord injury
JOA	Japanese Orthopedic Association
JOACMEQ	Japanese Orthopedic Association Cervical Myelopathy Evaluation Questionnaire
LPA	latent profile analysis
MCID	minimal clinically important difference
MDI	Myelopathy Disability Index
MJOA	modified JOA
NDI	Neck Disability Index
NISCI	Nogo Inhibition in cervical SCI
PROMIS	Patient-Reported Outcomes Measurement Information System
PROMs	patient-reported outcome measures
QOL	quality of life
QuickDASH	Quick Disabilities of the Arm, Shoulder, and Hand
ROC	receiver operating characteristic
SCI	spinal cord injury
SCIM	Spinal Cord Independence Measure
SCI-QOL	Spinal Cord Injury Quality of Life
SF-36	Short Form-36
tSSEP	tibial somatosensory evoked potentials

incidence in the sixth and seventh decades) and usually presents with slowly progressive neurologic decline and less autonomic involvement. Common manifestations of DCM include gait disturbance, upper-extremity dysfunction, (particularly fine motor impairment), and sensory deficits, while in SCI spinal cord syndromes, including incomplete and complete para- and tetraplegia prevails. In acute SCI, many patients cannot voluntarily control micturition and bowel emptying and suffer from cardiorespiratory dysfunction. The insidious onset of DCM often delays diagnosis and treatment, increasing the risk of irreversible neurologic injury.[6–9]

Assessment of SCI has evolved from a primarily clinician-reported outcome measures (CROMs) to include patient-reported outcome measures (PROMs) capturing functional independence, quality of life (QoL), and perceived disability, alongside increasingly emphasized objective approaches such as neurophysiological testing, advanced neuroimaging biomarkers, and instrumented performance measures for improved sensitivity and reproducibility.[1,2,10,11] Outcome measures are central across the continuum of SCI care, supporting diagnosis (particularly in DCM), monitoring disease progression, prognostication, treatment selection, and evaluation of recovery.[2,12] In research and regulatory contexts, standardized, validated outcome measures are essential for assessing treatment efficacy, enabling cross-study comparison, supporting data aggregation, and demonstrating meaningful patient-relevant benefit for approval and reimbursement decisions.[1,12,13]

Despite these advances, substantial challenges persist in outcome measurement for SCI. Current assessment in DCM relies predominantly on subjective questionnaires, with 92% of outcome measures being survey-based and only 8% incorporating objective neurologic testing in a recent review.[2] Many commonly used instruments lack psychometric validation in SCI and DCM patients, particularly with respect to content validity, structural validity, and responsiveness. Additionally, key domains, including pain, autonomic function, sensory pathway integrity (especially dorsal column function), and bowel, bladder, and sexual function, remain inadequately assessed in both clinical practice and research.[1,2,14] Heterogeneity in outcome measure selection and reporting has further limited evidence synthesis and consensus guideline development. For DCM alone, 29 different outcome instruments have been identified, with no single instrument evaluated across all relevant measurement properties and fewer than half assessed for reliability, validity, and responsiveness[1,2] highlighting the need for standardized, feasible core outcome sets that better capture the multidimensional nature of spinal cord dysfunction.

This narrative review outlines outcome measures for traumatic and nontraumatic SCI, with emphasis on tools designed to address limitations of existing assessments. We synthesize advances in patient-reported outcomes, functional measures, global and focal neurologic assessments, and objective quantitative approaches, highlighting their psychometric properties, clinical utility, and research applications. The goal is to inform clinical practice, guide future research, and support the development of consensus-based approaches to outcome measurement in spinal cord injury.

QUALITY-OF-LIFE OUTCOME MEASURES

SCI and DCM are distinct pathologies (as summarized in **Fig. 1**) with significant impact on QoL; therefore, QoL assessment plays an increasingly important role in evaluating outcomes for patients, reflecting a shift toward patient-centered, multidimensional evaluation beyond neurologic impairment alone. Both generic and condition-specific instruments are used to capture the physical, emotional, and social impact of these conditions.

Short Form-36

The Short Form-36 (SF-36) is a QoL instrument with physical and mental components, with

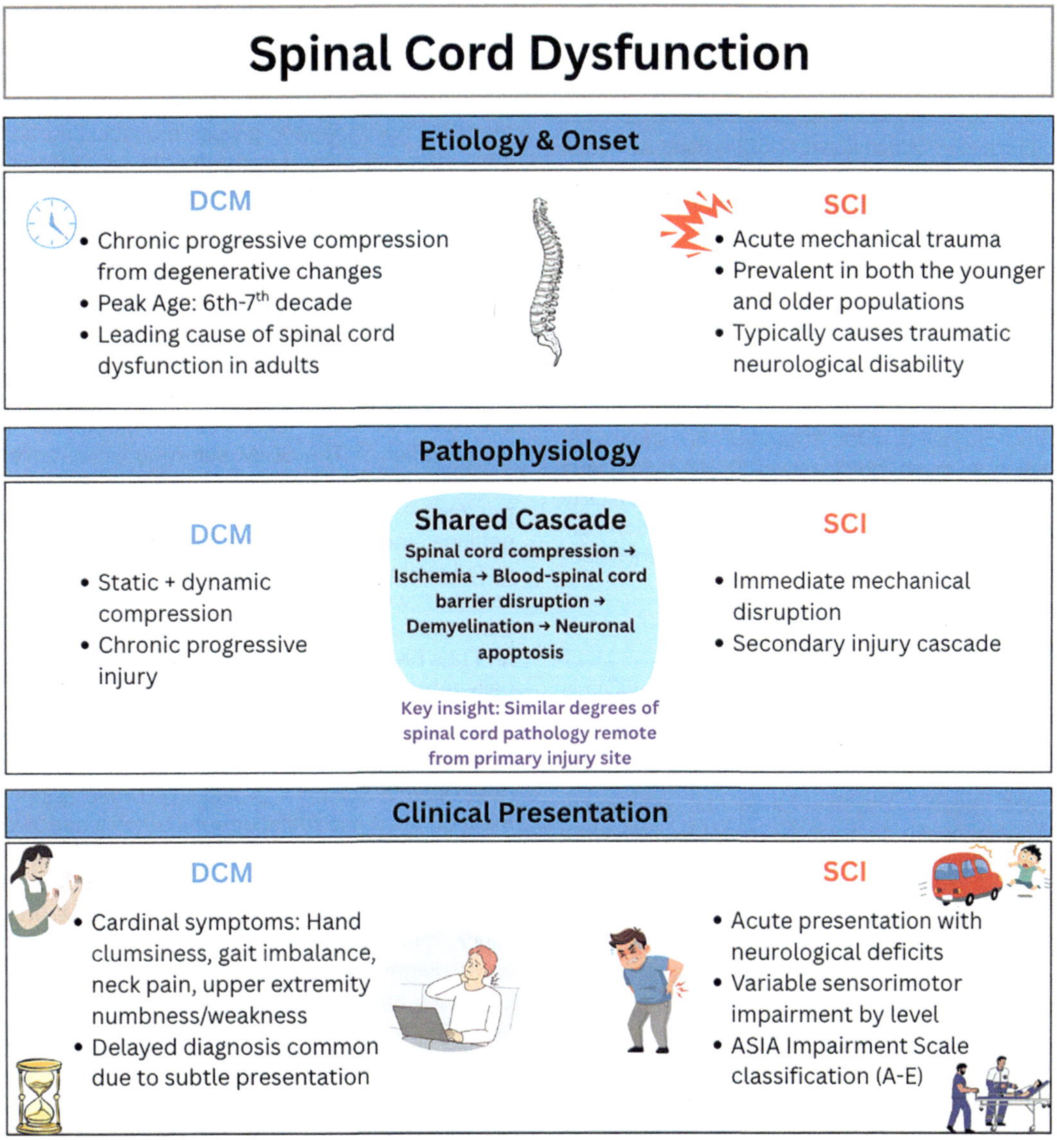

Fig. 1. *Comparative overview of degenerative cervical myelopathy and traumatic SCI: key clinical distinctions.* This figure contrasts DCM and traumatic SCI across 4 key domains. Despite different etiologies and onset patterns, both conditions share similar secondary pathophysiological mechanisms including ischemia, blood-spinal cord barrier disruption, and neuronal apoptosis.

moderate sensitivity and specificity for each component.[15] The SF-36 has demonstrated decreased QoL in all domains, impacting emotional health in DCM patients.[16] However, limitations include inconsistent reporting of the SF-36 version (SF-36v1, SF-36v2, or RAND-36) occurring in 84% of studies, limiting cross-study comparability,[17] with ceiling and floor effects in SCI populations despite a modified version (SF-36 Walk-Wheel) addressing floor effects to improve responsiveness in tetraplegic patients (standardized response mean increased from 0.11 to 0.58).[17] The SF-36 shows moderate responsiveness (effect sizes 0.57–0.93), and good internal consistency (Cronbach's α 0.73–0.85).[18]

EuroQol-5 Dimension

The EuroQol-5 Dimension (EQ-5D) is used for health economic analyses and quality-adjusted life year calculations.[19] In acute SCI, the EQ-5D-5L demonstrates severity-dependent utility values.[20,21] Utility scores at discharge were significantly higher in AIS D patients compared to more severe injury classifications.[20] However, the injury level and AIS grade do not consistently influence utility scores, suggesting limited sensitivity to neurologic impairment.[19] Comparative studies of preference-based measures (EQ-5D-5L, HUI-3, AQoL-8D,and SF-6D) show wide variation in mean index values (0.248–0.605) and only poor to moderate agreement.[19] This variability underscores the challenges of cross-study comparison and the importance of careful instrument selection in economic evaluations.

Spinal Cord Injury Quality of Life

The Spinal Cord Injury Quality of Life (SCI-QOL) is SCI-specific PROM developed to address the shortage of psychometrically sound assessment tools in SCI rehabilitation, covering physical-medical health, physical-functional, emotional, and social health domains.[22] Content validity was ensured through extensive qualitative input from individuals with SCI and clinicians.[22,23] A major strength is computer adaptive testing (CAT), which delivers high precision with minimal burden; for example, the Resilience CAT administers 4 to 6 items in less than 1 minute while maintaining excellent reliability (0.89), with no ceiling effect and minimal floor effect (3%).[22,23] The instruments demonstrate unidimensionality within each domain, appropriate item fit, and linking to other major measurement systems including PROMIS (Patient-Reported Outcomes Measurement Information System) and Neuro-QOL to facilitate cross-population comparisons.[22,23]

FUNCTIONAL OUTCOME MEASURES

Functional outcome measures represent a critical component of comprehensive assessment in SCI and DCM, capturing the impact of neurologic impairment on activities of daily living and independence. For SCI and DCM, the recommended timeline of when each outcome measure discussed in this review be administered is summarized in **Table 1**.

Spinal Cord Injury

Spinal Cord Independence Measure

Spinal Cord Independence Measure (SCIM) is SCI-specific functional scale more sensitive to functional changes than generic disability scales. SCIM IV has updated scoring definitions, addressing limitations of SCIM III,[24,25] demonstrating excellent psychometric properties, including high inter rater reliability, strong internal consistency, and Rasch model fit supporting interval level measurement.[24–27] SCIM is significantly more responsive than the Functional Independence Measure (FIM), capturing an additional 26% of changes missed by FIM, with greater sensitivity in respiration, sphincter management, and indoor and outdoor mobility.[24,27] It has broader operational range than FIM motor scale, supporting SCIM use for assessing functional independence in rehabilitation.[28] The SCIM self-report was developed to support longitudinal assessment of independence in individuals with SCI in home settings, reducing reliance on in-person professional evaluation. It demonstrates strong criterion validity, with high correlations to clinician-administered SCIM III scores (r=0.87, ICC=0.90), and has been identified as the most psychometrically robust PROM for SCI.[29]

Functional Independence Measure

FIM is a generic disability scale used in acute and rehabilitation SCI care, providing a broad assessment of, but it has limitations, including a narrower operational range than SCIM, item redundancy within the motor scale, and ceiling effects in cognitive subscales among patients without brain injury. Nonetheless, FIM remains useful for cross-diagnostic comparisons and for mandated insurance and regulatory reporting.[28,30] Moderate convergent validity between FIM and SCIM III has been demonstrated (r = 0.79–0.80).[26,31]

Degenerative Cervical Myelopathy

Japanese Orthopedic Association Score and Modified Japanese Orthopedic Association

The Japanese Orthopedic Association (JOA) score and modified JOA (mJOA) are the most widely

Table 1
Recommended timeline for outcome measure assessment in SCI and DCM

Clinical Phase	Timepoint	SCI Outcome Measures	DCM Outcome Measures	References
Diagnosis/Severity Assessment	SCI: Admission (0–10 d) DCM: Preoperative	ISNCSCI/ASIA SCIM III GRASSP (tetraplegia) SF-36, EQ-5D SCI-QOL	mJOA NDI SF-36v2 (PCS/MCS) EQ-5D SAVES2	61,84,100
Early Recovery	SCI: 1 mo DCM: 35 d	ISNCSCI/ASIA SCIM III GRASSP	mJOA NDI Safety/adverse events	101,102
Subacute	3 mo	ISNCSCI/ASIA SCIM III GRASSP 10MWT, 6MWT Berg Balance Scale	mJOA NDI SF-36v2 EQ-5D 10MWT, 6MWT	25,61,101,102
Primary Endpoint	6 mo	ISNCSCI/ASIASCIM III/SCIM-SR GRASSP SF-36, EQ-5D SCI-QOL 10MWT, 6MWT	mJOA (primary) NDI SF-36v2 EQ-5D SAVES2	26,61,84,101
Long-term	12 mo	ISNCSCI/ASIASCIM III/SCIM-SR GRASSP SF-36, EQ-5D SCI-QOL	mJOA NDI SF-36v2 EQ-5D JOACMEQ	32,61,101
Extended	24 mo	SCIM-SR SF-36, EQ-5D SCI-QOL	mJOA NDI SF-36v2 EQ-5D	61,103

This table summarizes the recommended timing for outcome measure assessment across clinical phases of SCI and DCM management. Timepoints are based on international consensus guidelines (AO Spine RECODE-DCM), major clinical trial protocols (CSM-Protect, STASCIS), and established registry practices (EMSCI, RHSCIR, NACTN).

Abbreviations: ASIA, american spinal injury association; SAVES2, symptom assessment for visual extremity symptoms.

used CROM of functional status in DCM. The mJOA assesses four weighted domains for a total score of 0 to 18, with higher scores indicating less myelopathy.[32–34] The original JOA score, still commonly used in East Asia, has a maximum of 17 points and slightly different weighting.[35,36] The minimal clinically important difference (MCID) for the mJOA has been established at 1 to 3 points, with variation depending on baseline myelopathy severity.[32] Using receiver operating characteristic (ROC) analysis with the Neck Disability Index (NDI) as an anchor, the MCID was determined to be 1 point for mild myelopathy (mJOA 15–17), 2 points for moderate myelopathy (mJOA 12–14), and 3 points for severe myelopathy (mJOA <12).[32] For the original JOA, the MCID and minimum detectable change are both 2.5 points, with a patient acceptable symptom state of 14.5 and a recovery-rate MCID of 52.8%.[36]

The mJOA is widely used worldwide, in clinical and research settings, and clinical practice guideline (CPG) recommendations[37] for treatment are based on mJOA validated severity categories.[34] Psychometric evaluation shows moderate internal consistency for the mJOA (Cronbach's $\alpha = 0.63$), strong convergent validity with the Nurick grade ($r = -0.625$), and excellent responsiveness (effect size = 1.0).[38] While total JOA and mJOA scores correlate well ($\rho = 0.87$), agreement in recovery rates is lower (Spearman's $\rho = 0.75$), with Bland–Altman analysis demonstrating wide limits of agreement, indicating the 2 instruments should not be used interchangeably.[35]

Neck Disability Index

NDI is scored from 0 to 50 (or 0%–100%) with higher scores indicating greater disability.[39–41] Psychometric evaluation demonstrates good to excellent internal consistency (Cronbach α 0.723–0.897) and test–retest reliability (ICC 0.79–0.90).[40,42,43] Exploratory factor analysis in preoperative DCM patients identified 2 factors, Physical and Mental, with Physical factors (standardized $\beta = 0.724$, $P < .001$) exerting a stronger impact on NDI scores than Mental factors (standardized $\beta = 0.409$, $P < .001$).[39] Numbness in the hand (standardized $\beta = 0.338$, $P < .001$) and pain in the neck (standardized $\beta = 0.202$, $P = .035$) were significant variables influencing the Physical factor, while numbness in the hand (standardized $\beta = 0.485$, $P < .001$) and pain in the head (standardized $\beta = 0.374$, $P<.001$) impacted the Mental factor.[39]

Although early systematic reviews found no DCM-specific validity or responsiveness data for the NDI through 2013,[11] more recent studies demonstrate diagnostic utility (Youden Index 63%),[44] and show that NDI percentage change is among the most accurate PROMs for detecting postoperative improvement in DCM, with approximately 60% of patients achieving the MCID at 12 months.[45]

Japanese Orthopedic Association Cervical Myelopathy Evaluation Questionnaire

The Japanese Orthopedic Association Cervical Myelopathy Evaluation Questionnaire (JOACMEQ) is a disease-specific PROM developed to assess disability and QoL in DCM.[24,36,43,46] Psychometric validation demonstrates excellent overall internal consistency (Cronbach α >0.9), good domain-level reliability including lower extremity ($\alpha = 0.823$) and QoL ($\alpha = 0.875$),[43] stable factorial structure across language versions,[47] and good to excellent test–retest reliability (ICC 0.695–0.905).[43,47,48]

JOACMEQ shows strong concurrent validity with established measures including the SF-36, NDI, and EQ-5D-5L,[35,43] with particularly strong correlation between the QoL domain and the Chinese NDI ($\rho = -0.76$).[48] It also demonstrates good discriminatory ability for detecting myelopathy (AUC 0.75–0.82) and satisfactory responsiveness,[48] with significant improvement observed from preoperative to 2-year postoperative assessments, particularly in recovery rate metrics.[47]

Myelopathy Disability Index

Myelopathy Disability Index (MDI) assesses functional disability of DCM,[11,49,50] and demonstrates good psychometric properties in DCM populations,[11] with validated severity cut-offs derived using ROC analysis with acceptable sensitivity and specificity.[49,50] Increasing MDI severity is associated with significantly worse performance on objective measures including the 30-m Walking Test and Nine-Hole Peg Test, and correlates strongly with Nurick grade categories, supporting its construct validity.[49]

Nurick grade

The Nurick grade is an older scale, classifying DCM severity primarily based on gait impairment and employment status.[11,51–53] It demonstrates good correlation with the mJOA, particularly with the lower limb mJOA component (Spearman $\rho = 0.901$ preoperatively and 0.886 postoperatively), compared to moderate correlation with total mJOA ($\rho = 0.846$ and 0.862).[52] Recovery rates correlate more strongly with lower limb mJOA recovery ($\rho = 0.840$) than with total mJOA recovery ($\rho = 0.793$).[52] However, a significant limitation is that at follow-up evaluation after surgery, there was disagreement between Nurick scale and lower limb mJOA in 11.8% of patients, with one major reason being the ability of patients to regain employment without improvement in the lower limb mJOA score.[52] Nurick scale has undergone limited psychometric evaluation in DCM (only one study to date) and has fallen out of favor.[11,34]

NEUROLOGIC OUTCOME MEASURES—GLOBAL

Spinal Cord Injury

International Standards for Neurologic Classification of spinal cord injury

International Standards for Neurologic Classification of spinal cord injury (ISNCSCI) is the gold-standard for assessing neurologic impairment after SCI,[54] comprising sensory, motor, and anorectal examinations from which neurologic level and AIS grade are derived.[54,55] It demonstrates strong reliability and validity across traumatic and nontraumatic SCI populations, with high inter-rater agreement and supportive correlations with functional outcomes such as SCIM.[56] The standards continue to evolve, with major updates incorporated into the 2019 revision, and international e-learning programs.[20] Electronic ISNCSCI tools and computerized classification algorithms have improved standardization, education, and data quality across SCI registries.[57]

Despite its strengths, ISNCSCI has limitations that reduce sensitivity in clinical trials. Nonlinear scoring limits detection of subtle neurologic change and reliance on single variables may misrepresent overall recovery.[58] To address this, the Integrated Neurologic Change Score aggregates normalized motor and sensory changes and shows improved correlation with functional independence (SCIM) in tetraplegia.[59] Additional limitations include omission of neurologic examination elements, such as deep tendon reflexes and proprioception, as ISNCSCI focuses only on components required for AIS classification.[54] The training-dependent reliability with inconsistent validity findings, requires further refinement.[60]

Degenerative Cervical Myelopathy

While DCM lacks a single validated global neurologic assessment comparable to ISNCSCI in SCI, several patient-reported and clinician-administered tools serve this function. The AO Spine RECODE-DCM consensus identified 4 outcome instruments for the Core Measurement Set: mJOA, NDI, SF-36v2, and SAVES2, with a recommendation for trials evaluating outcomes after surgery to include baseline measurement and at 6 months from surgery.[61] SAVES2 (Spinal Adverse Events Severity System, Version 2) is primarily an adverse event reporting system that has demonstrated almost-perfect interobserver reliability (Gwet's AC2 = 0.94 for neurosurgeons, 0.81 for registrars) in grading severity of adverse events.[62] However, a novel global neurologic outcome measure system has been developed which we will discuss next.

Degenerative cervical myelopathy subjective and outcome severity score

Degenerative cervical myelopathy subjective and outcome severity score (DCM-SOS) is a severity assessment scale, developed as a novel hybrid outcome measure integrating a PROM with a structured CROM to address the limitations of mJOA in the current practice.[44,63] It expands beyond the mJOA with the subjective component capturing neck pain, arm pain, hand clumsiness, arm/hand weakness and numbness, gait imbalance, and urinary dysfunction, while the objective component includes standardized testing of bilateral upper-extremity muscle strength, reflexes, C5–T1 light-touch sensation, and a scored 10-step tandem gait test.[63] Scoring is weighted according to patient-priority studies highlighting pain and ambulation as key recovery targets.[63,64]

Methodologically, DCM-SOS is developed using prospective cohort data and literature synthesis, and a modified Delphi process involving 42 multidisciplinary expert panel achieving unanimous consensus. Resulting strengths include improved content validity over mJOA through inclusion of pain and asymmetry, backward compatibility with mJOA domains, standardization of a focused and practical neurologic examination, and strong face validity grounded in both psychometric evidence and patient-defined priorities.[63]

NEUROLOGIC OUTCOME MEASURES—FOCAL

Focal neurologic assessments provide detailed evaluation of specific functional domains affected by SCI and DCM, complementing global neurologic scales with targeted measurement of upper extremity, lower extremity, and gait function.

Upper Extremity Assessment

Graded Redefined Assessment of Strength, Sensibility, and Prehension

Graded Redefined Assessment of Strength, Sensibility, and Prehension (GRASSP) assesses upper-limb function in individuals with complete and incomplete tetraplegia.[65] It provides a comprehensive functional profile,[65,66] while demonstrating excellent psychometric performance, with inter-retest and test-retest reliability ranging from 0.84 to 0.96 and 0.86 to 0.98, respectively, and approximately 50% greater sensitivity than ISNCSCI for upper-limb sensorimotor assessment. Strong concurrent validity has been shown with the SCIM self-care subscale (r = 0.57–0.83) and upper-extremity–specific questionnaires[65,66]

GRASSP-myelopathy (GRASSP-M)

GRASSP-myelopathy (GRASSP-M) is an adaptation designed for DCM, reflecting the distinct upper-limb impairment pattern seen in this population and simplified for shorter assessment.[67] In validation studies, strength, sensation, and dexterity declined with increasing DCM severity, with hand dexterity showing superior discrimination between mild, moderate, and severe disease. GRASSP-M demonstrates excellent intra-rater and inter-rater reliability (intraclass correlation coefficient [ICC] > 0.75) and strong construct and concurrent validity. Importantly, GRASSP-M identified objective impairment in patients (particularly those with mild DCM) who underreported disability, supporting its utility for early diagnosis, monitoring progression, and surgical decision-making.[67]

Grip dynamometry and Quick Disabilities of the Arm, Shoulder, and Hand

Grip dynamometry and the QuickDASH (Quick Disabilities of the Arm, Shoulder, and Hand) are commonly used ancillary upper-extremity measures.[67] In DCM, QuickDASH scores correlate with objective measures of strength, sensation, and dexterity, with symptom duration significantly influencing perceived disability, suggesting adaptation in patients with longer-standing mild disease[68]

Lower Extremity and Gait Assessment

Berg balance scale

Berg balance scale (BBS) is a performance-based assessment of static and dynamic balance. For myelopathy, the BBS demonstrates excellent test–retest and inter-rater reliability (ICC > 0.80) and strong correlation with the mJOA, but substantial ceiling effects (>80% easy items) limit its utility in patients with mild disease.[69] In SCI populations, the BBS shows excellent reliability (total score ICC = 0.95) and strong correlations with mobility, strength, and fear of falling,[70,71] and can distinguish ambulators with and without walking aids (AUC > 0.86).[70] However, it performs poorly for fall prediction and exhibits ceiling effects in approximately 28% of chronic SCI patients.[71,72] A ceiling effect is present in 28% of chronic SCI participants.[70] Evidence suggests the Brief BESTest is preferred over BBS for DCM due to better discriminative ability and shorter administration time.[69]

Walking tests

Timed walking tests provide objective evaluation of gait speed and endurance. The 10-m walk test (10MWT) assesses short-distance walking velocity, while the 6-min walk test (6MWT) measures endurance and distance.[73,74] In SCI, the two tests correlate strongly with each other (r > 0.88) and moderately with the Walking Index for SCI (r > 0.60),[74] yet are not interchangeable, as error increases with faster gait speeds and agreement varies by functional level.[73] Different thresholds and MCIDs are therefore required for each test.

The 10MWT speeds are generally faster than 6MWT speeds, and significant differences exist across SCI Functional Ambulation Inventory walking mobility categories (Wilcoxon sign rank test $P < .001$).[73] The concurrent validity between 10MWT and 6MWT varies by functional level: excellent correlation in patients with FIM-Locomotor score 7 (r = 0.83), good correlation with FIM-L6 (r = 0.74), but poor correlation with FIM-L5 (r = 0.31).[75] In DCM populations, 6MWD is significantly reduced (309.34 ± 116.71 m) compared to healthy controls (464.30 ± 52.59 m, $P < .01$).[76] The 6MWD correlates significantly with all clinical scales except VAS, with the strongest correlation to the Cooper Myelopathy Scale lower extremity score (r = −0.794, $P < .01$). **Table 2** summarizes the outcome measures discussed in this review, outlining their reliability, validity, and clinical utility.

MULTIDIMENSIONAL ASSESSMENT USING THE GLOBAL STATISTICAL TEST

Traditional clinical trials in SCI and DCM often rely on single primary endpoints. However, this approach may fail to capture the full therapeutic impact in heterogeneous conditions where recovery occurs across multiple domains, such as neurologic function, physical capacity, and quality of life.[77,78] global statistical test (GST) addresses this by providing a unified conclusion on treatment superiority through the simultaneous evaluation of multiple trial endpoints.[77] Using a multivariate nonparametric approach (such as a modified O'Brien rank-sum test), the GST integrates diverse measures into a composite assessment.[77,79] Higher summed ranks represent better global outcomes, and the overall probability of improvement is calculated as the global treatment effect (GTE).[77] This methodology is particularly valuable when individual measures show positive trends that fail to reach independent statistical significance due to small sample sizes or high patient variability.[77,79] The utility of the GST has been notably demonstrated in landmark trials, such as the RISCIS trial and cervical spondylotic myelopathy (CSM)-PROTECT trial, where it provided a more robust evaluation of functional recovery.[78–80]

CLUSTERING OF OUTCOMES TO DEFINE UNIQUE RECOVERY TRAJECTORIES

The inherent heterogeneity of both traumatic SCI and DCM presents a significant challenge for predicting individual recovery, as traditional analyses often rely on group averages that mask distinct patterns of improvement or decline. To address this, machine learning-based cluster analysis has emerged as a powerful tool to identify unique patient *phenotypes* and recovery trajectories.[81,82] Data-driven approaches, such as latent profile analysis (LPA) and k-means clustering, allow for the grouping of patients based on multi-domain baselines rather than single scores. For instance, a landmark study of over 1000 DCM patients identified 4 distinct phenotypes, ranging from *mild impairment* to *severe multidimensional impairment*, which differed not only in baseline severity but also in specific combinations of pain, motor/sensory deficits, and frailty.[81,82] Beyond static snapshots, longitudinal clustering can map how patients change over time, identifying *rapid responders*, *slow/steady improvers*, and *nonresponders* who may require alternative therapeutic interventions.[81,83]

INTEGRATED ASSESSMENT FRAMEWORKS: BEYOND FUNCTIONAL SCALES

The clinical complexity of SCI and DCM necessitates a shift away from isolated metrics toward a multidimensional assessment framework. While mJOA remains the gold standard for classifying

Table 2
Psychometric properties and clinical utility of outcome measures for spinal cord injury and degenerative cervical myelopathy

Domain	Instrument	Population	Reliability (Intraclass Correlation Coefficient)	Validity	Responsiveness (Minimal Clinically Important Difference)	Evidence Level
Quality of Life	SF-36 PCS/MCS	SCI, DCM	NR	Moderate correlation with mJOA, NDI; α = 0.73–0.85	MCID: 4 points (PCS), 4 points (MCS)	●●●
	EQ-5D	SCI, DCM	NR	Strong correlation with NDI (ρ = 0.83); moderate with mJOA	MCID: 0.05	●●●
	SCI-QOL	SCI	Good	Strong psychometric properties; CAT administration	Domain-specific MCIDs	●●●
Functional (SCI)	SCIM III/IV	SCI	Inter-rater: >0.94; α > 0.96	r = 0.79–0.80 with FIM; 50% more sensitive than FIM	Varies by subscale and injury severity	●●●
	SCIM-SR	SCI	ICC = 0.90 with SCIM III	r = 0.87 with SCIM III; subscales r = 0.81–0.87	Most validated SCI PROM	●●●
Functional (DCM)	mJOA	DCM	Inter-rater: 0.63–0.88	r = −0.63 with Nurick; Sens 93.5%, Spec 67.3% (DCM-SOS)	MCID: 2.5 points; Effect size = 1.0	●●●
	NDI	DCM	NR	Strong correlation with mJOA, SF-36, EQ-5D (ρ = 0.83)	MCID: 13.5–17.5 points (16% improvement)	●●●
	JOACMEQ	DCM	Test-retest: 0.85–0.95	Strong correlation with NDI (ρ = −0.85); α > 0.9	Responsive to surgery	●●
Neurological-Global	ISNCSCI/ASIA	SCI	High (values NR)	Content and construct validity established	Less sensitive than GRASSP for UE	●●●
	DCM-SOS	DCM	NR	Derived from mJOA items; AUC = 0.86	Emerging measure	
Neurological-Focal (UE)	GRASSP v1/v2	SCI	Inter-rater: 0.84–0.96; Test-retest: 0.86–0.98	r = 0.57–0.83 with SCIM self-care; 50% more sensitive than ISNCSCI	MDD: 3–4 points; SRM = 0.50–1.48	●●●
	GRASSP-M	DCM	Intra/inter-rater: >0.75	Discriminates mild/moderate/severe DCM	Detects mild dysfunction	●●

(continued on next page)

Table 2
(continued)

Domain	Instrument	Population	Reliability (Intraclass Correlation Coefficient)	Validity	Responsiveness (Minimal Clinically Important Difference)	Evidence Level
Neurological-Focal (LE)	Berg Balance Scale	SCI, DCM	Inter-rater/test-retest: >0.80	r = −0.83–0.93 with mobility; AUC > 0.86 for walkers	Ceiling effect in CSM (>80% easy items)	●●
	10MWT	SCI, DCM	NR	r > 0.88 with 6MWT; not redundant	Separate MCIDs for community ambulation	●●●
	6MWT	SCI, DCM	NR	r > 0.88 with 10MWT; r = −0.79 with Cooper LE (DCM)	Lower in DCM (309m) vs controls (464m)	●●●

This table summarizes the psychometric properties and clinical utility of commonly used outcome measures for SCI and DCM, organized by assessment domain. Reliability is reported as ICC for inter-rater and test-retest reliability, with Cronbach's alpha (α) for internal consistency. Validity includes construct validity (correlation coefficients with related measures) and diagnostic accuracy metrics where applicable. Responsiveness focuses on MCID values and effect sizes.

Evidence level reflects the extent of psychometric validation: ●●● indicates extensive validation with established psychometric properties and MCID values across multiple studies; ●● indicates moderate validation with some psychometric evidence but gaps in certain properties; ● indicates limited validation or emerging measures requiring further study.

Abbreviations: AUC, area under curve; LE, lower extremity; MDD, minimally detectable difference; NR, not reported; Sens, Sensitivity; Spec, Specificity; SRM, standardized response mean; UE, upper extremity; α, Cronbach's alpha.

functional impairment, it often fails to capture the full spectrum of the patient experience, particularly regarding pain and QoL. To address this, the AO Spine RECODE-DCM Core Outcome Set advocates for a standardized battery of instruments.[61] By combining CROM scales with PROM that track health-related QoL, researchers can mitigate *data silencing* and ensure that domains prioritized by patients—such as neuropathic pain and psychological well-being—are formally evaluated alongside motor function.

Furthermore, integrating ancillary outcome measures provides a more granular understanding of neurologic recovery that global scales may overlook.[11] Using specialized tools for upper limb dexterity, gait analysis, and sensory perception allows for the detection of subtle clinical changes that do not register as a full point shift on the mJOA. A comprehensive assessment strategy that intersects neurologic status, pain readouts, and functional independence creates a *hybrid* view of patient health. This holistic approach ensures that treatment success is not merely defined by radiographic decompression or gross motor gains but by the meaningful restoration of a patient's overall quality of life and social participation.

DISCUSSION

Strengths of Different Approaches

Comprehensive assessment of SCI and DCM necessitates multidimensional evaluation combining patient-reported, clinician-reported, and objective measures to capture the full spectrum of impairment and recovery. PROMs and CROMs provide complementary information that neither approach alone can capture.

Outcome measures vary substantially in sensitivity, specificity, and responsiveness across instruments and clinical contexts. In SCI populations, SCIM is approximately 50% more sensitive than FIM for detecting functional change, with superior responsiveness in respiration/sphincter management and mobility domains.[28,30] Among upper-extremity assessments, GRASSP demonstrates roughly 50% greater sensitivity than ISNCSCI in capturing sensorimotor integrity, with established MCID that vary by injury severity.[65,84] For DCM, systematic review evidence indicates that no instrument has been evaluated for all 10 measurement properties, and fewer than 50% have assessments across all 3 psychometric domains (reliability, validity, and responsiveness).[1]

The utility of outcome measures also varies by clinical setting and population. Acute care requires feasible instruments suited to limited endurance and evolving neurologic status, whereas rehabilitation and community settings support more comprehensive assessment batteries.[30] Moreover, most outcome measures were developed and validated in traumatic SCI populations, limiting their applicability to DCM and other nontraumatic etiologies characterized by distinct impairment patterns, slower progression, and older age at onset.[2,13]

Limitations and Knowledge Gaps

A fundamental limitation is the lack of a single gold-standard measure with full psychometric validation across all domains of spinal cord function,[11] necessitating the use of multiple instruments.[2] Important clinical domains, including dorsal column sensory function and respiratory, bowel, bladder, sexual, and autonomic systems, remain underrepresented in current assessment paradigms, particularly in DCM, where reliance on subjective questionnaires may fail to capture subtle or evolving neurologic deficits.[2,85] Psychosocial domains, while captured by generic QoL measures, lack disease-specific instruments that address the unique challenges of living with SCI.[86]

Nontraumatic SCI and DCM populations are also underrepresented in psychometric validation studies, limiting the generalizability of many commonly used tools.[2,67] Furthermore, substantial heterogeneity in outcome selection and reporting continues to impair cross-study comparability, with wide variability in reported recovery rates for the same patient cohorts based on the chosen instrument.[51,87]

Although this review evaluates widely used SCI and DCM outcome measures, it does not cover all the instruments included in the International SCI Data Sets—such as those addressing autonomic, bowel/bladder, cardiovascular, pulmonary, psychological, pain, skin/thermoregulation, sexual function, socio-demographics, and QOL—which provide globally endorsed frameworks for harmonized SCI data collection.[88]

Future Directions

The development of new and composite outcome measures is a critical priority. Digital health technologies offer transformative potential for continuous, objective monitoring of activity, gait, cardiovascular health, and sleep in real-world settings.[89,90] In SCI trials, wearable inertial sensors have demonstrated greater sensitivity than traditional clinical scales, detecting treatment-related changes in energy expenditure not captured by conventional measures.[91] However, challenges include validating algorithms for atypical movement patterns, balancing research-grade and consumer devices, and ensuring accessibility for individuals with severe impairments.[89,92]

In SCI, neurophysiology was proven to be valuable for increasing accuracy of outcome prediction complementing ISNCSCI and functional tests. For instance, it was shown that ISNCSCI together with tibial somatosensory evoked potentials (tSSEP), motor evoked potentials, and nerve conduction studies more correctly identified SCIM scores of patients with cervical SCI than ISNCSCI alone.[93] Another study in tetraplegics demonstrated utility of tSSEP in addition to lower extremity motor scores for predicting ambulatory outcomes.[94] More recently, tSSEP were shown to be beneficial for clinical trial stratification, as they helped identifying treatment responders in the randomized, placebo-controlled, phase 2b Nogo Inhibition in cervical SCI (NISCI) trial.[95]

Integration of neurophysiological and imaging biomarkers holds promise for early diagnosis, prognosis, and monitoring. Techniques such as diffusion tensor imaging, magnetization transfer, and MR spectroscopy quantify microstructural spinal cord changes,[96–98] with metabolite ratios demonstrating diagnostic value in mild–moderate DCM,[96] and dynamic MRI revealing early reversible injury patterns.[97] However, no multimodal prediction models yet integrate clinical, imaging, and electrophysiological data.[13]

AO Spine RECODE-DCM now provides a minimum data set—including a core outcome set, core data elements, and standardized timepoints—intended to reduce heterogeneity and improve comparability across studies.[61,87(p20),99] Adoption of these frameworks should be coupled with multidimensional assessment batteries in clinical practice[11,44,100] and with policy support for developing validated measures in underrepresented domains such as autonomic function, sensory pathways, and nontraumatic SCI.[2] Finally, Integrating digital biomarkers and advanced imaging into trials will require interdisciplinary collaboration, consistent reporting standards, and attention to equity and patient-centered design.[89,90,92]

SUMMARY

Outcome measurement, particularly in DCM, has evolved substantially but remains fragmented, with no single instrument fully capturing the multidimensional nature of spinal cord dysfunction. This review highlights that traditional clinician-reported scales and patient-reported questionnaires, while foundational, are limited by incomplete domain coverage, variable psychometric validation, and inconsistent responsiveness across disease severities and settings. Emerging tools, such as hybrid instruments that integrate patient-reported, clinician-reported, and objective performance-based measures, along with advances in digital health, imaging, and neurophysiological biomarkers, represent important steps toward more comprehensive and sensitive assessment.

CLINICS CARE POINTS

- The AO Spine RECODE-DCM consensus recommends a core measurement set of mJOA, NDI, SF-36v2, and SAVES2 with baseline and 6-month postoperative assessment as the minimum standard for DCM surgical trials, and adoption of this framework can reduce reporting heterogeneity and improve cross-study comparability.
- When using preference-based quality-of-life instruments (eg, EQ-5D-5L, SF-6D) for health economic analyses in SCI, clinicians should recognize that mean index values can vary widely (0.248–0.605) across instruments with only poor to moderate agreement, making cross-study comparisons unreliable without consistent instrument selection.
- No single outcome measure has been validated across all psychometric domains (reliability, validity, responsiveness) for DCM; clinicians and researchers should use multidimensional assessment batteries combining patient-reported, clinician-reported, and objective performance-based measures to capture the full spectrum of impairment.
- The modified Japanese Orthopaedic Association (mJOA) score remains the most widely used measure for degenerative cervical myelopathy (DCM) severity grading and guides surgical decision-making, but clinicians should be aware that its minimal clinically important difference (MCID) varies by baseline severity: 1 point for mild (mJOA 15–17), 2 points for moderate (mJOA 12–14), and 3 points for severe (mJOA <12) disease.
- The Spinal Cord Independence Measure (SCIM) is approximately 50% more sensitive than the Functional Independence Measure (FIM) for detecting functional change after spinal cord injury (SCI), particularly in respiration, sphincter management, and mobility domains; SCIM should be preferred over FIM when SCI-specific functional assessment is the primary goal.

FUNDING

C.M. Zipser reports funding from Swiss National Science Foundation, Switzerland (No. 10002350) and Swiss Paraplegia Foundation, Switzerland (Foko 09_2023).

DISCLOSURE

The authors share no conflict of interest related to the materials presented in this study.

REFERENCES

1. Yanez Touzet A, Bhatti A, Dohle E, et al. Clinical outcome measures and their evidence base in degenerative cervical myelopathy: a systematic review to inform a core measurement set (AO spine RECODE-DCM). BMJ Open 2022;12(1):e057650.
2. Soufi KH, Perez TM, Umoye AO, et al. How is spinal cord function measured in degenerative cervical myelopathy? A systematic review. JCM 2022;11(5):1441.
3. Martin AR, De Leener B, Cohen-Adad J, et al. Can microstructural MRI detect subclinical tissue injury in subjects with asymptomatic cervical spinal cord compression? A prospective cohort study. BMJ Open 2018;8(4):e019809.
4. Kovalova I, Kerkovsky M, Kadanka Z, et al. Prevalence and imaging characteristics of nonmyelopathic and myelopathic spondylotic cervical cord compression. Spine 2016;41(24):1908–16.
5. Smith SS, Stewart ME, Davies BM, et al. The prevalence of asymptomatic and symptomatic spinal cord compression on magnetic resonance imaging: a systematic review and meta-analysis. Glob Spine J 2021;11(4):597–607.
6. Nouri A, Cheng JS, Davies B, et al. Degenerative cervical myelopathy: a brief review of past perspectives, present developments, and future directions. JCM 2020;9(2):535.
7. Nouri A, Tetreault L, Singh A, et al. Degenerative cervical myelopathy: epidemiology, genetics, and pathogenesis. Spine 2015;40(12):E675–93.
8. Badhiwala JH, Ahuja CS, Akbar MA, et al. Degenerative cervical myelopathy — update and future directions. Nat Rev Neurol 2020;16(2):108–24.
9. Tetreault L, Goldstein CL, Arnold P, et al. Degenerative cervical myelopathy: a spectrum of related disorders affecting the aging spine. Neurosurgery 2015;77(Supplement 1):S51–67.
10. David G, Mohammadi S, Martin AR, et al. Traumatic and nontraumatic spinal cord injury: pathological insights from neuroimaging. Nat Rev Neurol 2019;15(12):718–31.
11. Kalsi-Ryan S, Singh A, Massicotte EM, et al. Ancillary outcome measures for assessment of individuals with cervical spondylotic myelopathy. Spine 2013;38:S111–22.
12. Wilson JR, Tetreault LA, Kim J, et al. State of the art in degenerative cervical myelopathy: an update on current clinical evidence. Neurosurgery 2017;80-(3S):S33–45.
13. Jannelli G, Nouri A, Molliqaj G, et al. Degenerative cervical myelopathy: review of surgical outcome predictors and need for multimodal approach. World Neurosurg 2020;140:541–7.
14. Singh A, Tetreault L, Casey A, et al. A summary of assessment tools for patients suffering from cervical spondylotic myelopathy: a systematic review on validity, reliability and responsiveness. Eur Spine J 2015;24(S2):209–28.
15. Badhiwala JH, Witiw CD, Nassiri F, et al. Minimum clinically important difference in SF-36 scores for use in degenerative cervical myelopathy. Spine 2018;43(21):E1260–6.
16. King JT, McGinnis KA, Roberts MS. Quality of life assessment with the medical outcomes study short Form-36 among patients with cervical spondylotic myelopathy. Neurosurgery 2003;52(1):113–21.
17. Whitehurst DGT, Engel L, Bryan S. Short form health surveys and related variants in spinal cord injury research: a systematic review. J Spinal Cord Med 2014;37(2):128–38.
18. Zhang Y, Zhou F, Sun Y. Assessment of health-related quality of life using the SF-36 in Chinese cervical spondylotic myelopathy patients after surgery and its consistency with neurological function assessment: a cohort study. Health Qual Life Outcome 2015;13(1):39.
19. Whitehurst DGT, Noonan VK, Dvorak MFS, et al. A review of preference-based health-related quality of life questionnaires in spinal cord injury research. Spinal Cord 2012;50(9):646–54.
20. Koga R, Sasaki T, Ideta R, et al. The EQ-5D-5L in patients admitted to a hospital in Japan with recent spinal cord injury: a descriptive study. Spinal Cord 2019;57(11):960–5.
21. Kirshblum SC, Burns SP, Biering-Sorensen F, et al. International standards for neurological classification of spinal cord injury (revised 2011). J Spinal Cord Med 2011;34(6):535–46.
22. Tulsky DS, Kisala PA, Victorson D, et al. Overview of the spinal cord injury – quality of life (SCI-QOL) measurement system. J Spinal Cord Med 2015;38(3):257–69.
23. Tulsky DS, Kisala PA, Victorson D, et al. Methodology for the development and calibration of the SCI-QOL item banks. J Spinal Cord Med 2015;38(3):270–87.
24. Catz A, Itzkovich M, Agranov E, et al. SCIM – spinal cord independence measure: a new disability scale for patients with spinal cord lesions. Spinal Cord 1997;35(12):850–6.
25. Catz A, Itzkovich M, Rozenblum R, et al. A multicenter international study on the spinal cord independence measure, version IV: rasch

psychometric validation. J Spinal Cord Med 2024;47(5):681–91.
26. Anderson KD, Acuff ME, Arp BG, et al. United States (US) multi-center study to assess the validity and reliability of the Spinal Cord Independence Measure (SCIM III). Spinal Cord 2011;49(8):880–5.
27. Itzkovich M, Gelernter I, Biering-Sorensen F, et al. The Spinal Cord Independence Measure (SCIM) version III: reliability and validity in a multi-center international study. Disabil Rehabil 2007;29(24):1926–33.
28. Maritz R, Fellinghauer C, Brach M, et al. A rasch-based comparison of the functional Independence measure and spinal cord Independence measure for outcome and quality in the rehabilitation of persons with spinal cord injury. JRM 2022;54:jrm00262.
29. Nuuttila E, Saarimäki SM, Hautala AJ, et al. Patient-Reported Outcome Measures for assessing functioning, disability, and health of people with spinal cord injury – a scoping review. J Spinal Cord Med 2025;1–21. https://doi.org/10.1080/10790268.2025.2477364.
30. Furlan JC, Noonan V, Singh A, et al. Assessment of disability in patients with acute traumatic spinal cord injury: a systematic review of the literature. J Neurotrauma 2011;28(8):1413–30.
31. Itzkovich M, Shefler H, Front L, et al. SCIM III (Spinal Cord Independence Measure version III): reliability of assessment by interview and comparison with assessment by observation. Spinal Cord 2018;56(1):46–51.
32. Tetreault L, Nouri A, Kopjar B, et al. The minimum clinically important difference of the modified Japanese orthopaedic association scale in patients with degenerative cervical myelopathy. Spine 2015;40(21):1653–9.
33. Ghogawala Z, Terrin N, Dunbar MR, et al. Effect of ventral vs dorsal spinal surgery on patient-reported physical functioning in patients with cervical spondylotic myelopathy: a randomized clinical trial. JAMA 2021;325(10):942.
34. Tetreault L, Kopjar B, Nouri A, et al. The modified Japanese Orthopaedic Association scale: establishing criteria for mild, moderate and severe impairment in patients with degenerative cervical myelopathy. Eur Spine J 2017;26(1):78–84.
35. Kato S, Oshima Y, Oka H, et al. Comparison of the Japanese Orthopaedic Association (JOA) Score and modified JOA (mJOA) Score for the assessment of cervical myelopathy: a multicenter observational Study. PLoS One 2015;10(4):e0123022. Fehlings M, ed.
36. Kato S, Oshima Y, Matsubayashi Y, et al. Minimum clinically important difference and patient acceptable symptom State of Japanese orthopaedic association score in degenerative cervical myelopathy patients. Spine 2019;44(10):691–7.
37. Fehlings MG, Tetreault LA, Riew KD, et al. A Clinical Practice Guideline for the management of patients with degenerative cervical myelopathy: recommendations for patients with mild, moderate, and severe disease and nonmyelopathic patients with evidence of cord compression. Glob Spine J 2017;7(3 Suppl):70S–83S.
38. Kopjar B, Tetreault L, Kalsi-Ryan S, et al. Psychometric properties of the modified Japanese orthopaedic association scale in patients with cervical spondylotic myelopathy. Spine 2015;40(1):E23–8.
39. Mizoguchi Y, Akasaka K, Suzuki K, et al. Psychometric evaluation of the Japanese neck disability index by exploratory factor analysis in preoperative patients with cervical spondylotic myelopathy: impact of pain and numbness. Spine J 2024;24(11):2172–80.
40. Bobos P, MacDermid JC, Walton DM, et al. Patient-reported outcome measures used for neck disorders: an overview of systematic reviews. J Orthop Sports Phys Ther 2018;48(10):775–88.
41. Danielsen E, Ingebrigtsen T, Gulati S, et al. Patient characteristics associated with worsening of neck pain–related disability after surgery for degenerative cervical myelopathy: a nationwide study of 1508 patients. Neurosurgery 2024;95(1):158–70.
42. Lemeunier N, Da Silva-Oolup S, Olesen K, et al. Reliability and validity of self-reported questionnaires to measure pain and disability in adults with neck pain and its associated disorders: part 3—a systematic review from the CADRE collaboration. Eur Spine J 2019;28(5):1156–79.
43. Cheung PWH, Wong CKH, Lau ST, et al. Psychometric validation of the adapted traditional Chinese (Hong Kong) version of the Japanese Orthopaedic Association Cervical Myelopathy Evaluation Questionnaire (JOACMEQ). Spine 2018;43(4):E242–9.
44. Soufi K, Ortuno O, Castillo JA, et al. Assessing the diagnostic accuracy of symptoms and signs of degenerative cervical myelopathy: a prospective study. Sci Rep 2025;15(1):37043.
45. Mjåset C, Zwart JA, Kolstad F, et al. Clinical improvement after surgery for degenerative cervical myelopathy; A comparison of patient-reported outcome measures during 12-month follow-up. PLoS One 2022;17(3):e0264954. Fehlings MG, ed.
46. Ramírez Valencia M, Haddad S, Pons Carreto A, et al. Translation, adaptation, and validation of a Spanish version of the Japanese orthopaedic association cervical myelopathy questionnaire. Spine 2024;49(5):E50–7.
47. Zhou F, Li S, Zhang Y, et al. Japanese Orthopaedic Association Cervical Myelopathy Evaluation Questionnaire (JOACMEQ) in mainland China: an

investigation of reliability, validity, and responsiveness. Health Qual Life Outcome 2020;18(1):349.
48. Chien A, Lai DM, Cheng CH, et al. Translation, cross-cultural adaptation, and validation of a Chinese version of the Japanese orthopaedic Association cervical myelopathy evaluation questionnaire. Spine 2014;39(12):963–70.
49. Pons CA, Ramírez Valencia M, De García Frutos A, et al. Myelopathy disability index: establishing criteria for mild, moderate and severe impairment in patients with degenerative cervical myelopathy. Eur Spine J 2023;32(2):584–9.
50. Davies BM, Nourallah B, Venkatesh A, et al. Establishing mild, moderate and severe criteria for the myelopathy disability index in cervical spondylotic myelopathy. Br J Neurosurg 2023;37(5): 1018–22.
51. Dalitz K, Vitzthum HE. Evaluation of five scoring systems for cervical spondylogenic myelopathy. Spine J 2019;19(2):e41–6.
52. Revanappa KK, Rajshekhar V. Comparison of nurick grading system and modified Japanese orthopaedic association scoring system in evaluation of patients with cervical spondylotic myelopathy. Eur Spine J 2011;20(9):1545–51.
53. Gibson J, Nouri A, Krueger B, et al. Degenerative cervical myelopathy: a clinical review. Yale J Biol Med 2018;91(1):43–8.
54.. Schroeder G, Vaccaro A, Welch W. Best Practices Guidelines spine injury. Chicago (IL): American College of Surgeons; 2022. Available at: https://www.facs.org/media/k45gikqv/spine_injury_guidelines.pdf.
55. Kirshblum S, Snider B, Rupp R, et al, International Standards Committee of ASIA and ISCoS. Updates of the international standards for neurologic classification of spinal cord injury. Phys Med Rehabil Clin 2020;31(3):319–30.
56. Lena E, Baroncini I, Pavese C, et al. Reliability and validity of the international standards for neurological classification of spinal cord injury in patients with non-traumatic spinal cord lesions. Spinal Cord 2022;60(1):30–6.
57. Walden K, Schuld C, Noonan VK, et al. Computer international standards for neurological classification of spinal cord Injury (ISNCSCI) algorithms: a review. Spinal Cord 2023;61(2):125–32.
58. Zipser CM, Cragg JJ, Guest JD, et al. Cell-based and stem-cell-based treatments for spinal cord injury: evidence from clinical trials. Lancet Neurol 2022;21(7):659–70.
59. Grassner L, Garcia-Ovejero D, Mach O, et al. A new score based on the international standards for neurological classification of spinal cord injury for integrative evaluation of changes in sensorimotor functions. J Neurotrauma 2022;39(9–10): 613–26.
60. Hales M, Biros E, Reznik JE. Reliability and validity of the sensory component of the international standards for neurological classification of spinal cord injury (ISNCSCI): a systematic review. Top Spinal Cord Inj Rehabil 2015;21(3):241–9.
61. Davies BM, Yang X, Khan DZ, et al. A minimum data set—Core outcome set, core data elements, and core measurement set—For degenerative cervical myelopathy research (AO spine RECODE DCM): a consensus study. PLoS Med 2024;21(8): e1004447.
62. Castle-Kirszbaum MD, Danks A, Xenos C, et al. Interobserver reliability of spinal adverse events severity system - neuro (SAVES-N): a prospective adverse event reporting system for neurosurgical cases. World Neurosurg 2018;116:e882–8.
63.. Soufi K, Ortuno O, Castillo J, et al. The degenerative cervical myelopathy subjective and objective severity (DCM-SOS) score: a data-driven outcome measure derived by a modified Delphi process. Global Spine J 2025;15(2_Suppl):413S–792S.
64. Davies B, Mowforth O, Sadler I, et al. Recovery priorities in degenerative cervical myelopathy: a cross-sectional survey of an international, online community of patients. BMJ Open 2019;9(10): e031486.
65. Kalsi-Ryan S, Curt A, Verrier MC, et al. Development of the Graded Redefined Assessment of Strength, Sensibility and Prehension (GRASSP): reviewing measurement specific to the upper limb in tetraplegia. SPI 2012;17(Suppl1):65–76.
66. Kalsi-Ryan S, Beaton D, Curt A, et al. The graded redefined assessment of strength sensibility and prehension: reliability and validity. J Neurotrauma 2012;29(5):905–14.
67. Kalsi-Ryan S, Riehm LE, Tetreault L, et al. Characteristics of upper limb impairment related to degenerative cervical myelopathy: development of a sensitive hand assessment (graded redefined assessment of strength, sensibility, and prehension version myelopathy). Neurosurg 2020;86(3):E292–9.
68. Kalsi-Ryan S, Clout J, Rostami P, et al. Duration of symptoms in the quantification of upper limb disability and impairment for individuals with mild degenerative cervical myelopathy (DCM). PLoS One 2019;14(9):e0222134. Hawryluk GWJ, ed.
69. Chiu AYY, Pang MYC. Assessment of psychometric properties of various balance assessment tools in persons with cervical spondylotic myelopathy. J Orthop Sports Phys Ther 2017;47(9):673–82.
70. Jørgensen V, Opheim A, Halvarsson A, et al. Comparison of the berg balance scale and the Mini-BESTest for assessing balance in ambulatory people with spinal cord injury: validation study. Phys Ther 2017;97(6):677–87.
71. Wirz M, Müller R, Bastiaenen C. Falls in persons with spinal cord injury: validity and reliability of

the berg balance scale. Neurorehabilitation Neural Repair 2010;24(1):70–7.
72. Abou L, Ilha J, Romanini F, et al. Do clinical balance measures have the ability to predict falls among ambulatory individuals with spinal cord injury? A systematic review and meta-analysis. Spinal Cord 2019;57(12):1001–13.
73. Forrest GF, Hutchinson K, Lorenz DJ, et al. Are the 10 meter and 6 minute walk tests redundant in patients with spinal cord injury? PLoS One 2014;9(5): e94108. Fehlings M, ed.
74. Van Hedel HJ, Wirz M, Dietz V. Assessing walking ability in subjects with spinal cord injury: validity and reliability of 3 walking tests. Arch Phys Med Rehabil 2005;86(2):190–6.
75. Amatachaya S, Naewla S, Srisim K, et al. Concurrent validity of the 10-meter walk test as compared with the 6-minute walk test in patients with spinal cord injury at various levels of ability. Spinal Cord 2014;52(4):333–6.
76. Fu W, Xu R, Wang X, et al. Can the 6-minute walking test assess ambulatory function impairment in patients with cervical spondylotic myelopathy? Spine 2024;49(21):1497–503.
77. Fehlings MG, Pedro KM, Alvi MA, et al. The sodium-glutamate antagonist riluzole improves outcome after acute spinal cord injury: results from the RISCIS randomised controlled trial analysed using a global statistical analytic technique. eBioMedicine 2025;118:105863.
78. Fehlings MG, Moghaddamjou A, Harrop JS, et al. Safety and efficacy of Riluzole in acute spinal cord injury Study (RISCIS): a Multi-Center, randomized, Placebo-Controlled, double-blinded trial. J Neurotrauma 2023;40(17–18):1878–88.
79. Fehlings MG, Badhiwala JH, Ahn H, et al. Safety and efficacy of riluzole in patients undergoing decompressive surgery for degenerative cervical myelopathy (CSM-Protect): a multicentre, double-blind, placebo-controlled, randomised, phase 3 trial. Lancet Neurol 2021;20(2):98–106.
80. Fehlings MG, Pedro KM, Alvi MA, et al. Riluzole for degenerative cervical myelopathy: a secondary analysis of the CSM-PROTECT trial. JAMA Netw Open 2024;7(6):e2415643.
81. Pedro KM, Alvi MA, Hejrati N, et al. Machine learning-based cluster analysis identifies four unique phenotypes of patients with degenerative cervical myelopathy with distinct clinical profiles and long-term functional and neurological outcomes. eBioMedicine 2024;106:105226.
82. Badhiwala JH, Witiw CD, Nassiri F, et al. Patient phenotypes associated with outcome following surgery for mild degenerative cervical myelopathy: a principal component regression analysis. Spine J 2018;18(12):2220–31.
83. Al-Shawwa A, Cadotte DW. Advancing precision medicine in degenerative cervical myelopathy. JCM 2025;14(23):8344.
84. Kalsi-Ryan S, Balbinot G, Wang JZ, et al. Minimal clinically important difference of graded redefined assessment of strength, sensibility, and prehension version 1 in acute cervical traumatic Spinal Cord injury. J Neurotrauma 2022;39(23–24):1645–53.
85. Mulcahey MJ, Thielen CC, Sadowsky C, et al. Despite limitations in content range, the SCIM-III is reproducible and a valid indicator of physical function in youths with spinal cord injury and dysfunction. Spinal Cord 2018;56(4):332–40.
86. Tulsky DS, Kisala PA, Victorson D, et al. Developing a contemporary patient-reported outcomes measure for spinal cord injury. Arch Phys Med Rehabil 2011;92(10):S44–51.
87. Davies BM, McHugh M, Elgheriani A, et al. Reported outcome measures in degenerative cervical myelopathy: a systematic review. PLoS One 2016; 11(8):e0157263. Ahmad F, ed.
88. Biering-Sørensen F. The guttmann lecture 2025: standardization of data collection in individuals with spinal cord injury. Spinal Cord 2026;64(1): 96–102.
89. Zhao F, Balthazaar S, Hiremath SV, et al. Enhancing spinal cord injury care: using wearable technologies for physical activity, sleep, and cardiovascular health. Arch Phys Med Rehabil 2024;105(10): 1997–2007.
90. Bi CL, Kurland DB, Ber R, et al. Digital biomarkers and the evolution of spine care outcomes measures: smartphones and wearables. Neurosurgery 2023;93(4):745–54.
91. Giagiozis M, Lerch I, Linke AD, et al. Feasibility and sensitivity of wearable sensors for daily activity monitoring in spinal cord injury trials. Neurorehabilitation Neural Repair 2025;39(10):814–25.
92.. Delgado AD, Balthazaar SJT, Soltesz AE, et al. Using machine learning with wearable devices to advance research and patient care using spinal cord injury as a model. Arch Phys Med Rehabil 2026;107(5):1148–60.
93. Hupp M, Pavese C, Bachmann LM, et al. Electrophysiological multimodal assessments improve outcome prediction in traumatic cervical spinal cord injury. J Neurotrauma 2018;35(24):2916–23.
94. Zörner B, Blanckenhorn WU, Dietz V, et al, EM-SCI Study Group. Clinical algorithm for improved prediction of ambulation and patient stratification after incomplete spinal cord injury. J Neurotrauma 2010; 27(1):241–52.
95. Scheuren PS, Schubert M, Hubli M, et al. Enhanced clinical trial stratification in spinal cord injury: the value of electrophysiology. Brain 2025; awaf354. https://doi.org/10.1093/brain/awaf354.

96.. Ramachandran K, Thippeswamy PB, Shetty AP, et al. Deciphering the role of glial cel l-specific metabolites as biomarkers in early cervical myelopathy-insights from in vivo MRS study. Spine J 2026;26(2):423–33.
97. Berberat J, Andereggen L, Gruber P, et al. A diagnostic biomarker for cervical myelopathy based on dynamic magnetic resonance imaging. Spine 2023;48(15):1041–6.
98. Khan AF, Mohammadi E, Haynes G, et al. Evaluating tissue injury in cervical spondylotic myelopathy with spinal cord MRI: a systematic review. Eur Spine J 2024;33(1):133–54.
99. Davies BM, Yanez Touzet A, Mowforth OD, et al. Development of a core measurement set for research in degenerative cervical myelopathy: a study protocol (AO spine RECODE-DCM CMS). BMJ Open 2022;12(6):e060436.
100. Eaton R, Duff J, Wallace M, et al. The value of the whole picture: rehabilitation outcome measurement using patient self-report and clinician-based assessments after spinal cord injury. Spinal Cord 2022;60(1):71–80.
101.. Foschi CVS, De Lima A, Michaelsen SM, et al. Spinal cord independence measure evidence-based recommendation: a systematic review of measurement properties. Spinal Cord 2026;64:113–25.
102. Catz A, Itzkovich M, Elkayam K, et al. Reliability validity and responsiveness of the spinal cord Independence measure 4th version in a multicultural setup. Arch Phys Med Rehabil 2022;103(3):430–40.e2.
103.. Baidya J, Ng M, Green WA, et al. Delayed yet durable functional recovery following posterior cervical decompression and fusion for mild degenerative cervical myelopathy spine. Spine (Phila Pa 1976) 2025. https://doi.org/10.1097/BRS.0000000000005590. Online ahead of print.

Artificial Intelligence and Machine Learning in Spinal Cord Injury

Mohammed Ali Alvi, MD, MS[a,b,c], Karlo M. Pedro, MD[a,b,c],
Michael G. Fehlings, MD, PhD, FRCSC, FRSC, FCAHS[a,b,c,*]

KEYWORDS

• Artificial intelligence • Machine learning • Innovation • Technology • Heterogeneity • Deep learning • Prognostication • Modeling

KEY POINTS

- SCI is highly heterogeneous, with substantial variability in injury severity, biological response, and recovery trajectories, making individualized, data-driven approaches essential for diagnosis and treatment.
- AI and ML can integrate imaging, clinical and longitudinal data to improve injury characterization, prognostication, and prediction of functional recovery after SCI.
- AI-driven imaging tools enable automated segmentation, quantitative biomarker extraction, and advanced radiomic analysis, supporting more objective assessment of spinal cord injury severity and recovery potential.
- Machine learning models outperform many traditional statistical approaches in predicting neurologic and functional outcomes by capturing nonlinear relationships within complex multimodal spinal cord injury datasets.
- Emerging applications of AI in regenerative therapies and rehabilitation may enable optimized patient selection, adaptive treatment strategies, and integrated precision medicine approaches for SCI patients.

INTRODUCTION

Burden of Spinal Cord Injury: Incidence, Disability, and Economic Impact

Spinal cord injury (SCI) remains a major global health problem, with consequences that extend well beyond physical disability to include mental health, social participation, and economic burden.[1] Clinically, SCI can result in profound and often permanent functional deficits, including paraplegia or quadriplegia, bowel and bladder dysfunction, chronic pain syndromes, and autonomic dysregulation.[2,3]

Data from the Global Burden of Disease initiative has shown that in 2019, an estimated 20.6 million individuals worldwide were living with SCI, representing a substantial increase in both prevalence and incidence compared to 1990.[4] The economic burden is particularly striking in high-income settings. In the United States, the annual direct cost of SCI is estimated to exceed US$9.7 billion,[5] with approximately 17,000 new cases each year

[a] Division of Neurosurgery & Spine Program, Department of Surgery, University of Toronto, Toronto, Ontario, Canada; [b] Institute of Medical Science, University of Toronto, Toronto, Ontario, Canada; [c] Division of Neurosurgery, Krembil Neuroscience Centre, Toronto Western Hospital, University Health Network, Toronto, Ontario, Canada
* Corresponding author. Toronto Western Hospital, 399 Bathurst Street, Suite 4WW-449, Toronto ONM5T 2S8, Canada.
E-mail address: Michael.fehlings@uhn.ca

Neurosurg Clin N Am 37 (2026) 523–533
https://doi.org/10.1016/j.nec.2026.05.003

Abbreviations	
AI	artificial intelligence
AIS	ASIA Impairment Scale
CNNs	convolutional neural networks
CT	computed tomography
ML	machine learning
NLP	natural language processing
SCI	spinal cord injury

and lifetime costs per patient ranging from US$1.1 to US$4.7 million.[6] In China, the average hospitalization cost for traumatic SCI is approximately US$11,500, with daily costs around US$700.[7] Taken together, these data highlight the significant and growing socioeconomic burden associated with SCI.

Fundamental Challenge: Heterogeneity

After SCI, the secondary injury cascade that ensues is complicated, and the complexity reflects something basic about SCI itself, the condition is heterogeneous by nature.[8–10] For that reason, it is hard to imagine one therapy meaningfully covering the entire range of mechanisms at play. By comparison, combined approaches that hit more than 1 biological pathway stand a better chance of producing a real clinical effect.[11]

This growing awareness of heterogeneity has been driven, in part, by what keeps happening in clinical trials, especially acute trials of new therapies. Differences between patients create major statistical "noise," so larger cohorts are needed to get stable estimates and limit bias. Yet acute SCI trials repeatedly run into recruitment bottlenecks, and many have ended up delayed, paused, or stopped entirely because enrollment could not be completed within required windows. A more coordinated, network-style approach to identifying eligible patients and enrolling them is likely part of what is needed.

Trial design itself also needs work. With SCI, between-person variability is substantial, so tighter inclusion windows and greater reliance on objective biological indicators of injury severity could improve patient selection. Paired with better prognostic models, these changes could produce more uniform cohorts and, in turn, make study results easier to interpret and more likely to succeed.

Limitations of Traditional Paradigms

The ASIA Impairment Scale (AIS) remains the central tool for classifying SCI, but its shortcomings are well recognized. AIS grades do not reliably map onto outcomes that matter functionally, and they often miss small but clinically relevant neurologic shifts. On top of that, patients grouped under the same AIS grade can look very different, with recovery paths that diverge widely even when their starting grades match.[12,13]

Taken together, these issues point to a wider problem in SCI care, dependence on generalized, one-size approaches. SCI varies at multiple levels, injury morphology, biological response, and recovery potential. Even in cohorts that appear clinically similar, outcomes can swing dramatically, which keeps pointing back to the same need: individualized, data-driven diagnosis, prognostication, and treatment.[14]

Emergence of Artificial Intelligence/Machine Learning to Quantify Injury, Predict Outcomes, and Personalize Treatment

Artificial intelligence (AI) refers broadly to computational systems designed to perform tasks that typically require human intelligence, including pattern recognition, decision-making, and prediction. In health care, these systems are applied to analyze complex datasets, identify clinically relevant patterns, and support decision-making across diagnostic, prognostic, and therapeutic domains.

Machine learning (ML) represents a subset of AI focused on algorithms that learn relationships directly from data rather than relying on predefined rules. These models are trained on datasets to identify patterns and make predictions, with performance improving as additional data are incorporated. ML approaches can be broadly categorized into supervised learning, where models are trained using labeled outcomes, unsupervised learning, which identifies patterns or groupings without predefined labels, and reinforcement-based approaches that optimize decisions through iterative feedback.

AI and ML are increasingly being used to deal with SCI's inherent complexity and variability. Across the care pathway, these tools support objective injury quantification through automated imaging and clinical data analysis, prediction of neurologic and functional outcomes, and tailoring of treatment strategies. Recent research shows ML models can classify injury features and pull clinically useful signals from routine inputs, including MRI and neurologic examinations.[15] Data-driven models have also performed strongly when predicting recovery patterns and functional outcomes, often doing better than conventional statistical methods because they can learn from high-dimensional, multimodal datasets.[16,17]

These predictions are not just descriptive. They can translate into decisions, informing early care choices, setting rehabilitation targets, and flagging patients most likely to benefit from advanced or regenerative options.[18] Overall, the field is moving away from AI as a retrospective tool and toward AI as a driver of precision, data-led, individualized SCI management.

In the current review, the authors summarize the emerging role of ML and AI in the context of diagnosis, prognostication, phenotyping, and novel therapeutics in the field of SCI (**Table 1**).

WHY SPINAL CORD INJURY IS UNIQUELY SUITED FOR APPLICATIONS OF ARTIFICIAL INTELLIGENCE

SCI stands out as one of the more complex clinical conditions because injury patterns, biological response, and functional recovery vary so widely. That built-in heterogeneity, paired with rich multimodal data and persistent uncertainty in day-to-day decisions, makes SCI a strong match for AI-driven approaches. Unlike conditions with more predictable courses, SCI pushes against traditional frameworks at almost every point in care, which strengthens the case for integrative, data-based models.

Data Richness in Spinal Cord Injury

For all its complexity, SCI generates a large amount of structured and semistructured data across the full care timeline. Imaging is central from the beginning and remains important throughout follow-up. MRI can detail cord pathology, edema, hemorrhage, lesion length, and preserved tissue bridges, while computed tomography (CT) defines bony injury and mechanical stability. Quantitative measurements drawn from these images have been linked to neurologic and functional outcomes.[19,20]

Neurologic assessment is another key stream. Standardized examinations, including the International Standards for Neurological Classification of Spinal Cord Injury (ISNCSCI), give reproducible motor and sensory measures that are collected routinely in both practice and research.[21] Many datasets also include longitudinal follow-up, which makes it possible to chart recovery trajectories in detail.

SCI research is also pulling in newer data types. Genomic and transcriptomic studies are starting to map biological responses at a systems level, and metabolomic plus proteomic work adds information on downstream cellular processes.[22,23] Wearables and mobile health tools now allow continuous tracking of movement, activity, and physiologic measures in everyday settings, supporting "digital phenotyping."[24] The result is a data-rich environment, but the information is high-dimensional, varied, and hard to merge with standard methods. That is exactly where AI and ML can have the most impact.

Clinical Decision Uncertainty

Even with guidelines and standardized assessments, SCI decision-making often carries a high degree of uncertainty. A long-running debate involves surgical decompression timing. Early surgery is generally linked with better outcomes, yet the best timing for a given patient still depends on factors like severity, imaging, and comorbidities.[25]

Table 1
Key applications of artificial intelligence across the spinal cord injury care continuum

Domain	AI Applications	Data Inputs	Clinical Impact
Acute diagnosis	Fracture detection and injury classification	Computed tomography and MRI	Improved diagnostic accuracy and reduced interobserver variability
Imaging analytics	Segmentation, lesion quantification, and tissue bridge analysis	MRI	Objective injury characterization and biomarker development
Prognostication	Outcome prediction and recovery modeling	Clinical + imaging	Improved prediction of motor recovery, function, and survival
Phenotyping	Clustering and trajectory analysis	Longitudinal clinical data	Identification of subgroups and personalized care pathways
Regenerative therapy	Patient selection, graft monitoring, and biomaterial optimization	Multimodal	Improved targeting and evaluation of advanced therapies

Selecting patients for specific interventions remains difficult as well. Two individuals with the same neurologic classification can recover in very different ways, making it hard to predict who will benefit most from surgery, rehabilitation, or emerging therapies. That variability reflects biological differences that current classification systems do not fully capture.

Prognosis is also inconsistent. Large cohort study shows that patients who look similar at baseline can still end up with markedly different functional outcomes, especially in incomplete injuries.[26–28]

ARTIFICIAL INTELLIGENCE IN ACUTE SPINAL CORD INJURY DIAGNOSIS AND CLASSIFICATION

AI is being applied more often at the earliest stages of SCI care, where diagnostic uncertainty and assessment variability can ripple through later management. In acute SCI, getting injury severity, morphology, and neurologic status right matters, but interpretation of imaging and clinical findings can be subjective. ML approaches can help standardize and strengthen these assessments by extracting objective signals from imaging and clinical data, improving diagnostic precision and supporting more refined classification systems.

Imaging-based Diagnosis

Computer vision progress has made it possible to apply deep learning models, including convolutional neural networks (CNNs) and vision transformer–based architectures, to spinal imaging.

In traumatic spinal injury, multiple studies show CNNs can detect vertebral fractures on CT with high accuracy. Zhang and colleagues,[29] for instance, built a deep learning model that automatically detects and classifies vertebral body fractures on CT and showed strong diagnostic performance across diverse datasets. Deep learning has also been applied to MRI to identify SCI severity and segment intramedullary lesions, producing quantitative measurements that go beyond what visual reads alone can provide.[30,31]

These models can also be trained to classify injuries using established systems such as the arbeitsgemeinschaft für osteosynthesefragen (AO) spine classification of upper cervical injuries or the AO spine thoracolumbar injury classification system. Automated classification could reduce interobserver variation, a persistent limitation in spine trauma assessment.[32] Standardized interpretation may improve diagnostic consistency and support more uniform decisions across centers.

Equally important, AI methods can extract quantitative imaging measures, lesion volume, cord compression, preserved tissue, that correlate with neurologic outcomes and may describe injury severity more finely than standard qualitative descriptors.[19]

NLP and Clinical Data Extraction

Alongside imaging approaches, natural language processing (NLP) is being used to pull clinically relevant details from unstructured electronic records. In SCI, much of the neurologic examination and clinical documentation sits in free text, including examination narratives, operative reports, and progress notes.

Recent research shows NLP models can extract key examination elements and reconstruct standardized scoring systems. ML-based text tools have been able to derive components of ISNCSCI from clinical notes with good accuracy, enabling automated estimates of neurologic severity.[33] Beyond scoring, these methods can track longitudinal narratives and capture symptom changes, complications, and treatment responses over time. Turning free text into analyzable variables matters in SCI because so much clinically meaningful information would otherwise stay outside conventional datasets.

Toward Objective Spinal Cord Injury Classification

Traditional classification systems offer a shared language for injury severity, yet they still struggle to represent the full biological and functional variation seen in SCI. AI-based methods are increasingly being investigated as a way to move from fixed categories toward objective, data-driven phenotyping.

Imaging-informed models are a leading example. Quantitative MRI features, including lesion characteristics and preserved tissue measures, have been built into ML models to improve prediction of neurologic and functional outcomes.[20,34] This study suggests imaging biomarkers can add information beyond the neurologic examination and improve stratification.

Multimodal models that combine clinical, imaging, and other inputs have recently begun emerging. By combining domains, these frameworks aim to capture SCI's multidimensional profile and identify patient subgroups that standard classifications miss. Early studies suggest ML can find clinically meaningful patterns and improve prognostic accuracy compared with single-domain strategies.[15]

ARTIFICIAL INTELLIGENCE IN SPINAL CORD INJURY IMAGING: FROM QUALITATIVE TO QUANTITATIVE

Image Reconstruction and Acquisition

AI is also being used at the start of the imaging pipeline, during acquisition and reconstruction. Deep learning reconstruction can speed up MRI by generating high-quality images from undersampled data. Prospective studies report scan time reductions of roughly 30% to 40% while maintaining, or even improving, image quality measures such as signal-to-noise and contrast resolution.[35,36] This matters in acute SCI, where discomfort, motion, and instability can make long scans unrealistic.

Deep learning has also been applied to improve low-dose CT. These methods can reduce noise while preserving detail, allowing lower radiation exposure without sacrificing diagnostic usefulness.[37]

Automated Segmentation

A major AI contribution in SCI imaging has been automated segmentation. Manually outlining cord anatomy, lesions, and surrounding structures takes time and varies across raters, which limits usability in clinical care and large studies.

Deep learning segmentation models can identify spinal cord anatomy and intramedullary lesions on MRI with accuracy similar to expert raters.[30,38] This supports rapid, high-throughput analysis and more consistent measurement of injury features.

The Spinal Cord Toolbox is a widely used open-source platform combining automated segmentation with standardized templates and quantitative tools.[39] Newer versions include deep learning modules for spinal cord, gray matter, and lesion segmentation, helping with reproducible feature extraction across datasets.

Quantitative Imaging Biomarkers

Moving from qualitative reads to quantitative imaging has supported development of imaging biomarkers, objective measures linked to injury severity and recovery potential. Lesion length and volume are among the most studied and have been associated with neurologic impairment and longer term outcomes.[19,20]

Tissue bridges, preserved tissue spanning the lesion, are another key biomarker. Quantifying dorsal and ventral tissue bridges has been tied to motor and sensory recovery, suggesting they reflect remaining functional connectivity.[19]

Radiomics adds another layer by extracting high-dimensional features related to texture, intensity, and spatial structure that are not visible on standard inspection. Early findings suggest radiomic signatures might improve outcome prediction when combined with clinical variables, though stronger validation is still needed.[15,34]

ARTIFICIAL INTELLIGENCE FOR PROGNOSTICATION AND OUTCOME PREDICTION IN SPINAL CORD INJURY

Clinical variables help frame recovery expectations, but they often cannot capture the nonlinear relationships that drive neurologic and functional outcomes in SCI. ML approaches have gained traction because they can improve prediction by learning from high-dimensional, multimodal data.

Traditional versus Machine Learning Approaches

Most traditional SCI prognostic models have used regression methods. They are easy to interpret and statistically feasible, but they depend on certain assumptions like linearity, variable independence, and limited interaction effects. In a condition as heterogeneous as SCI, those assumptions often do not fit well, which can limit accuracy and generalizability.

ML methods are built to model nonlinear effects and complex interactions across many variables. They can absorb high-dimensional information and combine heterogeneous inputs, including clinical findings, imaging, and longitudinal outcomes. Comparative studies report that ML can outperform traditional statistics for SCI outcome prediction, particularly when data are complex or multimodal.[40,41]

Supervised Learning Models

Multiple supervised ML algorithms have been applied in SCI outcome prediction. Tree-based methods, random forests and gradient boosting, are common because they capture nonlinear relationships and variable interactions. These models have predicted motor recovery and functional outcomes using clinical and imaging inputs.

Neural networks have also shown promise, especially where datasets are large. They can learn hierarchical representations and have been used to predict neurologic improvement and functional independence with strong accuracy.[17,42]

Across the literature, ML models have been used to predict motor recovery, independence in daily activities, and survival. Some models trained on large clinical datasets have performed well at predicting functional outcomes at rehabilitation admission and discharge, supporting their possible role in early planning.[17]

Trajectory Modeling

Many prognostic approaches focus on static endpoints, for example, neurologic status at a set time. Recovery after SCI is dynamic, and patients follow different paths. ML-based trajectory modeling addresses this by learning recovery patterns from longitudinal data.

Clustering and trajectory methods have been used to identify distinct recovery profiles, grouping patients with similar neurologic and functional changes over time. These models can also highlight early predictors of long-term trajectories that baseline measures may not reveal.[43,44]

Focusing on trajectories instead of single endpoints offers a more realistic view of recovery and could support more adaptive, individualized treatment planning. This is particularly relevant because timing and degree of recovery vary widely between patients.

Multimodal Models

A central advance in ML prognostication has been multimodal modeling. Instead of relying on one data stream, these models combine clinical variables, imaging features, and increasingly other measures such as wearable-derived metrics.

Research integrating clinical and imaging data has shown improved predictive performance compared with single-domain models. For instance, models combining MRI features with clinical assessments have improved prediction of neurologic recovery and functional outcomes.[34,45]

This approach fits SCI's multidimensional profile and aligns with precision medicine goals. By combining complementary signals about injury and recovery, multimodal models can offer more accurate and more individualized prognostic estimates.

UNSUPERVISED LEARNING AND PHENOTYPING IN SPINAL CORD INJURY

Concept of Spinal Cord Injury Phenotypes

AIS and related systems provide standardized descriptions, but they do not capture the full multidimensional nature of SCI. Within the same AIS grade, patients can differ in injury morphology, preserved pathways, comorbidities, and biological response, all of which influence recovery.

This has driven interest in data-driven phenotypes, patient subgroups defined not by preset categories but by patterns that emerge from the data. The aim is to represent SCI heterogeneity more faithfully and offer a finer-grained view of trajectories.

Trajectory studies already show that similar baseline status can still lead to distinct recovery pathways, reinforcing the limits of static classification and supporting more dynamic, data-based strategies.[43,44]

Clustering Approaches

Unsupervised learning is central to phenotype discovery. Unlike supervised prediction, clustering methods look for structure without outcome labels.

Common options include k-means, which partitions patients by similarity across chosen variables, and density-based methods like (Density-Based Spatial Clustering of Applications with Noise [DBSCAN]), which find clusters based on how points are distributed. Dimensionality reduction tools such as (Uniform Manifold Approximation and Projection UMAP]) have also been used to visualize high-dimensional clinical and imaging data and make underlying structure easier to detect.

These methods fit SCI datasets well because the data often mix clinical, imaging, and longitudinal variables. By capturing nonlinear patterns and interactions, clustering can reveal subgroups that conventional analysis misses.

Applications in neurologic and spine populations show that these techniques can identify clinically meaningful subgroups, including distinct recovery patterns and symptom profiles.[46,47]

Clinical Applications

Data-driven phenotypes have direct clinical relevance. One key use is identifying responder subgroups, patients more likely to benefit from a given intervention. This matters in SCI because treatment effects can vary widely.

Clustering can also support personalized rehabilitation by grouping patients with similar functional profiles and recovery trajectories. That makes it possible to plan therapy around expected patterns rather than defaulting to generalized protocols.

For clinical trials, phenotype-based stratification offers 1 route around heterogeneity. Enriching trials with more uniform subgroups could improve detection of treatment effects and reduce the risk of negative or ambiguous results, influencing how future SCI interventional studies are designed.

Implications for Precision Medicine

Unsupervised learning in SCI fits into a broader move toward precision medicine. Instead grouping patients under certain categories, the goal is to characterize individuals using multidimensional data and tailor care accordingly.

By combining clinical information, imaging, and longitudinal measures, phenotype-based frameworks give a more complete picture of patient status and recovery potential. They also provide a structure for linking biology to outcomes. As more modalities, imaging biomarkers, molecular profiles, are incorporated, these approaches could help connect underlying pathophysiology with observed recovery patterns.

ARTIFICIAL INTELLIGENCE IN REGENERATIVE AND EXPERIMENTAL THERAPIES IN SPINAL CORD INJURY

Effective SCI repair needs to address cell loss, structural disruption, and functional disconnection at the same time. Regenerative strategies, especially stem cell–based therapies, have grown out of that need. As these therapies develop, AI is being used to tackle practical barriers to development and clinical translation.

A major limitation in stem cell approaches is variability, in cell quality, differentiation capacity, and therapeutic behavior. Data-driven models can be trained to predict these properties before transplantation, improving consistency and lowering the chance of weak or unpredictable effects.

AI is also being used in biomaterial and scaffold design. Traditional biomaterials work is often iterative and slow. Computational methods can test design choices more quickly, scaffold structure, biochemical composition, and other parameters, helping speed up improvement of environments meant to support survival and axonal growth.

Neural Stem Cell-based Regeneration

Neural stem cells and induced pluripotent stem cell–derived progenitors can address multiple aspects of SCI pathology. They can differentiate into neurons and glia, remyelinate injured axons, and contribute to rebuilding neural circuits.[48]

Preclinical studies have clarified mechanisms. Kadoya and colleagues[49] reported that transplanted neural stem cells can extend axons across lesions into distal spinal pathways, forming organized projections that reconnect disrupted circuits. Ceto and colleagues[50] then showed graft-derived neurons can be functionally active, forming synaptic networks that integrate with host circuitry and support signal transmission across the injury.

Beyond structural repair, neural stem cells can also affect inflammation by changing the inflammatory environment, supporting tissue preservation, and limiting secondary damage.[51] Early clinical work has started translating these findings, and initial trials suggest stem cell transplantation can be feasible and safe in subacute and chronic settings.[52,53]

Role of Artificial Intelligence in Monitoring and Evaluating Regenerative Processes

After stem cell transplantation, measuring regeneration and integration is still difficult. AI-enabled imaging and analysis can quantify these processes more precisely. Automated morphometric tools have been used to assess axonal structure and white matter organization, producing objective measures of remodeling and repair.[54]

These tools support detailed assessment of graft survival, axonal growth, and circuit formation, replacing subjective impressions with reproducible quantitative outputs. That level of consistency is crucial in clinical trials and translational research.

Clinical Integration: Patient Selection and Therapeutic Optimization

Clinically, one of the most valuable roles of AI may be improving patient selection and intervention timing. Given the heterogeneous nature of SCI, selecting patients most likely to benefit from regenerative interventions remains challenging.

ML models trained on clinical and functional datasets have predicted recovery potential and functional improvement, offering a basis for more informed decisions.[55,56] These tools could help determine when to intervene and which patients have the best chance of benefiting.

Neuromodulation is also increasingly being paired with regenerative strategies. AI-based tuning of stimulation parameters has been proposed to strengthen emerging circuits and improve signal transmission, potentially enhancing functional recovery.[57]

Toward Integrated, Artificial Intelligence-driven Regenerative Systems

Regenerative therapy in SCI is likely to move toward tighter integration of biological and computational approaches. Emerging frameworks aim to merge imaging, electrophysiology, molecular measures, and clinical variables into unified patient-specific models.[58]

Instead of acting as isolated interventions, regenerative therapies are increasingly being viewed within broader interconnected systems, predictive modeling, adaptive rehabilitation, and real-time monitoring. In that setting, AI is not just an analysis tool, it becomes a coordinating component that helps refine complex strategies.

Table 2
Future directions in artificial intelligence-driven spinal cord injury care

Area	Emerging Direction	Potential Impact
Imaging	Quantitative MRI biomarkers and radiomics	Early detection and improved stratification
Prognostication	Multimodal predictive models	Personalized recovery forecasting
Regenerative therapy	AI-guided stem cell and scaffold optimization	Enhanced repair and integration
Rehabilitation	Adaptive, AI-driven therapy systems	Real-time personalization of recovery
Clinical trials	Phenotype-based stratification	Reduced heterogeneity and improved power
Precision medicine	Integration of clinical + imaging + omics	Fully individualized treatment pathways

Together, these trends point to a more integrated, individualized care model, with regenerative interventions guided and iterated through data-driven approaches that match the underlying complexity of SCI.

KEY POINTS AND TAKE-HOME MESSAGES

SCI presents a uniquely complex clinical challenge, defined by substantial heterogeneity in injury characteristics, biological response, and recovery trajectories. AI offers a framework to address this complexity by integrating diverse data sources and uncovering patterns that are not accessible through traditional approaches. Across the care continuum, these methods are enabling more objective characterization of injury, improving prediction of outcomes, and supporting more individualized treatment strategies.

Importantly, the value of these approaches lies not in replacing clinical judgment, but in augmenting it. By combining quantitative imaging biomarkers, longitudinal clinical data, and emerging data streams such as wearable-derived metrics, AI has the potential to reduce uncertainty in key clinical decisions and improve patient selection for both conventional and advanced therapies.

At the same time, significant challenges remain, including the need for robust external validation, standardization of data inputs, and integration into clinical workflows (**Table 2**). Addressing these limitations will be essential to ensure that these tools translate into meaningful improvements in patient care.

Taken together, the application of AI in SCI reflects a broader shift toward data-driven, individualized care. The continued integration of these approaches into clinical practice, imaging, rehabilitation, and regenerative therapies will likely play a central role in advancing outcomes in this field.

SUMMARY

AI is rapidly evolving within SCI care, moving beyond its initial role as a retrospective analytical tool toward active participation in clinical decision-making and, increasingly, therapeutic integration. What began as efforts to analyze imaging and clinical datasets has progressed to models that inform prognosis, guide treatment selection, and support real-time clinical decisions. More recently, these approaches are being incorporated into the design and optimization of therapeutic strategies, including regenerative interventions and rehabilitation programs.

SCI represents a particularly well-suited model for precision medicine. The condition is defined by substantial heterogeneity in injury characteristics, biological response, and recovery trajectories, yet it is also supported by rich, multimodal data collected longitudinally across the continuum of care. This combination of complexity and data availability creates an environment in which data-driven approaches can meaningfully enhance understanding and management of disease.

Looking forward, the most impactful advances are likely to arise from the convergence of multiple domains. AI will increasingly be integrated with quantitative imaging biomarkers that provide objective measures of injury and recovery, regenerative therapies that aim to restore neural structure and function, and adaptive rehabilitation systems that respond dynamically to patient progress. Rather than functioning as isolated innovations, these components are expected to operate within interconnected frameworks that support continuous assessment, prediction, and optimization of care.

CLINICS CARE POINTS

- Pearls: ML models, particularly tree-based methods and neural networks, consistently outperform traditional regression for SCI outcome prediction when data are high-dimensional or multimodal. Clinicians should know these tools are moving from research settings into practical prognostication.

- Quantitative MRI biomarkers (lesion volume, lesion length, dorsal/ventral tissue bridges) carry independent prognostic value beyond the neurological exam.
- Automated segmentation tools like Spinal Cord Toolbox now make reproducible extraction feasible in research workflows.
- Deep learning reconstruction can cut MRI scan time by roughly 30 to 40% without degrading image quality, a meaningful gain in acute SCI patients who are in pain, hemodynamically unstable, or unable to hold still for long acquisitions.
- NLP tools can reconstruct ISNCSCI scoring from free-text clinical notes with reasonable accuracy, opening the door to large-scale retrospective cohort analyses without manual chart review.
- Patients sharing the same AIS grade at admission can follow very different functional trajectories. Trajectory-based ML models capture this better than static classification and are better suited to individualized rehabilitation planning.
- Pitfalls: AIS grade alone is a poor surrogate for outcome. Grouping patients by AIS for trial enrollment or prognostication without incorporating imaging or biological variables risks masking the heterogeneity that drives recovery differences.
- Most published ML models in SCI have been trained on single-center or registry data with limited external validation. Applying these models outside the development cohort should be done cautiously until multi-center validation exists.
- Radiomics and multimodal models can overfit when sample sizes are small relative to the number of features. High reported accuracy in discovery datasets does not guarantee generalizability.
- Automated segmentation tools perform well on standard acquisitions but degrade with poor image quality, off-protocol sequences, or artifact-heavy scans common in acute trauma settings. Outputs should be reviewed before being used in clinical decisions.
- AI-assisted patient selection for regenerative or experimental therapies remains largely investigational. Using predictive models to include or exclude patients from emerging interventions requires careful validation before being adopted into clinical or trial practice.

ACKNOWLEDGMENT

MGF was supported by the Robert Campeau Family Foundation/Dr C.H. Tator Chair in Brain and Spinal Cord Research at UHN.

DISCLOSURE

The authors have nothing to disclose.

DECLARATION OF AI AND AI-ASSISTED TECHNOLOGIES IN THE WRITING PROCESS

During the preparation of this work the author(s) used grammerly and quillbot to refine the written content. AFter using this tool/service, the authors reviewed and edited the content as needed and take full responsibility for the content of the publication.

REFERENCES

1. Quadri SA, Farooqui M, Ikram A, et al. Recent update on basic mechanisms of spinal cord injury. Neurosurg Rev 2020;43(2):425–41.
2. Hersh AM, Davidar AD, Weber-Levine C, et al. Advancements in the treatment of traumatic spinal cord injury during military conflicts. Neurosurg Focus 2022;53(3):E15.
3. Müller-Jensen L, Ploner CJ, Kroneberg D, et al. Clinical presentation and causes of non-traumatic spinal cord injury: an observational study in emergency patients. Front Neurol 2021;12:701927.
4. GBD Spinal Cord Injuries Collaborators. Global, regional, and national burden of spinal cord injury, 1990-2019: a systematic analysis for the global burden of disease study 2019. Lancet Neurol 2023;22(11):1026–47.
5. GBD 2017 US Neurological Disorders Collaborators, Feigin VL, Vos T, Alahdab F, et al. Burden of neurological disorders across the US from 1990-2017: a global burden of disease study: a global burden of disease study. JAMA Neurol 2021;78(2):165–76.
6. Spinal cord injury (SCI) 2016 facts and figures at a glance. J Spinal Cord Med 2016;39(4):493–4.
7. Zhou H, Lou Y, Chen L, et al. Epidemiological and clinical features, treatment status, and economic burden of traumatic spinal cord injury in China: a hospital-based retrospective study. Neural Regen Res 2024;19(5):1126–33.
8. Charles Aidemise O. Secondary injury mechanisms in traumatic spinal cord injury: a nugget of this multiply Cascade. Acta Neurobiol Exp 2011;71(2):281–99.
9. Li C, Wu Z, Zhou L, et al. Temporal and spatial cellular and molecular pathological alterations with single-cell resolution in the adult spinal cord after injury. Signal Transduct Targeted Ther 2022;7(1):65.

10. Anwar MA, Al Shehabi TS, Eid Ali H. Inflammogenesis of secondary spinal cord injury. Front Cell Neurosci 2016;10:98.
11. Hu X, Xu W, Ren Y, et al. Spinal cord injury: molecular mechanisms and therapeutic interventions. Signal Transduct Targeted Ther 2023;8(1):245.
12. Aimetti AA, Kirshblum S, Curt A, et al. Natural history of neurological improvement following complete (AIS A) thoracic spinal cord injury across three registries to guide acute clinical trial design and interpretation. Spinal Cord 2019;57(9):753–62.
13. Roberts TT, Leonard GR, Cepela DJ. Classifications in brief: american spinal injury association (ASIA) impairment scale. Clin Orthop Relat Res 2017; 475(5):1499–504.
14. van Middendorp JJ, Goss B, Urquhart Su, et al. Diagnosis and prognosis of traumatic spinal cord injury. Glob Spine J 2011;1(1):1–8.
15. Jeong S, Kang SH, Ko MJ, et al. Determination of diagnosis and prognosis in spinal cord injury using machine learning. Korean J Nutr 2025;21(4):228–36.
16. Håkansson S, Tuci M, Bolliger M, et al. Data-driven prediction of spinal cord injury recovery: an exploration of current status and future perspectives. Exp Neurol 2024;380(114913):114913.
17. Kato C, Uemura O, Sato Y, et al. Functional outcome prediction after spinal cord injury using ensemble machine learning. Arch Phys Med Rehabil 2024; 105(1):95–100.
18. Zhong L, Huang Q, Zhang H, et al. Predicting spinal cord injury prognosis using machine learning: systematic review and meta-analysis. JMIR AI 2025;4-(v4i11e66233):e66233.
19. Freund P, Seif M, Weiskopf N, et al. MRI in traumatic spinal cord injury: from clinical assessment to neuroimaging biomarkers. Lancet Neurol 2019;18(12): 1123–35.
20. Mummaneni N, Burke JF, DiGiorgio AM, et al. Injury volume extracted from MRI predicts neurologic outcome in acute spinal cord injury: a prospective TRACK-SCI pilot study. J Clin Neurosci 2020;82(Pt B):231–6.
21. Kirshblum SC, Biering-Sørensen F, Betz R, et al. International standards for neurological classification of spinal cord injury: cases with classification challenges. Top Spinal Cord Inj Rehabil 2014;20(2):81–9.
22. Ahuja CS, Wilson JR, Nori S, et al. Traumatic spinal cord injury. Nat Rev Dis Primers 2017;3(1):17018.
23. Patel M, Deng AJ, Hasoon J, et al. A review of pathophysiology, molecular mechanisms, and omics approaches of spinal cord injury. Int J Mol Sci 2025; 26(16):7895.
24. Dunn J, Runge R, Snyder M. Snyder Michael. Wearables and the medical revolution. Per Med 2018; 15(5):429–48.
25. Fehlings MG, Vaccaro A, Wilson JR, et al. Early versus delayed decompression for traumatic cervical spinal cord injury: results of the surgical timing in acute spinal cord injury study (STASCIS). PLoS One 2012;7(2): e32037.
26. Burns AS, Lee BS, Ditunno JF Jr, et al. Patient selection for clinical trials: the reliability of the early spinal cord injury examination. J Neurotrauma 2003;20(5): 477–82.
27. Kirshblum S, Snider B, Eren F, et al. Characterizing natural recovery after traumatic spinal cord injury. J Neurotrauma 2021;38(9):1267–84.
28. Punjani N, Deska-Gauthier D, Hachem LD, et al. Neuroplasticity and regeneration after spinal cord injury. N Am Spine Soc J 2023;15(100235):100235.
29. Zhang J, Liu F, Xu J, et al. Automated detection and classification of acute vertebral body fractures using a convolutional neural network on computed tomography. Front Endocrinol 2023;14:1132725.
30. McCoy DB, Dupont SM, Gros C, et al. Convolutional neural network-based automated segmentation of the spinal cord and contusion injury: deep learning biomarker correlates of motor impairment in acute spinal cord injury. AJNR Am J Neuroradiol 2019; 40(4):737–44.
31. Artha WI, Gusti LNA, Kristian Y, et al. A deep learning approach for cervical cord injury severity determination through axial and sagittal magnetic resonance imaging segmentation and classification. Eur Spine J 2024;33(11):4204–13.
32. Dalen V, Vegsgaard OA-S, Jerome C-P, et al. Low diagnostic accuracy and inter-observer agreement on CT and MRI in diagnosis of spinal fractures in multiple myeloma. Hematol Rep 2021; 13(3):9037.
33. Fernandes MB, Valizadeh N, Alabsi HS, et al. Classification of neurologic outcomes from medical notes using natural language processing. Expert Syst Appl 2023;214(119171):119171.
34. Shimizu T, Inomata K, Suda K, et al. A multimodal machine learning model integrating clinical and MRI data for predicting neurological outcomes following surgical treatment for cervical spinal cord injury. Eur Spine J 2025;34(9):3747–55.
35. Bash S, Johnson B, Gibbs W, et al. Deep learning image processing enables 40% faster spinal MR scans which match or exceed quality of standard of care : a prospective multicenter multireader study: a prospective multicenter multireader study. Clin Neuroradiol 2022;32(1):197–203.
36. Yoo H, Yoo R-E, Choi SH, et al. Deep learning-based reconstruction for acceleration of lumbar spine MRI: a prospective comparison with standard MRI. Eur Radiol 2023;33(12):8656–68.
37. Daiki T. Review: noise and artifact reduction for MRI using deep learning. arXiv [eessIV] 2020. https://doi.org/10.48550/arXiv.2002.12889.
38. Naga KE, McGinnis J, Wurm R, et al. Automatic segmentation of spinal cord lesions in MS: a robust

tool for axial T2-weighted MRI scans. Imaging Neurosci (Camb) 2025;3. https://doi.org/10.1162/IMAG.a.45.

39. De Leener B, Lévy S, Dupont SM, et al. SCT: spinal cord toolbox, an open-source software for processing spinal cord MRI data. Neuroimage 2017;145(Pt A):24–43.
40. Karhade AV, Thio Quirina CBS, Ogink Paul T, et al. Development of machine learning algorithms for prediction of 30-day mortality after surgery for spinal metastasis. Neurosurgery 2019;85(1):E83–91.
41. Merali ZG, Witiw CD, Badhiwala JH, et al. Using a machine learning approach to predict outcome after surgery for degenerative cervical myelopathy. PLoS One 2019;14(4):e0215133.
42. Brüningk SC, Bourguignon L, Lukas LP, et al. Prediction of segmental motor outcomes in traumatic spinal cord injury: advances beyond sum scores. Exp Neurol 2024;380(114905):114905.
43. Jaja BNR, Badhiwala J, Guest J, et al. Trajectory-based classification of recovery in sensorimotor complete traumatic cervical spinal cord injury. Neurology 2021;96(22):e2736–48.
44. Badhiwala JH, Wilson JR, Kulkarni AV, et al. A novel method to classify cervical incomplete spinal cord injury based on potential for recovery: a group-based trajectory analysis. J Neurotrauma 2022;39(23–24):1654–64.
45. Zhang Z, Li N, Ding Y, et al. Establishment and validation of a ResNet-based radiomics model for predicting prognosis in cervical spinal cord injury patients. Sci Rep 2025;15(1):9163.
46. Gao CX, Dwyer D, Zhu Y, et al. An overview of clustering methods with guidelines for application in mental health research. Psychiatry Res 2023;327-(115265):115265.
47. Pedro KM, Alvi MA, Hejrati N, et al. Machine learning-based cluster analysis identifies four unique phenotypes of patients with degenerative cervical myelopathy with distinct clinical profiles and long-term functional and neurological outcomes. EBioMedicine 2024;106(105226):105226.
48. Hosseini SM, Borys B, Karimi-Abdolrezaee S. Neural stem cell therapies for spinal cord injury repair: an update on recent preclinical and clinical advances. Brain 2024;147(3):766–93.
49. Kadoya K, Lu P, Nguyen K, et al. Spinal cord reconstitution with homologous neural grafts enables robust corticospinal regeneration. Nat Med 2016;22:479–87. - references - scientific research publishing. Available at: https://www.scirp.org/(S(351jmbntvnsjtlaadkozje))/reference/referencespapers?referenceid=3910132. Accessed April 4, 2026.
50. Ceto S, Sekiguchi KJ, Takashima Y, et al. Neural stem cell grafts form extensive synaptic networks that integrate with host circuits after spinal cord injury. Cell Stem Cell 2020;27(3):430–40. e5.
51. Donnelly DJ, Popovich Phillip G. Inflammation and its role in neuroprotection, axonal regeneration and functional recovery after spinal cord injury. Exp Neurol 2008;209(2):378–88.
52. Smriti M. Paralysed man stands again after receiving “reprogrammed” stem cells. Nature 2025;640(8057):18–9.
53. Martin JR, Cleary D, Abraham ME, et al. Long-term clinical and safety outcomes from a single-site phase 1 study of neural stem cell transplantation for chronic thoracic spinal cord injury. Cell Rep Med 2024;5(12):101841.
54. Abdollahzadeh A, Belevich I, Jokitalo E, et al. Automated 3D axonal morphometry of white matter. Sci Rep 2019;9(1):6084.
55. Rasoolinejad M, Say I, Wu PB, et al. Machine learning predicts improvement of functional outcomes in spinal cord injury patients after inpatient rehabilitation. Front Rehabil Sci 2025;6(1594753):1594753.
56. Bugajska J, Lukas Louis P, Rupp R, et al. Reassessing the role of machine learning in clinical prediction: a benchmark of predicting walking function after spinal cord injury. J Neurotrauma 202508977151251386008. https://doi.org/10.1177/08977151251386008.
57. Prunskis JV, Masys T, Pyles ST, et al. The application of artificial intelligence to enhance spinal cord stimulation efficacy for chronic pain management: current evidence and future directions. Curr Pain Headache Rep 2025;29(1):85.
58. Şerban M, Toader C, Covache-Busuioc RA. Covache-Busuioc Răzvan-Adrian. CRISPR and artificial intelligence in neuroregeneration: closed-loop strategies for precision medicine, spinal cord repair, and adaptive neuro-oncology. Int J Mol Sci 2025;26(19):9409.

Central Cord Syndrome

A Reconsideration from Clinical Phenotype to Mechanism-Based Classification

Joshua I. Chalif, MD, PhD, Emmanuel O. Mensah, MD, Yi Lu, MD, PhD*

KEYWORDS

- Central cord syndrome • Spinal cord injury • Incomplete cervical injury • Structural instability
- Surgical decompression • Hyperextension injury • Cervical spondylosis
- Degenerative cervical myelopathy

KEY POINTS

- Despite being the most common incomplete cervical spinal cord injury, central cord syndrome remains poorly defined, with marked heterogeneity in presentation, management, and prognosis.
- The syndrome is best understood, not as a discrete anatomic lesion, but as a clinical phenotype arising from distinct pathophysiologic mechanisms.
- Management decisions should be driven by structural stability, injury severity, and underlying cord substrate rather than age or traditional textbook definitions.

INTRODUCTION: THE "PROBLEM" WITH CENTRAL CORD SYNDROME

Spinal cord injury (SCI) is a debilitating condition with profound societal, economic, and personal impacts. Globally, as many as 500,000 people suffer from SCI each year, and approximately 15 million people are living with sequalae from SCI.[1,2] The vast majority of clinical SCI is incomplete, leaving some residual white and gray matter intact—though associated disabilities in motor, sensory, and autonomic function continue to severely affect patients, particularly when hand and upper-extremity deficits are present. Among incomplete SCI, central cord syndrome (CCS) is the most commonly applied diagnostic label.[3,4] Despite this, CCS remains surprisingly difficult to define with precision. There is no true consensus regarding its diagnostic criteria.[5–8] Instead, the syndrome is usually characterized by historical or inconsistent definitions that do not fully reflect the heterogeneity seen in modern clinical practice.

Traditionally, CCS has been characterized by disproportionately greater weakness in the upper extremities (UEs) than in the lower extremities (LEs), often in the setting of cervical spondylosis and a hyperextension mechanism.[9–11] Attempts have therefore been made to codify the syndrome using differences in upper extremity motor score (UEMS) and lower extremity motor score (LEMS).[12–14] However, this has introduced somewhat arbitrary thresholds that do not always reliably distinguish CCS from other forms of incomplete cervical SCI.[6,8] Indeed, even incomplete SCI with the same pathophysiological mechanisms might not fulfill the rigid UEMS and LEMS difference. To further complicate the diagnosis, CCS often has significant overlap with other pathophysiological processes, including degenerative cervical myelopathy (DCM) and unstable cervical

Department of Neurosurgery, Mass General Brigham and Harvard Medical School, Boston, MA, USA
* Corresponding author. Department of Neurosurgery, Mass General Brigham 60 Fenwood Road, Boston, MA, 02115.
E-mail address: yilu1945@gmail.com

Neurosurg Clin N Am 37 (2026) 535–544
https://doi.org/10.1016/j.nec.2026.05.004

Abbreviations	
CCS	central cord syndrome
DCM	degenerative cervical myelopathy
OPLL	ossification of the posterior longitudinal ligament
LE	lower extremity
LEMS	Lower extremity motor score
SCI	Spinal cord injury
UE	upper extremity
UEMS	upper extremity motor score

trauma with "central cord" features. As a result, the term "CCS" is used broadly to describe a clinical pattern, even when the underlying anatomy, mechanism of injury, and radiographic findings vary considerably—and even when those factors are vital to the management of patients with CCS.

CCS may therefore be better understood, not as a discrete anatomic lesion, but as a clinical phenotype that arises from distinct pathophysiologic mechanisms. Management should not be driven by traditional textbook definitions, but instead by structural stability, the degree of ongoing cord compression, and the severity of neurologic injury, as these factors most directly determine urgency and ultimate prognosis.

HISTORY: THE EVOLUTION OF CENTRAL CORD SYNDROME PATHOPHYSIOLOGY

Schneider and colleagues originally proposed a pathophysiology model of CCS in 1954.[9] This model—which was expanded in 1958,[10] and ultimately became the classic framework that is still taught today—described CCS as a hyperextension-type cervical injury producing a central intramedullary lesion. The lesion was conceptualized as central cord destruction or hematomyelia, causing disproportionately greater weakness in the UE compared to the LE. The understanding at the time was that the somatotopy of the corticospinal tract was lamellar, such that arm is medial and leg is lateral; the central destruction was thought to disrupt arm more than leg fibers, causing this clinical picture.[15] Therefore, the term "central" implied a distinct anatomic lesion, and the phenotype was viewed as a localizing clue to the underlying pathology.

More recently, however, this model linking the injury site to the clinical phenotype has been substantially weakened by new clinicopathologic and neuroanatomical evidence. MRI imaging has shown that acute traumatic CCS is predominantly a white matter injury.[16] Furthermore, intramedullary hemorrhage is not uniformly or even routinely present.[16,17] Most importantly, CCS does not correlate with selective injury to the central gray matter at the level of hand motor neurons.[17] Surprisingly, high-resolution tract-tracing studies in macaques have also disrupted our understanding of lamellar somatotopy: instead, there appears to be extensive intermingling of arm/hand, shoulder, and leg corticospinal fibers through the craniocervical junction and cervical lateral corticospinal tract.[18–23] This finding directly challenges the somatotopic explanation for arm-predominant weakness proposed by Schneider and colleagues. Additional corticospinal studies have shown dense projections from primary motor cortex to hand and finger motor nuclei, likely reflecting the fine motor control of these muscles in humans.[24] This implies that the UE predominance in CCS more likely reflects the greater corticospinal dependence of dexterous arm and hand function, and resulting damage to these tracts, rather than a selectively injured "medial arm" tract.

In other words, "central" does not necessarily mean central gray injury. The phenotype alone does not localize the pathology.

DEFINITIONS: THE "PROBLEM"

CCS has no consistent definition or consensus diagnostic criteria.[5–7,12] Attempts to formalize the phenotype of UE > LE weakness using quantitative motor scores have also been limited.

Most modern definitions rely on a ≥10 or ≥5 point difference between total UEMS and LEMS.[12,14] However, these thresholds are arbitrary and inconsistently adopted across studies, producing heterogeneous patient cohorts under the same diagnostic label.[4,12–14,25,26] Studies can vary in their inclusion criteria. More importantly, the arithmetical structure of the ASIA motor scoring system creates intrinsic distortions. Total UEMS include intact myotomes above the neurologic level of injury, artificially inflating UE strength and biasing the UE–LE comparison. This effect becomes increasingly problematic in lower cervical injuries, where preserved proximal arm strength makes it mathematically difficult—and, in certain AIS configurations, effectively impossible—to meet both ASIA criteria and a required UEMS–LEMS difference. As a result, the lower the injury level, the greater the disparity required to qualify as "CCS," a gradient that reflects scoring mechanics rather than biology.

Clinical presentation further complicates definition.[12,27] Patients with distal hand-only weakness, mixed myotomal involvement, or predominantly sensory symptoms may share the same anterior–posterior compressive mechanism yet fail quantitative cutoffs. Mild injuries may not even meet a 5 or 10 point threshold, despite clearly fitting the mechanism; more severe incomplete injuries may be excluded because of the distortions noted above or when the injury is from a similar pathophysiological mechanism but is too severe to show a greater than 5 numerical difference in the UEMS and LEMS.[25,27] Overlaps with Brown-Sequard or mixed incomplete patterns further blur syndromic boundaries.[13] To further complicate the clinical presentation, numerous incomplete SCI patients sharing similar mechanisms are often not included in clinical studies due to the inability to meet the rigid UEMS/LEMS score difference.

Radiographically, the ambiguities persist. T2 central cord hyperintensity is common but not universal; hemorrhage is uncommon but may be present; mechanical instability may or may not be present.[16,28] However, instability significantly influences prognosis and management. Grouping stable degenerative hyperextension injuries with fracture-dislocation injuries that seemingly have a "CCS" phenotype under a single label conflates distinct pathophysiologic diseases requiring different therapeutic considerations.

In summary, the current "CCS" lacks a mechanistically grounded definition. It functions primarily as a descriptive phenotype—UE > LE weakness—rather than as an entity anchored in consistent anatomy, biomechanics, or prognosis. This definitional problem has contributed substantially to historical confusion in both clinical management and scientific study.

DISCUSSION: REFRAMING CENTRAL CORD SYNDROME —A MECHANISM-BASED MODEL

A more consistent approach to CCS—and to the classification of incomplete SCI, in general—is to classify these injuries based on the presence or absence of structural instability. Doing so would more directly reflect the underlying pathophysiology, while also clarifying clinical management and prognosis.

Central Incomplete Cervical Spinal Cord Injury with Structural Instability

This subset of CCS includes incomplete cervical injuries associated with fracture, dislocation, or facet subluxation resulting in mechanical instability. The injury mechanism is often high-energy trauma-producing displacement or translation, with cord damage arising from both the initial impact and persistent biomechanical compromise due to instability. Although patients may demonstrate the classic UE > LE phenotype, the defining feature is not motor score disparity but structural failure of the spinal column. Management implications are fundamentally different from so-called "stable CCS" (see further discussion). Regardless of whether the UE–LE motor difference meets a 5 or 10 point threshold, instability mandates early stabilization and likely decompression to prevent further neurologic deterioration and restore structural integrity. Grouping these injuries under the same category as stable hyperextension injuries obscures this critical distinction and has historically contributed to confusion in treatment algorithms.

Central Incomplete Cervical Spinal Cord Injury with Structural Stability

In contrast, this subset of CCS typically occurs in the setting of pre-existing DCM and spinal canal stenosis. Patients are often older and sustain low-energy hyperextension trauma.[29] There is no gross fracture dislocation or mechanical instability; instead, the cord experiences acute anterior–posterior compression superimposed on a chronically narrowed canal. The pathophysiology reflects an acute insult to a chronically hypoperfused or metabolically vulnerable cord.[30,31] Static compression from spondylosis, ligamentous thickening, and osteophytes produces a narrowed reserve space; hyperextension transiently increases anterior–posterior cord compression, and the central portion of the cord gets damaged. Importantly, there is no ongoing mechanical instability after the inciting event—and management in this group is therefore not dictated by instability. The efficacy of surgical decompression is dependent on neurologic severity, radiographic compression, recovery trajectory, and patient comorbidities. Some patients will improve substantially with non-operative management; others will benefit from surgical intervention.

Differentiating Progressive Degenerative Cervical Myelopathy from Central Incomplete Cervical Spinal Cord Injury with Structural Stability

Progressive DCM merits further discussion because it can be difficult to differentiate from central incomplete cervical SCI with structural stability. Progressive DCM is best understood as a form of chronic non-traumatic SCI, arising from chronic static and dynamic compression, microvascular compromise, and cumulative metabolic and axonal stress to the cord.[30–33] In contrast, acute central incomplete cervical SCI with structural stability reflects a traumatic insult to that vulnerable substrate: a low-energy hyperextension trauma or similar event produces abrupt neurologic worsening in a stenotic canal. These entities share important biological features—limited cord reserve, chronic compression, impaired perfusion, and selective vulnerability of hand and upper-extremity function—but they should not be conflated. In practice, the most useful discriminator is symptom chronology: acute-on-chronic injury is marked by a clear inciting event and an abrupt decline over minutes to hours, whereas progressive DCM typically evolves insidiously over weeks to months, sometimes with intermittent plateaus or stepwise worsening. MRI signal change may support cord vulnerability but does not by itself distinguish acute from chronic injury.

Age Is a Surrogate, not a Definition

The traditional bimodal age distribution of CCS reflects the differences in mechanism noted earlier. Younger patients are more likely to sustain high-energy trauma with fracture dislocation and instability. Older patients more commonly have low-energy hyperextension events associated with pre-existing stenosis. Age therefore correlates strongly with injury pattern—but it is the mechanism, not the patient's age, that determines pathophysiology and management. A mechanism-based classification—central incomplete cervical SCI with structural instability or with structural stability—preserves the familiar terminology while resolving longstanding confusion. It aligns classification with biology, clarifies treatment imperatives, and provides a more rational framework for future clinical investigation.

CURRENT EVIDENCE: SURGICAL TIMING—WHAT THE MODERN EVIDENCE ACTUALLY SHOWS

The strongest evidence favoring early decompression comes from broader traumatic SCI cohorts, rather than from studies confined to CCS. STASCIS remains the landmark study most commonly cited in support of surgery within 24 hours: in a heterogeneous cohort of patients with traumatic cervical SCI, early decompression was associated with greater meaningful neurologic improvement compared to delayed surgery.[34] More recent analyses of acute SCI populations have reinforced the same conclusion, suggesting that earlier decompression is associated with improved sensorimotor recovery across traumatic SCI as a whole.[35] However, these studies did not clearly separate patients with fracture dislocation, facet injury, or other forms of structural instability from patients with low-energy hyperextension injury in a stenotic but mechanically stable cervical spine. As a result, they are highly relevant to acute cervical SCI broadly, but only indirectly informative for the dichotomy of CCS presented in this article. The 2017 AO Spine clinical practice guideline did suggest that early decompression be considered in adult patients with traumatic CCS, but the recommendation was weak and the underlying evidence was judged low quality.[36] The guideline did not make a conclusion for CCS patients as a whole; rather, it acknowledged that early surgery is a reasonable option in a syndrome with heterogeneous mechanisms and an imperfect evidence base. In other words, surgical timing should be judged in the context of stability, severity, and ongoing compression.

The most informative modern CCS-specific study is a propensity-matched multicenter analysis by Badhiwala and colleagues, which compared decompression within 24 hours with later surgery in patients diagnosed with CCS. Early surgery was associated with improved UE motor recovery at 1 year, supporting the view that timing may matter within this phenotype.[14] Of note, the benefit was not uniform across neurologic severity. When patients were stratified by AIS grade, the clearest signal favoring early surgery was seen in AIS C injuries, whereas AIS D patients did not demonstrate the same consistent benefit. This suggests that the relevant question is not simply whether a patient has "CCS," but which type of CCS, with what degree of neurologic injury, and on what structural substrate.

Most SCI definitions in the literature stratify patients into AIS C and AIS D, which is unfortunately too crude to identify which patients are most likely to benefit from early decompressive surgery. In practice, the AIS D category contains substantial neurologic heterogeneity in patient presentation and neurologic examination. For example, a patient with very weak UE strength (1/5–2/5) but with preserved LE function likely has a very different prognosis and treatment urgency than a patient with stronger UE strength (eg, 4/5), yet both may be classified as AIS D. This grouping of patients obscures important classification differences that likely have meaningful impacts on the benefit of surgery. This becomes particularly important for patients in the stenosis-dominant population with stability. Ultimately, a more refined motor severity classification would be very helpful for future studies to help determine which patients truly benefit from early surgical decompression.

When patients present with structural instability the literature becomes most consistent. In patients with incomplete cervical SCI and clear mechanical instability—that is, central incomplete SCI with structural instability—the rationale for early decompression and stabilization is both biologically and surgically compelling.

Many surgical series show that early surgical intervention for patients with structural instability improves outcomes.[37–42] In modern surgical practice, structural instability itself drives urgency, regardless of whether the UE >LE pattern satisfies an arbitrary quantitative definition of CCS.

The evidence is much less definitive in stenosis-only injuries without structural instability. In these patients, decompression may still be beneficial—particularly when deficits are severe, compression is substantial, recovery plateaus, or neurologic deterioration continues. But the literature on this subset of SCIs is dominated by retrospective single-center series, heterogeneous diagnostic criteria, variable timing windows, and substantial treatment-selection bias.[41,43–46] Many reports include only surgically treated patients, making it difficult to determine whether early surgery is superior to delayed surgery or to initial conservative management.

Taken together, the modern evidence supports a stratified rather than uniform approach to surgical timing. Early decompression is well supported in acute traumatic SCI broadly and is most compelling in patients with structural instability, persistent cord compression, or more severe incomplete deficits (particularly AIS C patients).[14,34,35] In contrast, for stenosis-dominant injuries without structural instability—many of which fall into AIS D—the case for a universal less than 24 h mandate is much weaker. In that subgroup, the decision to operate and the urgency of surgery should be individualized according to injury severity, degree of radiographic compression, recovery trajectory, and the possibility of acute-on-chronic DCM. Thus, the current literature does not support applying a single timing algorithm to all patients diagnosed with CCS. The timing of surgical intervention should depend on injury mechanism and severity, rather than on the application of a uniform standard across a heterogeneous phenotype.

RECOMMENDATIONS: PRACTICAL MANAGEMENT FRAMEWORK

A practical management algorithm for patients presenting with CCS should begin with the variable that most clearly changes both pathophysiology and urgency: structural stability.

Step 1: Determine whether there is fracture dislocation, facet subluxation, translation, or other evidence of mechanical instability. If instability is present, the patient should be managed as an incomplete cervical SCI with structural instability, and early decompression with stabilization is indicated regardless of whether the UE > LE pattern satisfies a formal CCS definition.

Step 2: If the spine is structurally stable, assess neurologic severity. Patients with AIS C or worse, substantial hand dysfunction, or marked radiographic compression are the subset for whom the rationale and available evidence for early decompression are strongest. By contrast, mild AIS D patients without instability should not be subjected to a reflexive less than 24 h rule, as the evidence for uniform urgency in this population is considerably weaker than in broader traumatic SCI cohorts or unstable injuries. Patients with severe AIS D might also benefit from early surgery; however, further studies are needed to confirm that.

Step 3: Monitor neurologic trajectory. For patients with a stable spine who do not undergo urgent surgical decompression and are instead observed conservatively, progressive deficit, failure of early improvement, or persistent disabling weakness in the setting of compressive pathology should shift management toward surgery. On the other hand, neurologically stable patients with mild impairments may reasonably continue to undergo close observation and rehabilitation.

Step 4: Continue follow up. For patients that are initially determined to undergo observation and rehabilitation, a close follow up is still needed. Patient with myelopathic symptoms with DCM, chronic T2 signal change, or multilevel stenosis will likely need elective surgical decompression to prevent future neurologic function decline.

ILLUSTRATIVE CASE: SEVERE CENTRAL INCOMPLETE CERVICAL SPINAL CORD INJURY WITH STRUCTURAL STABILITY

A man in his late 50s presented after a low-energy fall down several stairs. Extremity examination showed full bilateral shoulder abduction and elbow flexion strength, bilateral elbow extension 3/4- (right/left), hand grip 1/2, hip flexion 1/2, knee extension 1/2, knee flexion 1/2, ankle dorsiflexion 1/2, and plantarflexion 1/2, with sensation intact to light touch. MRI and computed tomographic scans demonstrated severe C3–C5 cord compression with underlying ossification of the posterior longitudinal ligament (OPLL) (**Fig. 1**A,B). Although the clinical presentation was consistent with an acute central cord-type injury superimposed on a chronically stenotic cervical canal, the severity of his LE weakness meant that he

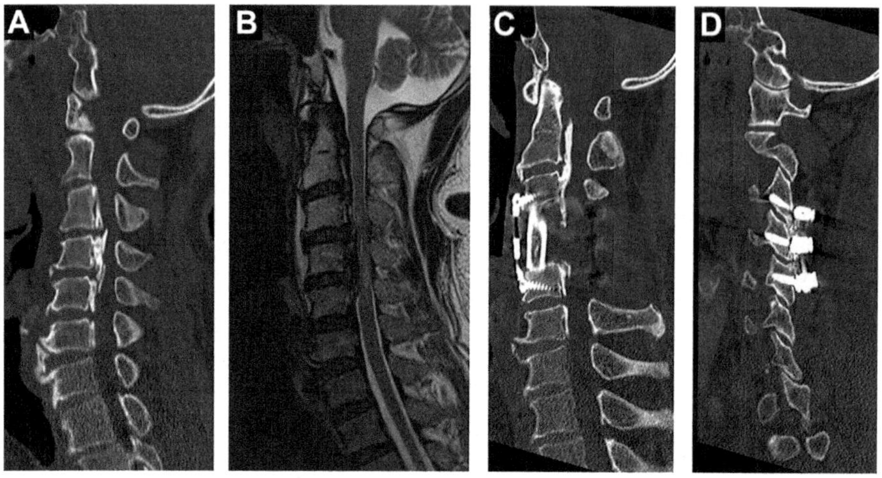

Fig. 1. Severe central incomplete cervical spinal cord injury with structural stability in the setting of OPLL. (*A*) Preoperative sagittal CT from a man in his late 50s who sustained a severe incomplete cervical SCI after a low-energy fall demonstrates multilevel cervical spondylosis with continuous ossification of the posterior longitudinal ligament, most severe from C3–C5. (*B*) Preoperative sagittal T2-weighted MRI shows severe cervical canal stenosis and cord compression at C3–C5 with intramedullary T2 signal change consistent with acute cord contusion/edema. (*C*) Postoperative sagittal CT following C4 corpectomy and C3–C5 anterior fusion demonstrates adequate anterior decompression and reconstruction. (*D*) Postoperative parasagittal CT demonstrates posterior C3–C5 instrumentation following staged posterior decompression and fusion.

would not satisfy traditional or quantitative definitions of CCS based on disproportionate upper versus lower extremity motor impairment.

Given the combination of severe neurologic deficit, marked ongoing cord compression, and his underlying OPLL he underwent staged circumferential decompression and stabilization. The first stage consisted of C4 corpectomy with C3–C5 anterior fusion to address the dominant ventral compression from OPLL (**Fig. 1**C), with the second stage a C3–C5 posterior laminectomy and (**Fig. 1**D). At follow-up, he regained strength with substantial left-sided strength (4+ or 5 throughout), but continued to have residual right-sided weakness with wrist extension 1/5, finger flexion 1/5, hand intrinsic strength 1/5, hip flexion 3/5, knee extension 3/5, ankle dorsiflexion 2/5, and plantarflexion 1/5.

This case highlights why CCS is better understood as a mechanism-based phenotype rather than a rigid motor-score diagnosis. Mechanistically, the injury fits the category of central incomplete cervical SCI with structural stability: an acute traumatic insult to a chronically compressed, vulnerable cord in the setting of OPLL. Yet phenotypically, the patient's severe bilateral LE involvement would exclude him from many traditional CCS definitions. The case therefore illustrates one of the central controversies in CCS classification: severe injuries may fail to appear "central" by arithmetical UE–LE motor-score criteria precisely because the cord injury is extensive. Management in such patients should be driven by structural stability, neurologic severity, and persistent compression—not by whether the presentation satisfies an arbitrary quantitative definition of CCS.

ILLUSTRATIVE CASE PAIR: HETEROGENEITY WITHIN AIS D CENTRAL CORD SYNDROME

Two patients with central cord-type presentations illustrate the limitations of using AIS grade alone to classify or study CCS. The first is a man in his late 70s who presented after a fall. His initial examination demonstrated profound UE weakness, with 3/5 biceps strength bilaterally and 0/5 strength in all other UE motor functions, while both LEs remained approximately 4+/5 throughout, with preserved sensation. CT did not demonstrate fracture or gross instability, but MRI showed severe C3–C4 cervical stenosis with cord signal change (**Fig. 2**A). Although this patient would still be classified as AIS D because of preserved LE motor strength, given his severe clinical presentation, he underwent urgent C3–C4 anterior cervical discectomy and fusion for decompression and stabilization.

In contrast, the second patient is a man in his early 80s who presented 2 weeks after a fall with stable mild bilateral hand numbness, mild clumsiness, and only trace intrinsic hand weakness with 4+/5 interosseous strength bilaterally,

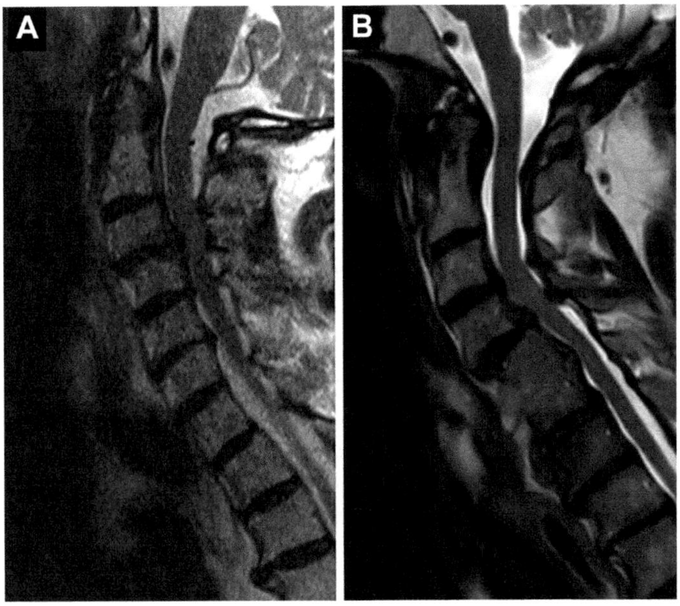

Fig. 2. Clinical heterogeneity within AIS D central cord syndrome. (*A*) Sagittal T2-weighted cervical MRI from a patient with severe AIS D injury demonstrating marked C3–C4 stenosis with cord compression and intramedullary T2 signal change. (*B*) Sagittal T2-weighted cervical MRI from a patient with mild AIS D injury demonstrating C4–C5 degenerative stenosis with focal intramedullary T2 signal change.

but otherwise preserved strength throughout. MRI demonstrated C4–C5 cord signal change in the setting of degenerative cervical disease, including an autofused C5–C6 segment and C4–C5 anterolisthesis (**Fig. 2**B). He ultimately underwent C4–C5 ACDF, but the clinical context was fundamentally different: this was a mild, stable AIS D presentation with limited hand dysfunction and no evidence of rapid deterioration, which prompted non-urgent intervention.

These cases demonstrate why AIS D is too broad a category for CCS classification. Both patients would be grouped together as motor-incomplete AIS D injuries, yet they represent very different clinical severities. The first patient had a severe injury with near-complete loss of UE function providing strong rationale for urgent decompression. The second had a mild, stable hand-predominant syndrome in which decompression was reasonable but not driven by the same degree of neurologic urgency. These cases illustrate the fundamental limitations using traditional AIS classifications to study CCS patients. Patients with CCS tend to have stronger LE strength meaning the traditional AIS classification can underestimate the severity of the SCI in certain patients. Grouping these patients together as AIS D obscures the relationship between injury severity, treatment timing, and outcome. Future studies of CCS should therefore subdivide AIS D patients by more refined motor severity classification, rather than treating AIS D as a uniform prognostic or therapeutic category.

SUMMARY: SHOULD CENTRAL CORD SYNDROME BE RECLASSIFIED?

The central conclusion of this review is that CCS should no longer be treated as a single, mechanistically coherent diagnosis. Rather, it is better understood as a clinical phenotype—typically, but not uniformly, UE-predominant weakness—produced by distinct anatomic and biomechanical substrates. Patients grouped under the CCS label span fundamentally different pathophysiological states, from unstable fracture dislocation injuries to stable stenosis-dominant acute-on-chronic cord injuries. In addition, the classic somatotopic explanation is difficult to sustain given modern neuroscientific evidence, and the quantitative motor-score definitions are distorted by ASIA scoring mechanics. The literature has therefore confounded different disease entities, making prognosis and management of CCS difficult. The problem is that phenotype-based labeling of CCS has obscured the variables of greatest clinical significance.

A more useful framework is mechanism-based: central incomplete cervical SCI with structural instability versus central incomplete cervical SCI with structural stability (**Fig. 3**). This distinction better captures the true therapeutic divide. Structural instability is the clearest discriminator of surgical urgency. In addition, neurologic severity, particularly AIS C and severe AIS D versus mild AIS D, informs the expected benefit of early decompression. The modern timing literature

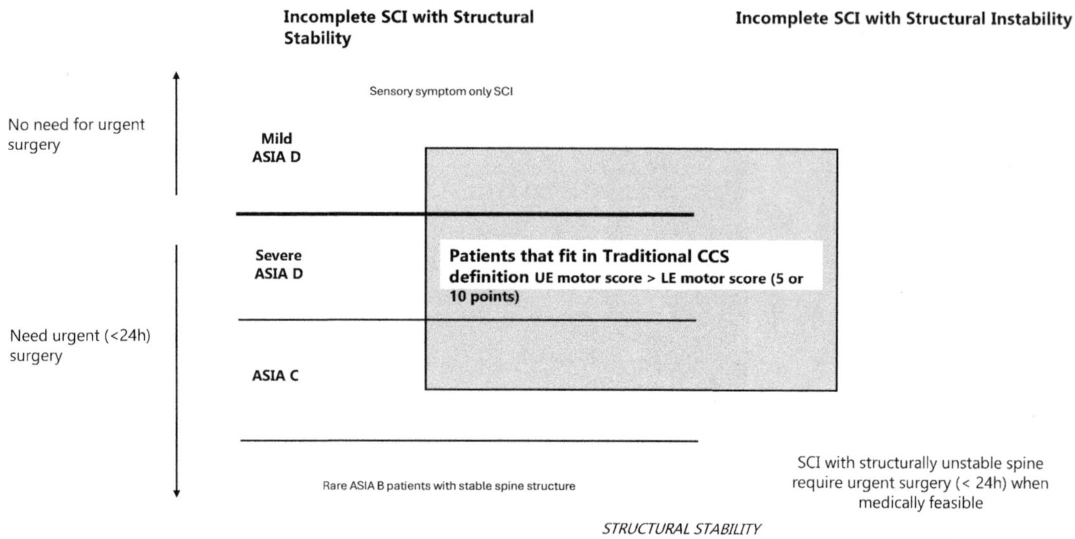

Fig. 3. Mechanism-based framework for central cord-type incomplete cervical spinal cord injury. Proposed classification emphasizing structural stability and neurologic severity to guide treatment urgency rather than traditional central cord syndrome definitions based only on upper extremity versus lower extremity motor score differences. Patients with incomplete cervical SCI and structural instability generally require urgent decompression and stabilization when medically feasible, regardless of neurologic severity. Among patients with structurally stable injuries, treatment urgency should be stratified by severity: AIS C and severe AIS D injuries with significant motor impairment and ongoing compression should be considered for urgent decompression, whereas mild AIS D injuries or sensory-predominant presentations might have a favorable recovery trajectory and might not need urgent decompression. Instead, they should managed more selectively according to neurologic trajectory, radiographic compression, comorbidities, and recovery. Traditional CCS definitions capture only a subset of patients with similar injury mechanisms and do not take structural stability into consideration.

supports this stratified view: early surgery is most compelling in unstable lesions and more severe incomplete injuries, but much less definitive in mild, stenosis-only stable cases. Future studies should therefore stratify patients by instability, neurologic severity (particularly within AIS D group), radiographic compression, chronic cord substrate, and recovery trajectory rather than by phenotype alone.

CLINICS CARE POINTS

- Patient with incomplete cervical spinal cord injury with structual instability should receive urgent surgery for decompression and stabilization when medically feasible.
- Patient with severe (ASIA C or severe ASIA D) incomplete spinal cord injury with structual stability could benefit from early surgical decompression.
- Patient with mild (mild ASIA D) incomplete spinal cord injury with structual stability could be initially observed. Elective surgery could be considered with persistent symptoms or with underlying cervical myelopathy.

DISCLOSURES

The authors have nothing to disclose.

REFERENCES

1. GBD 2016. Traumatic Brain Injury and Spinal Cord Injury Collaborators. Global, regional, and national burden of traumatic brain injury and spinal cord injury, 1990-2016: a systematic analysis for the Global Burden of Disease Study 2016. Lancet Neurol 2019;18(1):56–87.
2. Singh A, Tetreault L, Kalsi-Ryan S, et al. Global prevalence and incidence of traumatic spinal cord injury. Clin Epidemiol 2014;6:309–31.
3. Bosch A, Stauffer E, Nickel VL. Incomplete traumatic quadriplegia: a ten-year review. JAMA 1971;216: 473–8.
4. Engel-Haber E, Botticello A, Snider B, et al. Incomplete spinal cord syndromes: current incidence and Quantifiable criteria for classification. J Neurotrauma 2022;39:1687–96.
5. Avila MJ, Hurlbert RJ. Central cord syndrome Redefined. Neurosurg Clin 2021;32:353–63.
6. Smith É. Is it time to redefine or rename the term "Central Cord Syndrome". Spinal Cord 2021;59:935–6.

7. Badhiwala JH, Wilson JR, Fehlings MG. The case for revisiting central cord syndrome. Spinal Cord 2020; 58:125–7.
8. Engel-Haber E, Snider B, Kirshblum S. Central Cord Syndrome definitions, variables, and limitations. Spinal Cord 2023;61:579–86.
9. Schneider RC, Cherry G, Pantek H. The syndrome of acute central cervical spinal cord injury; with special reference to the mechanisms involved in hyperextension injuries of cervical spine. J Neurosurg 1954;11(6):546–77.
10. Schneider RC, Thompson JM, Bebin J. The syndrome of acute central cervical spinal cord injury. J Neurol Neurosurg Psychiatry 1958;21(3):216–27.
11. Charles A, Andrade K, Owolo E, et al. Central Cord Syndrome: mechanisms, clinical presentation, and management strategies. Seminars in Spine Surgery 2024;36(2).
12. Van Middendorp JJ, Pouw MH, Hayes KC, et al. Diagnostic criteria of traumatic central cord syndrome. Part 2: a questionnaire survey among spine specialists. Spinal Cord 2010;48:657–63.
13. Wirz M, Zörner B, Rupp R, et al. Outcome after incomplete spinal cord injury: central cord versus Brown-Sequard syndrome. Spinal Cord 2010;48:407–14.
14. Badhiwala JH, Wilson JR, Harrop JS, et al. Early vs late surgical decompression for central cord syndrome. JAMA Surg 2022;157:1024–32.
15. Shakil H, Santaguida C, Wilson JR, et al. Pathophysiology and surgical decision-making in central cord syndrome and degenerative cervical myelopathy: correcting the somatotopic fallacy. Front Neurol 2023;14:1276399.
16. Quencer RM, Bunge RP, Egnor M, et al. Acute traumatic central cord syndrome: MRI-pathological correlations. Neuroradiology 1992;34(2):85–94.
17. Collignon F, Martin D, Lénelle J, et al. Acute traumatic central cord syndrome: magnetic resonance imaging and clinical observations. J Neurosurg 2002;96(1 Suppl):29–33.
18. Morecraft RJ, Stilwell-Morecraft KS, Ge J, et al. Lack of somatotopy among corticospinal tract fibers passing through the primate craniovertebral junction and cervical spinal cord: pathoanatomical substrate of central cord syndrome and cruciate paralysis. J Neurosurg Published online October 2021;8.
19. Levi AD, Schwab JM A. Critical reappraisal of corticospinal tract somatotopy and its role in traumatic cervical spinal cord syndromes. J Neurosurg Spine 2022;36:653–9.
20. Morecraft RJ, Ge J, Stilwell-Morecraft KS, et al. Terminal distribution of the corticospinal projection from the hand/arm region of the primary motor cortex to the cervical enlargement in rhesus monkey. J Comparat Neurol 2013;521:4205–35.
21. Rosenzweig ES, Brock JH, Culbertson MD, et al. Extensive spinal decussation and bilateral termination of cervical corticospinal projections in rhesus monkeys. J Comparat Neurol 2009;513:151–63.
22. Soderblom C, Lee D-H, Dawood A, et al. 3d imaging of axons in transparent spinal cords from rodents and nonhuman primates1,2,3. Eneuro 2015; 2:2015.
23. Lemon RN, Griffiths J. Comparing the function of the corticospinal system in different species: organizational differences for motor specialization? Muscle Nerve 2005;32:261–79.
24. Maier MA, Armand J, Kirkwood PA, et al. Differences in the corticospinal projection from primary motor cortex and supplementary motor area to macaque upper limb motoneurons: an anatomical and electrophysiological study. Cereb Cortex 2002; 12(3):281–96.
25. Pouw MH, Van Middendorp JJ, Van Kampen A, et al. Diagnostic criteria of traumatic central cord syndrome. Part 3: descriptive analyses of neurological and functional outcomes in a prospective cohort of traumatic motor incomplete tetraplegics. Spinal Cord 2011;49:614–22.
26. Hayes KC, Hsieh JT, Wolfe DL, et al. Classifying incomplete spinal cord injury syndromes: algorithms based on the International standards for neurological and functional classification of spinal cord injury patients. Arch Phys Med Rehabil 2000;81:644–52.
27. Engel-Haber E, Snider B, Botticello A, et al. Clinical subsets of central cord syndrome: is it a distinct entity from other forms of incomplete tetraplegia for research? J Neurotrauma 2024;41(17–18):2133–45.
28. Song J, Mizuno J, Inoue T, et al. Clinical evaluation of traumatic central cord syndrome: emphasis on clinical significance of prevertebral hyperintensity, cord compression, and intramedullary high-signal intensity on magnetic resonance imaging. Surg Neurol 2006;65(2):117–23.
29. Aarabi B, Koltz M, Ibrahimi D. Hyperextension cervical spine injuries and traumatic central cord syndrome. Neurosurg Focus 2008;25(5):E9.
30. Akter F, Yu X, Qin X, et al. The pathophysiology of degenerative cervical myelopathy and the Physiology of recovery following decompression. Front Neurosci 2020;14:138.
31. Gooding MR, Wilson CB, Hoff JT. Experimental cervical myelopathy. Effects of ischemia and compression of the canine cervical spinal cord. J Neurosurg 1975;43(1):9–17.
32. Karadimas SK, Erwin WM, Ely CG, et al. Pathophysiology and Natural history of cervical Spondylotic myelopathy. Spine 2013;38(22 Suppl 1):S21–36.
33. Lebret A, Lévy S, Pfender N, et al. Investigation of perfusion impairment in degenerative cervical myelopathy beyond the site of cord compression. Sci Rep 2023;13(1):22660.
34. Fehlings MG, Vacarro A, Wilson J, et al. Early versus delayed decompression for traumatic cervical spinal

cord injury: results of the STASCIS. PLOS One 2012; 7(2):e32037.
35. Badhiwala JH, Wilson J, Witiw C, et al. The influence of timing of surgical decompression for acute spinal cord injury: a pooled analysis of individual patient data. The Lancet Neurology 2021;20(2):117–26.
36. Fehlings MG, Tetreault LA, Aarabi B, et al. A clinical practice guideline for the management of patients with acute spinal cord injury and central cord syndrome: recommendations on the timing of decompressive surgery. Global Spine Journal 2017;7(3 Suppl):195S–202S.
37. Guest J, Eleraky M, Apostolides P, et al. Traumatic central cord syndrome: results of surgical management. Journal of Neurosurgery 2002;97(1 Suppl):25–32.
38. Pollard ME, Apple DF. Factors associated with improved neurologic outcomes in patients with incomplete tetraplegia. Spine 2003;28:33–9.
39. Bose B, Northrup BE, Osterholm JL, et al. Reanalysis of central cervical cord injury management. Neurosurgery 1984;15:367–72.
40. Jug M, Kejžar N, Vesel M, et al. Neurological recovery after traumatic cervical spinal cord injury is superior if surgical decompression and instrumented fusion are performed within 8 hours versus 8 to 24 hours after injury: a single center experience. J Neurotrauma 2015;32:1385–92.
41. Yelamarthy PKK, Chhabra HS, Vaccaro A, et al. Management and prognosis of acute traumatic cervical central cord syndrome: systematic review and Spinal Cord Society-Spine Trauma Study Group position statement. Eur Spine J 2019;28:2390–407.
42. Divi S, Schroeder G, Oner F, et al. Management of acute traumatic central cord syndrome: a narrative review. Global Spine Journal 2019;9(1 Suppl): 89S–97S.
43. Aarabi B, Alexander M, Mirvis S, et al. Predictors of outcome in acute traumatic central cord syndrome due to spinal stenosis. Journal of Neurosurgery: Spine 2011;14(1):122–30.
44. Pouw MH, van Middendorp JJ, van Kampen A, et al. Diagnostic criteria of traumatic central cord syndrome. Part 1: a systematic review of clinical descriptors and scores. Spinal Cord 2010;48.
45. Wilson JR, Tetreault LA, Kwon BK, et al. Timing of decompression in patients with acute spinal cord injury: a systematic review. Global Spine J 2017; 7(3 Suppl):95S–115S.
46. Badhiwala JH, Witiw CD, Wilson JR, et al. Treatment of acute traumatic central cord syndrome: a study of North American trauma centers. Neurosurgery 2024; 94(4):700–10.

Management of Mild Degenerative Cervical Myelopathy

Current Evidence and Emerging Directions

Niccolò Innocenti, MD[a], Edoardo Maria Barbieri, MD[b], Octavian Vatavu, MD[b], Luca Mattioli, MD[b], Elio Mazzapicchi, MD[b], Francesco Costa, MD[a,b,*]

KEYWORDS

- Spinal cord compression • Degenerative cervical myelopathy • Mild myelopathy
- Spondylotic myelopathy • Surgical treatment

KEY POINTS

- Mild degenerative cervical myelopathy (DCM) often presents with subtle symptoms (eg, hand clumsiness and gait imbalance), requiring careful clinical assessment to avoid delayed diagnosis.
- Management of DCM may be conservative and surgical: both approaches are valid. Surgery can prevent progression, while selected stable patients may undergo supervised nonoperative management.
- Patients managed conservatively need regular neurologic and imaging follow-up to detect early deterioration. Worsening symptoms or functional decline should prompt transition to surgical decompression.
- Management should consider patient age, comorbidities, symptom severity, and individual preferences.

INTRODUCTION

Degenerative cervical myelopathy (DCM) is the leading cause of nontraumatic spinal cord dysfunction in adults and is increasingly common with population aging.[1,2] Mild DCM represents the earliest clinically apparent stage of a progressive spinal cord disorder arising from age-related degenerative changes in the cervical spine. These changes—including intervertebral disc degeneration, osteophyte formation, facet joint arthropathy, and ligamentous hypertrophy—contribute to progressive narrowing of the spinal canal and chronic mechanical compression of the cervical spinal cord. In this initial phase, neurologic impairment is often subtle and may manifest as reduced manual dexterity, intermittent sensory disturbances in the upper limbs, or mild gait instability, frequently without significant functional limitation. As a result, mild DCM can be easily overlooked despite its potential for progression.

Central to the definition and clinical characterization of mild DCM is the modified Japanese Orthopaedic Association (mJOA) scoring system, which provides a standardized and reproducible measure of disease severity (**Table 1**). The mJOA scale evaluates upper and lower extremity motor function, sensory deficits, and sphincter control, yielding a total score ranging from 0 to 18. Within this framework, mild DCM is defined by a score of 15 to 17, distinguishing it from moderate (12–14) and severe ($\leq$11) disease. This classification

[a] Spine Neurosurgery Unit, Department of Neurosurgery, Fondazione IRCCS Istituto Neurologico Carlo Besta, Via Giovanni Celoria 11, 20133, Milan, Italy; [b] University of Milan, Milan, Italy
* Corresponding author.
E-mail address: francesco.costa@istituto-besta.it

Neurosurg Clin N Am 37 (2026) 545–553
https://doi.org/10.1016/j.nec.2026.05.005

Abbreviations	
CSS	Cervical Surgical score
DCM	degenerative cervical myelopathy
GCSF	franulocyte colony-stimulating factor
mJOA	modified Japanese Orthopaedic Association
MT	magnetization transfer
NMSCC	nonmyelopathic spinal cord compression
OPLL	ossification of the posterior longitudinal ligament

is not merely descriptive but carries important clinical implications, as it informs both prognosis and management strategies. Patients classified as having mild DCM typically retain a high degree of functional independence; however, a proportion will experience neurologic decline over time. Consequently, accurate identification and stratification using the mJOA system are essential for guiding clinical decision-making, structuring follow-up, and determining the optimal timing for potential intervention.

EPIDEMIOLOGY

DCM is now framed as a chronic, age-linked spinal cord injury rather than a rare neurosurgical curiosity. Degeneration of discs, facet joints and ligaments gradually narrows the cervical canal, producing cord compression—and eventually—myelopathy in a subset of people.[1,3] This process accelerates with aging, so the burden of DCM is rising in parallel with demographic shifts.

Epidemiologically, there are 2 very different pictures. Hospital and surgical series suggest a relatively uncommon disease: in England and North America, hospitalization or surgically treated DCM sits around 4 to 8 per 100,000 person/years (incidence) and ≥60 per 100,000 in prevalence, with rates increasing over the last decade.[3–5] Men and people in their 50s to 70s predominate, and socioeconomic deprivation appears to increase risk, while Asian ethnicity is associated with lower odds of DCM among those with cervical spondylosis.[3,5,6]

MRI-based population work, however, reveals a much larger reservoir of disease. Cross-sectional meta-analysis finds degenerative spinal cord compression in ~24% of apparently healthy adults, rising to ~35% over 60, and clinical DCM in about 2% to 3%.[7] UK modeling that combines these data with hospital statistics estimates a *true* DCM prevalence around 2% overall and greater than 4% in the oldest age groups, compared with only 0.2% to 0.4% actually diagnosed, implying that most cases—especially mild, elderly presentations—never reach specialist care.[5,7–9]

People with mild DCM often present with nonspecific complaints—subtle hand clumsiness, difficulty with fine motor tasks, unsteadiness,

Table 1
Modified Japanese Orthopaedic Association score

	Score
I. Motor dysfunction score of the upper extremities	
Inability to move hands	0
Inability to eat with a spoon but able to move hands	1
Inability to button shirt but able to eat with a spoon	2
Able to button shirt with great difficulty	3
Able to button shirt with slight difficulty	4
No dysfunction	5
II. Motor dysfunction of the lower extremities	
Complete loss of motor and sensory function	0
Sensory preservation without ability to move legs	1
Able to move legs but unable to walk	2
Able to walk on flat floor with a walking aid (ie, cane or crutch)	3
Able to walk up and/or down stairs with hand rail	4
Moderate to significant lack of stability but able to walk up and/or down stairs without hand rail	5
Mild lack of stability but walk unaided with smooth reciprocation	6
No dysfunction	7
III. Sensation	
Complete loss of hand sensation	0
Severe sensory loss or pain	1
Mild sensory loss	2
No sensory loss	3
IV. Sphincter dysfunction	
Inability to urinate voluntarily	0
Marked difficulty with micturition	1
Mild to moderate difficulty with micturition	2
Normal micturition	3
Mild myelopathy	mJOA from 15 to 17
Moderate myelopathy	mJOA from 12 to 14
Severe myelopathy	mJOA from 0 to 11

increased falls, sleep disturbance—readily attributed to normal aging or peripheral joint disease[10,11] Primary care clinicians may not routinely look for myelopathic signs (eg, Hoffmann's and impaired tandem gait), delaying recognition. Epidemiologically, this means mild DCM is systematically underascertained.

DCM can be viewed as the clinical tip of a large iceberg of cervical degeneration and spinal cord compression. Imaging shows that structural risk is widespread in older adults; yet only a fraction develop overt myelopathy, and only a fraction of those receive a diagnosis. Aging populations, male sex, socioeconomic deprivation, and perhaps certain occupational exposures all contribute to increasing. The epidemiology of mild DCM is therefore best understood in terms of under-recognition: a common, progressive neurologic condition frequently mislabeled as *just getting old*, with important implications for early detection, counseling, and timely referral to spine services.[1,8,10,11]

DEFINITION AND NATURAL HISTORY OF MILD DEGENERATIVE CERVICAL MYELOPATHY

Clinical presentation ranges from subtle hand clumsiness and paresthesia to gait disturbance and sphincter dysfunction.[2,12] Mild DCM denotes symptomatic cord compression with limited functional impairment, usually quantified by mJOA 15 to 17.[13–15]

Natural history data show that DCM is generally progressive, but with marked variability. In symptomatic patients treated nonoperatively, 20% to 62% deteriorate neurologically over 3 to 6 years[8] and a small but real proportion suffer superimposed traumatic cord injury with resulting severe disability.[8,16] At the same time, most subjects with asymptomatic compression never progress, highlighting a difficult boundary between common age-related imaging findings and clinically important myelopathy.

For mild DCM specifically, some patients remain stable for long periods, whereas others experience stepwise decline.[8,15] A recent large prospective cohort of 140 patients with mild DCM initially managed conservatively found that at 1 year, mean mJOA remained essentially unchanged, with clinically meaningful deterioration ($\geq$2 point mJOA drop) in 13.3% and conversion to surgery in 12.1% over a mean of 3.4 years.[17] These data suggest that short to midterm stability is common, but a nontrivial minority deteriorates.

Asymptomatic or minimally symptomatic spinal cord compression (nonmyelopathic spinal cord compression [NMSCC]) is frequent: population estimates suggest prevalence around 24% in healthy individuals and over 35% in those greater than 60 years.[8] Among NMSCC patients, clinical radiculopathy and/or electrophysiological evidence of cord dysfunction markedly increases the risk of progressing to myelopathy.[8] Similarly, radiographic progression of incidental ossification of the posterior longitudinal ligament (OPLL) is common, and myelopathy develops in up to 61.5% over long-term follow-up in some series.

This poses a specific management dilemma because its natural history is heterogeneous and the risk–benefit balance of early surgery versus structured nonoperative care is less clear than in moderate–severe disease[13–15]

PATHOPHYSIOLOGY AND IMAGING CORRELATES RELEVANT TO MILD DISEASE

DCM encompasses cervical spondylotic myelopathy, OPLL, ligamentum flavum hypertrophy and other age-related degenerative processes that narrow the cervical canal and chronically compress the cord.[1,2,13] Pathogenesis reflects both static factors (degenerative stenosis, OPLL, osteophytes, disc herniation, and kyphotic deformity) and dynamic factors (abnormal motion, segmental instability, and repetitive shear) causing ischemia, demyelination, neuronal loss, and gliosis within the cord.[1,2,13] Even in mild DCM, histopathological injury may be substantial, which underpins the argument for timely decompression.

Conventional MRI demonstrates canal narrowing and cord signal change (**Fig. 1**). T2 hyperintensity and T1 hypointensity correlate with more advanced pathology and poorer surgical outcomes.[1,18] Recent AO Spine clinical practice recommendations highlight the prognostic value of diffusion-weighted and quantitative microstructural MRI, including diffusion tensor imaging and magnetization transfer (MT) imaging, which better quantify myelin and axonal integrity.[1,18]

A 2025 prospective study using advanced quantitative MRI (qMRI) in 49 patients with mild DCM followed for up to 2 years found neurologic deterioration in 38% of 6 month intervals; machine-learning models combining clinical and qMRI metrics predicted deterioration with 83% balanced accuracy (AUC 0.87).[19] Reduced MT ratio (indicative of demyelination) in dorsal and ventral funiculi above the maximal compression level, together with sensory deficits and gait imbalance, strongly predicted decline and may justify earlier surgery. These data support the concept that *mild* by mJOA may conceal substantial structural injury.

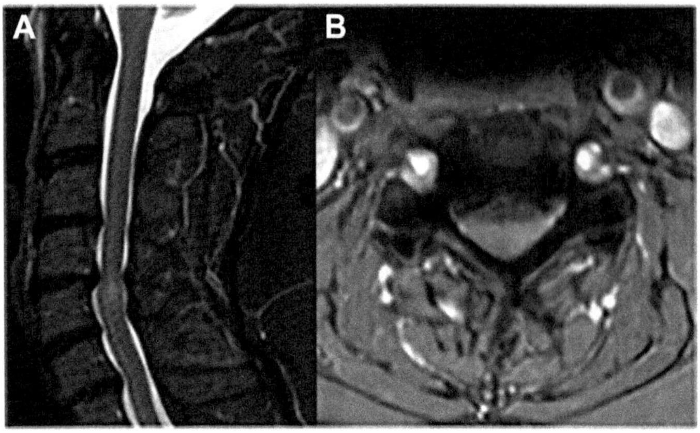

Fig. 1. Sagittal (*A*) and axial (*B*) T2-weighted MRI images showing a case of DCM.

CLINICAL GUIDELINES AND OVERALL MANAGEMENT FRAMEWORK

The 2017 AO Spine/Cervical Spine Research Society guideline remains the cornerstone for DCM management across severity grades.[14] Key recommendations relevant to mild DCM are the following:

- *Moderate–severe DCM (mJOA ≤14):* strong recommendation for surgical decompression.[1,2,14]
- *Mild DCM (mJOA 15–17):* suggest offering either of the following:
  - Immediate surgical decompression, or
  - A supervised trial of structured rehabilitation, with close follow-up; surgery is recommended if neurologic deterioration occurs and suggested if there is failure to improve.[14,18,20]
- *NMSCC without radiculopathy:* no prophylactic surgery; counsel about risk, educate regarding symptoms and follow clinically.
- *NMSCC with clinical radiculopathy:* either surgery or close observation/structured rehab; if myelopathy develops, manage as above.

Subsequent narrative reviews and consensus efforts (eg, RECODEDCM) broadly support this framework while emphasizing that current evidence for optimal management of mild disease is weak and practice is heterogeneous.[13,15,21–23] An international survey of 699 spine surgeons showed that most provide outpatient follow-up for mild DCM and asymptomatic cord compression, typically at 6 month intervals, but there is wide variation in imaging, functional assessments and thresholds for recommending surgery.[15] This highlights the need for standardized surveillance protocols and better prognostic tools.

MANAGEMENT OF MILD DEGENERATIVE CERVICAL MYELOPATHY

Conservative Management

Conservative management is typically reserved for the following categories:

- Mild DCM (mJOA ≥15) with nonprogressive or minimally progressive symptoms.
- Patients with significant comorbidities or surgical contraindications.
- Patients who decline surgery after counseling.

Nonoperative care includes supervised physical therapy, activity modification, cervical traction, and short-term use of collars, largely for symptomatic relief rather than disease modification.[12,24,25] Observational data suggest that patients with the following features may fare better with conservative treatment: early presentation (<1 year of symptoms), single level soft disc herniation rather than multilevel spondylosis, absence of circumferential cord compression on MRI, and preserved cervical lordosis.[24] However, evidence quality is low and no robust prediction rules exist.[8,23]

In the recent cohort of conservatively managed mild DCM, global function remained stable at 1 year, with modest improvements in quality of life and neck/arm pain, but 13.3% deteriorated neurologically and 12.1% eventually underwent delayed surgery with subsequent pain improvement.[17] This supports conservative care as an option, contingent on structured follow-up and rapid access to surgery if deterioration occurs.

Patients should be explicitly counseled that DCM is usually progressive, that deterioration may be stepwise, and that mild DCM carries an elevated risk of acute spinal cord injury after minor trauma compared with the general population. Recommendations usually include avoidance of high-risk activities (contact sports, extreme neck extension/

flexion) and prompt evaluation for any new weakness, gait change or sphincter disturbance.

- *Physiotherapy and exercise:* programs focusing on neck and scapular strengthening, posture, and balance may improve pain and function, but there is limited evidence they alter neurologic progression. There is also uncertainty about the safety of high velocity cervical manipulation; most experts discourage it in DCM.
- *Traction and collars:* intermittent traction or temporary immobilization may alleviate radicular pain, but long-term collars risk deconditioning and are not recommended as a primary DCM treatment.
- *Analgesics and symptomatic drugs:* nonsteroidal anti-inflammatory drugs (NSAIDs), neuropathic pain agents, and muscle relaxants are widely used for neck and radicular pain, but their effect on myelopathy specific deficits is unproven.

Surgical Management

Although surgery is unequivocally recommended in moderate–severe DCM, its role in mild disease has been more controversial. Over the past decade, multiple prospective studies and meta-analyses have demonstrated that surgical decompression halts disease progression and yields clinically meaningful improvements in function and quality of life even in mild DCM, with acceptable complication rates.[1,2,13,26]

The recent AO Spine practice recommendations explicitly state that surgery is a valid option in mild DCM, with favorable outcomes.[18] Long-term data suggest that earlier intervention, shorter symptom duration, and higher preoperative mJOA scores are associated with better postoperative recovery, supporting a strategy of timely, rather than delayed, decompression.[1,13] A narrative review on timing emphasizes that defining optimal timing in the *gray-zone* of mild or asymptomatic disease is a major unresolved issue, but convergence of evidence favors avoiding prolonged observation once there is evidence of progression, significant cord signal change or other high risk features.[8,22,27]

Approach selection is driven by pathology location, number of levels, sagittal alignment, and patient factors:

- Anterior approaches (anterior cervical discectomy and fusion [ACDF], corpectomy, and hybrid constructs):
  - Preferred for level 1 to 2 ventral compression, focal kyphosis, and OPLL with high canal occupying ratio.[2,13]
  - Provide direct decompression and superior restoration of lordosis, but may carry higher reoperation or dysphagia risk in multilevel disease.
- Posterior approaches (laminoplasty and laminectomy with fusion):
  - Favored for multilevel (≥3) dorsal or combined compression in a lordotic spine.
  - Laminoplasty preserves motion and may reduce adjacent segment disease; laminectomy with fusion provides robust stability, especially in kyphosis or instability.[2,13]
- Comparative studies generally show similar neurologic recovery between anterior and posterior strategies when both are technically feasible, but with differing complication profiles; a randomized trial found equipoise in physical function outcomes between ventral and dorsal surgery.[18]

A possible structured framework has been recently described in literature with the Cervical Surgical score (CSS) by Costa and colleagues[28,29] This tool that can be incorporated into the decision-making process for selecting the surgical approach in DCM, particularly in borderline cases such as mild disease. By combining key clinical and radiological variables—including age, comorbidities, extent and location of compression, alignment, and the mJOA score—it provides a standardized way to weigh factors that may influence the choice between anterior and posterior approaches (**Fig. 2**, **Table 2**). Available studies suggest that its application may influence surgical planning in a subset of *gray-zone* cases and that concordance with its recommendations has been associated with improved neurologic outcomes. In this context, the CSS can be considered among the elements that may help inform a more structured and individualized approach to surgical decision-making in mild DCM.

In mild DCM, less invasive anterior procedures (short segment ACDF) or motion preserving techniques (laminoplasty, selected arthroplasty) may be particularly attractive to minimize morbidity while achieving decompression.[1,2,13,26]

EMERGING TOOLS FOR CHARACTERIZATION AND RISK STRATIFICATION IN MILD DEGENERATIVE CERVICAL MYELOPATHY

Despite being widely accepted and clinically practical, subgrouping DCM patients into *mild*, *moderate* and *severe* classes based solely on neurologic decline, as assessed by the mJOA score, may offer a limited perspective; indeed, the heterogeneity of these patients' complaints, even within

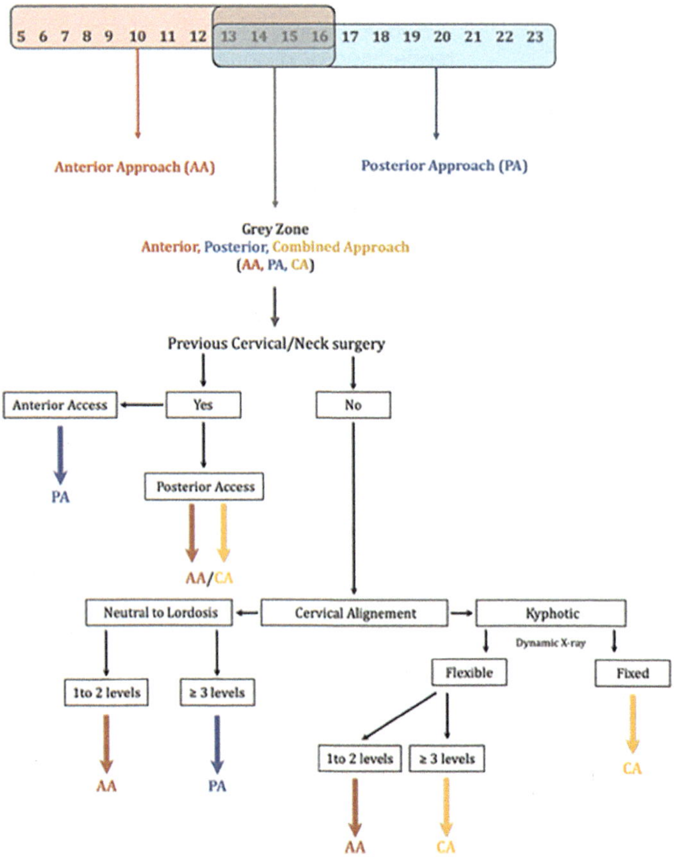

Fig. 2. Algorithm for decision making for surgical approach for DCM derived by the CSS. AA, anterior approach; CA, combined approach; PA, posterior approach.

the same subgroup, has been evident since the earliest reports and requires a more nuanced assessment.[30,31] To this regard, recent studies have exploited machine learning-based cluster analyses to identify 4 distinct clinical DCM phenotypes, namely (1) a *severe multimodal impairment* phenotype, (2) a *minimal impairment* phenotype, (3) a motor-dominant impairment phenotype, and (4) a *pain-dominant impairment* phenotype, whereby phenotypes 2 to 4 all fell within the mild DCM class when assessed with mJOA only.[32] Remarkably, each phenotype showed different postoperative recovery and pain trajectories.[32,33] Hence, a multidimensional framework approach becomes particularly relevant in the characterization of mild DCM patients, where precise delineation of expected outcomes is a key step influencing both management decisions and the outcomes themselves.[33] The adoption of refined multidimensional assessments is thus becoming a key step toward a personalized management of mild DCM.

Given the aforementioned heterogeneity, a major research priority also lies in identifying biomarkers and prediction models that distinguish patients likely to remain stable from those at high risk of deterioration.[8,21]

Promising avenues include the following:

- *Advanced MRI:* Quantitative microstructural techniques (diffusion tensor imaging [DTI], MT, and T2* mapping) detect demyelination and axonal loss beyond conventional T2 changes. Demyelination above the compression level, particularly in dorsal and ventral columns, predicts short-term deterioration in mild DCM.[1,19] Diffusion-weighted imaging changes have been recommended as a prognostic marker in AO Spine recommendations.[18]
- *Neurophysiology:* Prolonged somatosensory and motor evoked potentials, and electromyography (EMG) evidence of anterior horn cell involvement, are associated with myelopathy development in asymptomatic compression and may help guide early intervention.[13,20]
- *Clinical variables and frailty:* Age, baseline mJOA, symptom duration, gait disturbance, and medical frailty influence surgical outcome and may also relate to risk under nonoperative care.[18,21]

Table 2
Cervical surgical score

Cervical Score System	
Parameters	**Points**
Age	
≤70 y	1
71–79 y	2
≥80 y	3
N. of level/s (disc) of cervical pathology/ies	
1	1
2	2
3	3
≥4	5
N. of level/s of radiological myelopathy	
0	0
1	1
2	2
≥3	3
Extesion of compression	
Disc level	1
Disc and vertebral body	2
Predominance of site of compression/s	
Anterior	1
Both	2
Posterio	3
Type of compression	
Soft	1
Hard/calcified	2
Cervical alignment	
Kyphotic	0
Neutral	1
Lordotic	2
Grade of clinical myelopathy (mJOA)	
None	0
Mild (15–18)	1
Moderate (12–14)	2
Severe (≤11)	3

Total Score	Proposed Surgical Approach
5–12	Anterior approach
13–16	Gray zone: anterior/posterior/ combined approach
17–23	Posterior approach

- *Machine learning models:* Integration of clinical, imaging and electrophysiological data using machine learning has shown high accuracy for predicting deterioration in mild DCM and may soon support individualized decision making.[8,18,19]

PHARMACOLOGIC AND NEUROPROTECTIVE STRATEGIES

There is intense interest in pharmacologic agents to modify disease course in mild DCM, delay surgery or augment postoperative recovery. However, current evidence remains limited and largely preclinical.[20,24,34]

Key agents and findings include the following:

- *Riluzole:* effective in rat models but failed to improve mJOA outcomes in human DCM trials; not recommended as routine therapy.
- *Cerebrolysin:* neuroprotective in animal models; early human studies show mixed results and more randomized controlled trials (RCTs) are needed.
- *Limaprost alfadex (PGE1 analog):* improves motor function in animal models and showed encouraging results in a small clinical trial; a phase III study is ongoing).
- *Erythropoietin:* demonstrated neuroprotective effects in animals and some human data, but thromboembolic risks may limit use.
- *Granulocyte colony-stimulating factor (GCSF):* preserved neurologic function in animal DCM models; human data are limited.
- *Glucocorticoids:* no benefit and potential harm (impaired healing, infection); not recommended for chronic DCM.
- Various experimental agents (cilostazol, anti-Fas ligand antibody, Jingshu Keli, and stem cell–related strategies) show promise preclinically but lack robust human evidence.

A 2024 narrative review of all pharmacologic efforts concluded that current data rest mainly on small, low quality clinical studies and animal experimentation; neuroprotective drugs might eventually allow better nonoperative management of mild/stable DCM and optimization of surgical outcomes, but no pharmacologic therapy can currently replace decompression in patients with progressive disease.

RESEARCH GAPS AND FUTURE DIRECTIONS IN MILD DEGENERATIVE CERVICAL MYELOPATHY

Multiple reviews and RECODEDCM consensus workstreams have outlined key gaps specifically relevant to mild disease[8,13,21]:

1. *Natural history precision*: Current estimates of progression risk in mild DCM and NMSCC lack precision, especially beyond 5 years.[8]
2. *Defining structured rehabilitation:* Guidelines recommend rehab for mild DCM, but there

is no evidence based specification of content, intensity or duration, leading to practice variability.[1,4,14,15]

3. *Randomized trials*: Few high-quality RCTs directly compare early surgery versus nonoperative care in mild DCM; such trials are needed, ideally stratified by imaging and electrophysiological risk markers.[13,22,24]
4. *Standardized follow-up protocols*: Optimal frequency and nature of surveillance (clinical scales, imaging intervals, use of advanced MRI/neurophysiology) for patients under observation remain undefined.[8,15,22]
5. *Pharmacologic neuroprotection*: Large, rigorously designed RCTs of promising agents (eg, limaprost, erythropoietin, and GCSF combinations) are required, with attention to long-term safety and integration with surgery.[20,24,34]
6. *Patient centered outcomes and quality of life*: More work is needed on how mild DCM affects employment, mental health, and caregivers, and how different strategies (early surgery vs monitoring) shape these outcomes.[1,13,21]

SUMMARY

Mild DCM is common and clinically heterogeneous. Current evidence and guidelines support two broad strategies: early surgical decompression, which reliably halts progression and often improves function, and supervised structured nonoperative care with vigilant follow-up, recognizing that a meaningful minority (≈10%–20% over a few years) will deteriorate and ultimately require surgery. Choice between these approaches should be individualized, integrating symptom burden, imaging and neurophysiological risk markers, comorbidities, patient values and access to timely surgery. Rapid advances in microstructural MRI, neurophysiology, machine learning prediction models and neuroprotective pharmacology are poised to refine risk stratification and expand therapeutic options, but robust evidence specific to mild DCM is still emerging.

CLINICS CARE POINTS

- Mild DCM often presents with subtle symptoms that delay diagnosis.
- Neurological deterioration occurs in a meaningful proportion of conservatively treated patients, warranting careful clinical follow-up.
- Both early surgery and supervised conservative management are acceptable options.
- Quantitative MRI biomarkers and neurophysiology may improve risk stratification and treatment selection.
- Personalized management remains essential and should integrate clinical, imaging, and patient factors.

DISCLOSURE

The authors declare no competing interests.

REFERENCES

1. Badhiwala JH, Ahuja CS, Akbar MA, et al. Degenerative cervical myelopathy - update and future directions. Nat Rev Neurol 2020;16:108–24.
2. Choi SH, Kang C-N. Degenerative cervical myelopathy: pathophysiology and current treatment strategies. Asian Spine J 2020;14:710–20.
3. Nouri A, Tetreault L, Singh A, et al. Degenerative cervical myelopathy: epidemiology, genetics, and pathogenesis. Spine 2015;40:E675.
4. Boogaarts HD, Bartels RH. Prevalence of cervical spondylotic myelopathy. Eur Spine J 2015;24(Suppl 2):139–41.
5. Goacher E, Phillips R, Mowforth OD, et al. Hospitalisation for degenerative cervical myelopathy in England: insights from the National Health Service Hospital Episode Statistics 2012 to 2019. Acta Neurochir 2022;164:1535–41.
6. Shlykov MA, Giles EM, Kelly MP, et al. Evaluation of genetic and nongenetic risk factors for degenerative cervical myelopathy. Spine 2023;48:1117.
7. Smith SS, Stewart ME, Davies BM, et al. The prevalence of asymptomatic and symptomatic spinal cord compression on magnetic resonance imaging: a systematic review and meta-analysis. Glob Spine J 2021;11:597–607.
8. Nouri A, Tessitore E, Molliqaj G, et al. Degenerative cervical myelopathy: development and natural history [AO spine RECODE-DCM research priority number 2]. Glob Spine J 2022;12:39S–54S.
9. Grodzinski B, Stubbs DJ, Davies BM. Most degenerative cervical myelopathy remains undiagnosed, particularly amongst the elderly: modelling the prevalence of degenerative cervical myelopathy in the United Kingdom. J Neurol 2023;270:311–9.
10. Lannon M, Kachur E. Degenerative cervical myelopathy: clinical presentation, assessment, and natural history. J Clin Med 2021;10.
11. Balmaceno-Criss M, Singh M, Daher M, et al. Degenerative cervical myelopathy: history, physical examination, and diagnosis. J Clin Med 2024;13(23):7139.
12. Saunders LM, Sandhu HS, McBride L, et al. Degenerative cervical myelopathy: an overview. Cureus 2023;15.

13. Wilson JRF, Badhiwala JH, Moghaddamjou A, et al. Degenerative cervical myelopathy; A review of the latest advances and future directions in management. Neurospine 2019;16:494–505.
14. Fehlings MG, Tetreault LA, Riew KD, et al. A clinical practice guideline for the management of patients with degenerative cervical myelopathy: recommendations for patients with mild, moderate, and severe disease and nonmyelopathic patients with evidence of cord compression. Glob Spine J 2017;7:70S–83S.
15. Brannigan JFM, Davies BM, Mowforth OD, et al. Management of mild degenerative cervical myelopathy and asymptomatic spinal cord compression: an international survey. Spinal Cord 2024;62:51–8.
16. Tetreault LA, Karadimas S, Wilson JR, et al. The natural history of degenerative cervical myelopathy and the rate of hospitalization following spinal cord injury: an updated systematic review. Global Spine J 2017;7(3 Suppl):28S–34S.
17. Kögl N, Evaniew N, McIntosh G, et al. Outcome of patients with mild degenerative cervical myelopathy treated nonoperatively: an observational study from the Canadian spine outcome and research network. Neurosurgery 2022. https://doi.org/10.1227/neu.0000000000003803.
18. Fehlings MG, Evaniew N, Ter Wengel PV, et al. AO spine clinical practice recommendations for diagnosis and management of degenerative cervical myelopathy: evidence based decision making - a review of cutting edge recent literature related to degenerative cervical myelopathy. Glob Spine J 2025;15:2585–93.
19. Al-Shawwa A, Craig M, Ost K, et al. Spinal cord demyelination predicts neurological deterioration in patients with mild degenerative cervical myelopathy. BMJ Neurol. Open 2025;7.
20. Levett JJ, Georgiopoulos M, Martel S, et al. Pharmacological treatment of degenerative cervical myelopathy: a critical review of current evidence. Neurospine 2024;21:375–400.
21. Hejrati N, Pedro K, Alvi MA, et al. Degenerative cervical myelopathy: where have we been? Where are we now? Where are we going? Acta Neurochir 2023;165:1105–19.
22. Fasinella MR, Benato A, Creatura D, et al. Degenerative cervical myelopathy: timing of surgery. EFORT Open Rev 2025;10:403–15.
23. Rodriguez-Unda NA, Wu DS. Exoscope for upper extremity peripheral nerve surgery: revision carpal tunnel release with epineurolysis and hypothenar fat flap. Cureus 2022;14:e22539.
24. Ede O, Cheung JPY. Conservative and newer drug treatment for degenerative cervical myelopathy. J. Clin. Orthop. Trauma 2025;64:102972.
25. Kim MW, Kang C-N, Choi SH. Update of the natural history, pathophysiology, and treatment strategies of degenerative cervical myelopathy: a narrative review. Asian Spine J 2023;17:213–21.
26. Thompson K, Travers H, Ngan A, et al. Updates in current concepts in degenerative cervical myelopathy: a systematic review. J Spine Surg 2024;10(2):313–26.
27. Rodrigues-Pinto R, Montenegro TS, Davies BM, et al. Optimizing the application of surgery for degenerative cervical myelopathy [AO Spine RECODE-DCM Research Priority Number 10]. Global Spine J 2022;12(1_suppl):147S–58S.
28. Costa F, Restelli F, Mazzapicchi E, et al. Proposal of a new score system (Cervical Surgical Score) for management of degenerative cervical myelopathy. J Neurosurg Sci 2025;69.
29. Costa F, Mazzapicchi E, Granato LG, et al. Validation of a novel scoring system (Cervical Surgical Score) for the management of degenerative cervical myelopathy. Brain Spine 2025;5:104250.
30. Clarke E, Robinson PK. Cervical myelopathy: a complication of cervical spondylosis. Brain 1956;79(3):483–510.
31. Cook C, Brown C, Isaacs R, et al. Clustered clinical findings for diagnosis of cervical spine myelopathy. J Man Manip Ther 2010;18(4):175–80.
32. Pedro KM, Alvi MA, Hejrati N, et al. Machine learning-based cluster analysis identifies four unique phenotypes of patients with degenerative cervical myelopathy with distinct clinical profiles and long-term functional and neurological outcomes. EBioMedicine 2024;106:105226.
33. Wong R, Alvi MA, Quddusi AI, et al. Role of neck pain in defining clinical trajectories of outcomes in patients with degenerative cervical myelopathy: results of a novel machine learning algorithm. Glob Spine J 2026;16(1):218–29.
34. Ganau M, Holly LT, Mizuno J, et al. Future directions and new technologies for the management of degenerative cervical myelopathy. Neurosur Clin N Am 2018;29:185–93.

Imaging Biomarkers for Compressed Spinal Cord

Unlocking the Silent Injury in Early Myelopathy

Zachary A. Smith, MD, Fauziyya Muhammad, MD, PhD*

KEYWORDS

• Degenerative cervical myelopathy • Spinal cord compression • MRI biomarkers
• Magnetization transfer ratio • Spinal cord toolbox • Quantitative imaging

KEY POINTS

- Degenerative cervical myelopathy remains difficult to diagnose in early stages, with patients navigating an average of 5 physician visits and up to 46 months before receiving a correct diagnosis.
- Quantitative MRI techniques, including magnetization transfer ratio and diffusion tensor imaging, can detect microstructural spinal cord injury, including myelin damage and axonal loss, in tissues that appear normal on conventional imaging.
- Advances in standardized acquisition protocols, automated segmentation tools, and open-source analysis pipelines have brought quantitative spinal cord imaging closer to clinical implementation.
- Spinal cord morphometric measures derived from standard T2-weighted imaging, including cross-sectional area and cord shape descriptors, associate with neurologic deficits and predict surgical outcomes.
- Patients with "asymptomatic" spinal cord compression demonstrate measurable functional deficits and morphometric changes intermediate between healthy controls and symptomatic myelopathy, suggesting a prodromal state of early disease.

INTRODUCTION

Degenerative cervical myelopathy (DCM) is a progressive disease of canal narrowing that manifests as weakness, coordination loss, and hyperreflexia. When the disease progresses, surgical intervention becomes necessary to halt functional decline. Yet the trajectory of DCM is poorly understood. Sumi and colleagues[1] demonstrated that approximately 30% of patients experience stepwise functional decline over time, often unpredictably tilting toward deterioration. Given that cervical degeneration is exceedingly common and that surgery is primarily focused on preventing further injury, early identification of risk factors for progression has been a major focus of modern research.

Imaging assessment of spinal cord compression has historically relied on qualitative interpretation and manual measurement. The key qualitative changes observed on conventional imaging include canal narrowing, disk/osteophyte complex, cord edema (T2 signal change), and visualization of spinal cord compression. Often, an experienced surgeon can appraise these features. However, these qualitative changes are evaluated through a physician's subjective assessment and only loosely associate with neurological deficits. The optimal management of mild DCM remains

Department of Neurosurgery, University of Oklahoma Health Campus, 1000 N Lincoln Boulevard, Suite 4000, Oklahoma City, OK 73104, USA
* Corresponding author.
E-mail address: fauziyya-muhammad@ou.edu

Neurosurg Clin N Am 37 (2026) 555–565
https://doi.org/10.1016/j.nec.2026.05.006

Abbreviations

ADC	apparent diffusion coefficient
CSA	cross-sectional area
DCM	degenerative cervical myelopathy
DTI	diffusion tensor imaging
FA	fractional anisotropy
GM	gray matter
mJOA	modified Japanese Orthopedic Association
MS	multiple sclerosis
MSCC	Maximum Spinal Cord Compression
MTR	magnetization transfer ratio
NAWM	normal-appearing white matter
RIS	Radiologically Isolated Syndrome
WM	white matter

controversial because many patients present with nonspecific symptoms that may not correspond to the subtle or overt changes on the spinal MRI. There is limited evidence to support conservative management techniques, such as physical therapy, injections, or traction, in halting the progression of cord injury.[2] Current clinical practice guidelines support surgery for[3] both moderate and severe DCM, but there generally remains clinical equipoise with regard to surgical decision-making in mild disease.[4–6] As a result, improved evaluation tools that can elaborate the presence and accurate estimation of cord injury have been a focus of recent research.

Over the past 2 decades, there have been significant advances in MRI imaging that can improve the understanding and assessment of early DCM. These include techniques that measure microstructural injury in the cord, including diffusion tensor imaging (DTI) and magnetization transfer ratio (MTR)[4] as well as macrostructural measures such as cross-sectional area (CSA), intramedullary signal changes, and cord shape morphometrics.[7–9] There have additionally been important new advances in MRI acquisition, segmentation, and normalization methods.[3,4,10–13] Among these has been the development of a standardized acquisition protocol for quantitative MRI of the spinal cord, validated across 19 sites and 260 subjects.[3,10] This protocol addresses the large variability in imaging parameters that has been common between imaging sites—a major barrier for quantitative MRI. In addition, a major advance has been the development of key segmentation and analysis tools, such as the Spinal Cord Toolbox, which enables automatic segmentation and registration to a template space (PAM50).[13,14] This template allows for normalization and comparison across patients, establishing a baseline for detecting pathological change.

This review examines imaging biomarkers for the compressed spinal cord and is organized into 3 sections. First, we discuss what can be learned from other pathologies, particularly multiple sclerosis (MS), where the concept of normal-appearing white matter (NAWM) transformed research findings into clinical trial endpoints. Second, we trace the evolution of spinal cord imaging biomarkers from early manual methods through automated pipelines, addressing persistent barriers to clinical adoption. Third, we address the concept of a prodromal phase in DCM the silent injury that precedes overt myelopathy; and the emerging solutions that promise to transform early detection.

QUANTITATIVE MRI OF THE SPINAL CORD-TRACKING WHITE MATTER INJURY

Advanced MRI techniques evaluate the physical and chemical properties of spinal cord tissue, taking advantage of magnetic susceptibility and magnetization transfer to characterize cord integrity. The development of these techniques has been pioneered by researchers studying other spinal pathologies, particularly MS. While DCM and MS are distinct diseases, MS research has established fundamental principles for using this technology to monitor patients with cord disease.

Diffusion Tensor Imaging

DTI can detect spinal cord microstructural damage before obvious cord deformity or signal change is apparent on conventional MRI.[15–17] Histopathological changes associated with DCM including edema, myelomalacia, and gliosis alter the microstructural architecture of the spinal cord and disrupt the normal linear diffusion of water molecules within axons. DTI quantifies this disruption through 2 primary parameters: fractional anisotropy (FA), which measures the directionality of water molecule diffusion, and the apparent diffusion coefficient (ADC), which measures the mean magnitude of water molecule displacement.[16,17] In DCM, FA is reduced and ADC is increased at and adjacent to the level of compression, reflecting disrupted axonal organization.[17] Both FA and ADC have been shown to significantly correlate with modified Japanese Orthopedic Association (mJOA) scores and surgical outcomes.[15,16,18,19] Importantly, tract-specific DTI analysis has further demonstrated its ability to detect early cord injury in patients who do not yet meet criteria for clinical myelopathy on conventional MRI.[18]

Magnetization Transfer Imaging

Magnetization transfer imaging exploits the interaction between free water protons and protons bound to macromolecules, in particular myelin phospholipids. This technique involves application of an off-resonance radiofrequency pulse that saturates bound protons. The resulting magnetization transfer equates to the quantity of macromolecules in the spinal cord tissue, including myelin, cell membranes, and others. Through this technique, it is possible to calculate a quantitative value—the MTR—comparing MRI signals both with and without this radiofrequency pulse.[20] Higher MTR values reflect intact myelin, axonal membranes, and glial cell integrity. Conversely, a lower MTR may signify developing disease through demyelination, axonal loss, or inflammation.

Lessons from Multiple Sclerosis: The Clinical-Radiological Paradox

The application of magnetization transfer imaging in MS research led to the development of new principles applicable to other spinal cord pathologies.[21] Among these is the clinical-radiological paradox, where visible lesion burden on T2-weighted MRI did not associate well with patient disability.[21–23] Studies with histopathological correlation confirmed that reduced MTR in NAWM reflected demyelination, axonal loss, and inflammation.[24] When applied in patients with active demyelinating disease, spinal cord MTR values independently associated with clinical disability even after controlling for brain lesion load.[25] Further, when quantified, this technique can characterize and track long-term disease progression in MS.[26] The validation of MTR as an imaging biomarker has led to its use as an endpoint in multiple randomized clinical trials for MS treatment, with imaging outcomes in clinical trials for progressive MS more than doubling in the last two decades.[24]

Magnetization Transfer Ratio in Degenerative Cervical Myelopathy

The application of magnetization transfer imaging in the degenerative spine has demonstrated robust associations with clinical disease. Leveraging this technique, our group and others have shown that lower MTR values—suggesting myelin loss and microstructural damage—associate with lower mJOA and Nurick scale scores in patients diagnosed with DCM.[27] Tract-specific analysis has further refined these findings. Haynes and colleagues demonstrated in 27 patients and 20 age-matched controls that tract-specific MTR loss aligned with known DCM symptoms and predicted disease severity.[28] Filimonova and colleagues showed that MTR values were decreased particularly in the ventral columns and lateral funiculi, suggesting significant clinical association with descending white matter (WM) pathway injury.[29] Importantly, these values may also be predictive of surgical response. When MTR values were calculated in the anterior spinal cord of DCM patients, they were found to associate with mJOA recovery following decompression.[30] These clinical-imaging relationships suggest that MTR has potential as a marker of injury, prognosis, and treatment response in patients with cervical myelopathy.

BUILDING UPON IMPROVED METHODS

The modern use of quantitative spinal imaging is the result of progressive advancements in imaging acquisition, analysis, and standardization. Imaging the spinal cord presents unique challenges. The cervical spinal cord is affected by patient-specific lordosis, giving the cord unique curvatures that create challenges for obtaining quantitative results comparable from patient to patient.[10] Anatomy of interest, such as the spinal cord WM tracts, cannot be readily visualized on T2 cross-sectional imaging. In addition, images are commonly obtained from different MRI vendors with different acquisition protocols. As a result, the impact of new MRI techniques on clinical care has lagged behind discovery (**Table 1**).

Standardized Acquisition and Automated Segmentation

Recent advances have brought imaging discoveries closer to use in modern-day clinics. The 2021 publication of a standardized "spine-generic" protocol by Cohen-Adad and colleagues provided a standard procedure for obtaining key MRI sequences.[10] This protocol was validated across 19 sites and in 260 subjects and developed methods that could standardize imaging data across major MRI scanner types (Siemens, Philips, and GE).[3,10,12] This protocol supplemented the increasing use and refinement of open-source imaging analysis tools, including the Spinal Cord Toolbox.[11,14] This tool allows for automatic segmentation of the spinal cord and registration to the PAM50 template, enabling accurate quantitative analysis.[11,12] Numerous studies have used this tool to automatically extract key anatomic regions of interest in both healthy subjects and those with disease, improving upon previous hand-drawn analysis studies that were difficult to reproduce and prone to error.[8,11,34,36,37]

Table 1
Evolution of spinal cord imaging: from data acquisition to advanced analysis

Era	Acquisition	Segmentation and Analysis	Key Metrics	Limitations	Representative References
Early Manual Methods (pre-2015)	Non-standardized protocols Variable across sites and vendors	Hand-drawn regions of interest on axial slices	Whole-cord MTR Manual CSA measurement	Labor-intensive Poor reproducibility Operator-dependent variability	Levy et al,[31] 2015, Frostell et al,[32] 2016, De Leener et al,[14] 2017, Cloney et al,[27] 2018
Region- and Tract-Specific Refinement (2015–2020)	Improved 3T protocols Introduction of multi-parametric imaging	Semi-manual tract delineation using atlas overlays PAM50 template	Tract-specific MTR (ventral, lateral, dorsal) DTI fractional anisotropy	Required anatomic expertise Still operator-dependent limited cross-site comparability	Martin et al,[4] 2018, Cloney et al,[27] 2018, Grabher et al,[33] 2016, Haynes et al,[28] 2024
Standardized Acquisition (2021–present)	Spine-generic protocol validated across 19 sites, 260 subjects, 3 major vendors	Spinal Cord Toolbox Automatic segmentation PAM50 template registration	Normalized CSA, AP diameter, eccentricity, solidity, MSCC GM/WM ratio	Requires specific pulse sequences; Ongoing validation in disease populations	Cohen-Adad et al,[3] 2021, Valosek et al,[12] 2024, Bedard et al,[34] 2025
Automated Analysis and Open-Source Tools (2023–present)	Multi-vendor, multi-resolution Applicable to clinical-grade 1.5T and 3T	Fully automated segmentation; SCT, EPISeg); Open-source GitHub repositories	Automated morphometrics; intramedullary lesion volume and length Maximal axial damage ratio	Validation in large prospective cohorts ongoing Integration into clinical workflow pending	Muhammad et al,[8] 2024, Bedard et al,[34] 2025, Naga Karthik et al,[35] 2025, Naga Karthik et al,[9] 2025, Valosek et al,[12] 2024

Abbreviations: 3T, 3 Tesla; AP, anterior-posterior diameter; CSA, cross-sectional area; DCM, degenerative cervical myelopathy; DTI, diffusion tensor imaging; GM, gray matter; MSCC, maximum spinal cord compression; MTR, magnetization transfer ratio; SCT, spinal cord toolbox; WM, white matter.

Quantitative Morphometrics from Standard Imaging

As new methods become more consistent across centers and reproducible, the value of morphometric cord measures has taken on new importance. While MTR provides microstructural tissue characterization, standard T2-weighted imaging enables quantitative morphometric analysis of cord shape and compression.[8,34,38] This can reflect atrophy and compression severity. We have shown that spinal cord morphometrics, in particular CSA, associate with neurologic deficits and myelopathy scores in DCM patients.[8] Bedard and colleagues recently demonstrated that automatic MRI measures of spinal cord compression severity and morphometric injury predicted both clinical scores and therapeutic decision-making.[34] Both of these works additionally demonstrated that these measures predict surgical outcomes following intervention. This technique includes calculation of Maximum Spinal Cord Compression (MSCC) and shape descriptors, including eccentricity and solidity—measures of cord deformation.[8,34,39] Further, using T2w star signal intensity ratios, gray matter (GM) and WM volumes can be automatically and consistently calculated. An elevated GM-to-WM ratio has been shown to reflect early underlying spinal tissue injury in the compressed spine.[4] These T2-MRI-derived measures complement research-grade sequences such as MTR: morphometrics quantify the structural consequences of compression (cord shape, atrophy), whereas MTR captures the microstructural integrity of the cord (myelin and axon status).[29,30,38]

Radiomics and Machine Learning

Beyond standard morphometry, radiomics has emerged as a powerful method for high-dimensional tissue characterization using clinical MRI.[40] Radiomics involves the high-throughput extraction of quantitative features from segmented MRI volumes that describe the texture, shape, and intensity distribution of the spinal cord. These features are often imperceptible to human visual inspection.[41] This process typically utilizes open-source packages such as PyRadiomics to extract multiple feature classes, including first-order statistics (histogram-based), shape-based features, and texture-based matrices such as the gray-level co-occurrence matrix, gray-level size-zone matrix, and neighborhood gray-tone difference matrix (**Fig. 1**).[40–43]

Recent work by Arnest and colleagues has demonstrated that machine learning models leveraging these radiomic features can achieve an AUROC of 0.93 in discriminating DCM from healthy controls, showing superior diagnostic performance compared with both standard MRI and conventional morphometry.[44] These features, often derived from high-resolution 3D T1-weighted or T2-weighted scans, enable the generation of a case-level radiomics feature matrix that can effectively predict baseline neurologic function and classify disease severity. Wang and colleagues similarly demonstrated the utility of this approach in assessing cord function in patients with mild DCM.[41] While the inherent complexity of these models often leads to them being viewed as black boxes, they offer a reproducible, objective framework for identifying subtle imaging signatures of cord injury that could transform early detection and longitudinal monitoring.

Automated Quantification of Intramedullary Signal Change

The prognostic significance of cord signal change remains controversial. While some studies demonstrate this feature as a sensitive measure of developing myelopathy,[45] others cast doubt.[46] However, despite some uncertainty, most practicing surgeons consider this an important marker of injury. Building upon the aforementioned advances in methods, T2 intramedullary signal can now be reliably quantified. For example, Karthik and colleagues developed an automated segmentation tool (SCIseg) that can determine the presence of intramedullary signal change and also obtain lesion volume, lesion length, and calculate a maximal axial damage ratio in 191 patients with spinal cord injury.[9,47] Importantly, this technique was developed using various imaging manufacturers and with different image resolutions, including both isotropic and anisotropic scans.[47] This technique, like morphometric analysis, can be applied to other spinal pathologies, including DCM.

Open-Source Tools and Reproducibility

The transition from manual to automated methods represents a key step toward clinical implementation. Automation has removed manual region-of-interest variability—a significant source of potential error. Most recent advances in imaging applicable to DCM remain open-source and easily accessible, including algorithms from the Spinal Cord Toolbox and tools like SCIseg that are publicly available on GitHub.[7,48] This promotes reproducibility and more widespread adoption (**Fig. 2**).

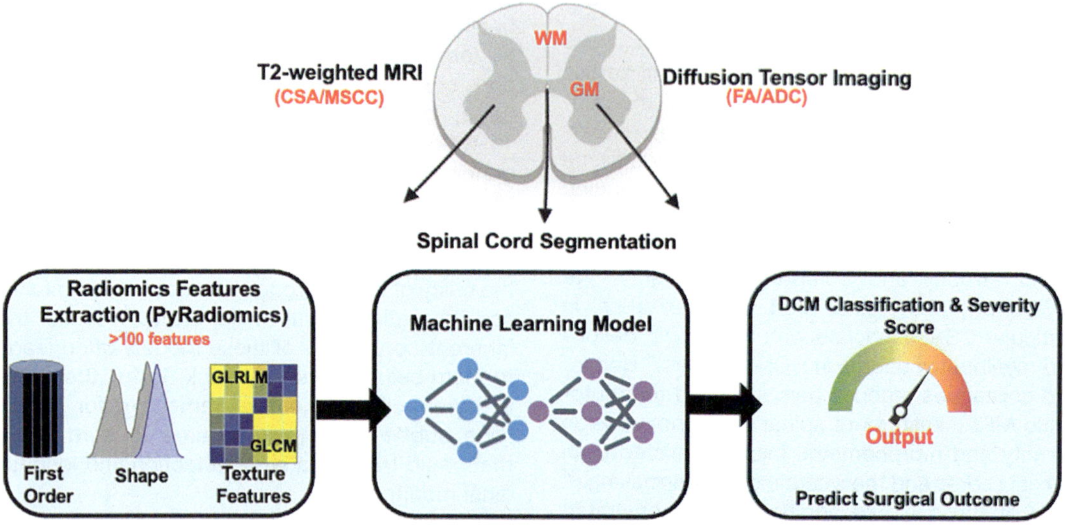

Fig. 1. Radiomics and machine learning pipeline for quantitative spinal cord analysis in DCM. Standard T2-weighted MRI and DTI sequences serve as dual inputs into an automated spinal cord segmentation pipeline. Following segmentation, radiomic features are extracted using PyRadiomics, encompassing 3 feature classes: first-order statistics (intensity histogram-based measures), shape descriptors (morphometric cord geometry), and texture features including GLRLM and GLCM. These high-dimensional features are then input into a machine learning model represented here as a multilayer neural network trained to distinguish DCM from healthy controls and to quantify disease severity. DCM, degenerative cervical myelopathy; DTI, diffusion tensor imaging; GLCM, gray-level co-occurrence matrix; GLRLM, gray-level run-length matrix. (*Adapted from* Refs.[41,44])

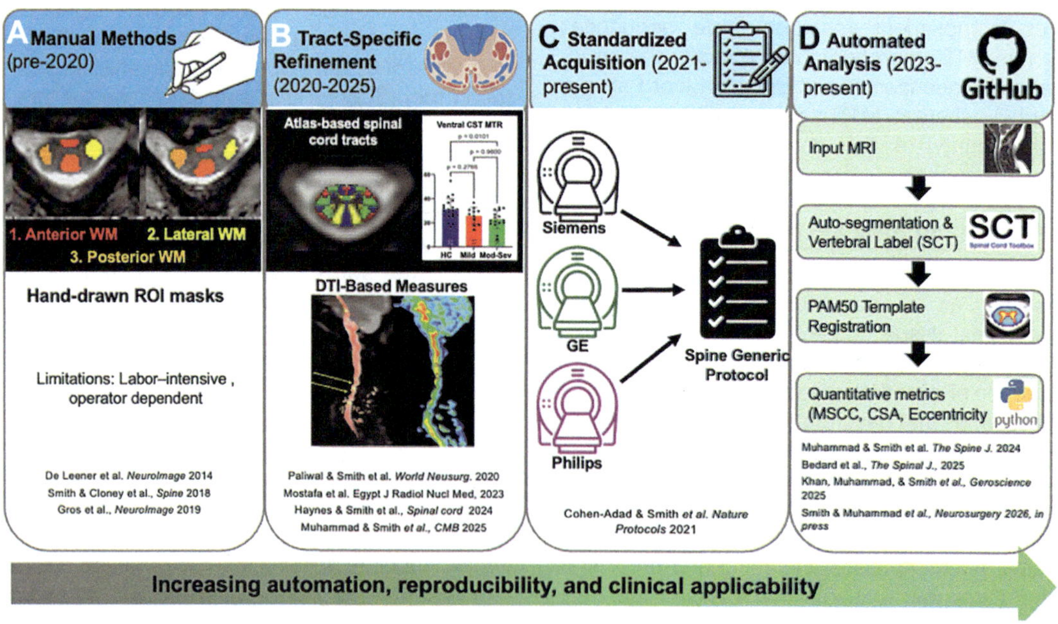

Fig. 2. Evolution of spinal cord imaging methodology for the compressed cord. Timeline illustrating the progression from (*A*) early manual region-of-interest methods requiring hand-drawn masks on axial slices with non-standardized acquisition, through (*B*) tract-specific refinement using atlas-guided analysis with improved 3T imaging, to (*C*) Standardized spine-generic acquisition protocols now enable cross-vendor, cross-site reproducibility (Siemens, GE, Philips). (*D*) Current automated pipelines leveraging the Spinal Cord Toolbox for automatic segmentation, PAM50 template registration, and normalization, while open-source analysis code on GitHub promotes widespread adoption and reproducibility.

Table 2
Key quantitative MRI techniques for evaluating the compressed spinal cord: mechanism, clinical associations, and implementation status

Technique	MRI Sequence	What It Measures	Key Clinical Associations in DCM	Strengths	Limitations
Magnetization Transfer Ratio (MTR)	MT-weighted gradient echo	Myelin and macromolecular integrity; bound proton pool	Decreased MTR associates with lower mJOA/Nurick scores; predicts surgical recovery; tract-specific loss maps to symptom profiles	Sensitive to early myelin damage; validated in MS trials; applicable at 1.5T and 3T	Requires dedicated MT pulse sequence; not universally available
Diffusion Tensor Imaging FA	EPI-based DWI	White matter tract coherence; axonal organization	Decreased FA in compressed segments correlates with disability; distinguishes HC from ASCC and DCM	Directionally sensitive; maps individual tracts; radiomics-compatible	Susceptibility artifacts; distortion at cord boundaries; vendor variability
DTI—&&MD/RD/AD	EPI-based DWI	Water diffusion magnitude and anisotropy; axonal vs myelin injury compartments	Increased MD/RD reflects demyelination and edema; increased AD may reflect axonal injury	Complements FA; multi-compartment sensitivity	Same limitations as FA; requires dedicated post-processing
MRI Radiomics/ Machine Learning	High-res 3D T1/T2; DTI	High-dimensional texture and shape features	Diagnose DCM (AUROC 0.93); predict baseline function and surgical outcomes	Superior to standard morphometry for diagnosis; objective and reproducible	Complex analysis; requires large training datasets; validation ongoing
Cross-Sectional Area	Standard T2-weighted	Cord atrophy; structural compression severity	Decreased CSA associates with mJOA scores and gait dysfunction; predicts surgical outcomes	Derived from clinical scans; fully automated with SCT; multi-vendor validated	Influenced by normal anatomic variation and lordosis
MSCC/Cord Shape (Eccentricity, Solidity)	Standard T2-weighted	Degree and geometry of cord deformation	MSCC and shape descriptors predict clinical scores and surgical decision-making	No additional sequences needed; reproducible and automated	Validated primarily in single-center studies
T2 Intramedullary Signal Change	Standard T2-weighted	Edema, gliosis, myelomalacia within cord parenchyma	ISC presence associated with more severe myelopathy; automated lesion volumetry emerging	Universally acquired; EPISeg tool enables automated quantification	Prognostic significance debated; qualitative-to-quantitative transition ongoing
GM/WM Ratio (T2-weighted)*	T2*-weighted (GRE)	Gray/white matter volume balance; early tissue injury	Elevated GM/WM ratio reflects early white matter loss in compressed cord	Sensitive early marker; aligns with histopathological injury	Requires T2*-weighted sequence; less widely available

Abbreviations: AD, axial diffusivity; ASCC, asymptomatic spinal cord compression; CSA, cross-sectional area; DCM, degenerative cervical myelopathy; DTI, diffusion tensor imaging; EPI, echo-planar imaging; FA, fractional anisotropy; GM, gray matter; GRE, gradient echo; HC, healthy controls; ISC, intramedullary signal change; MD, mean diffusivity; mJOA, modified Japanese Orthopedic Association scale; MS, multiple sclerosis; MSCC, maximum spinal cord compression; MT, magnetization transfer; MTR, magnetization transfer ratio; RD, radial diffusivity; SCT, Spinal Cord Toolbox; WM, white matter.

DELAYED DIAGNOSIS AND IDENTIFYING EARLY DEGENERATIVE CERVICAL MYELOPATHY

Diagnosing early DCM can be quite difficult. In the early stages of disease, classic symptoms such as gait instability and clumsiness are rarely present. Once these symptoms develop, like the accompanying physical examination findings, the diagnosis is typically straightforward.[49] However, this is rarely the case in early disease, when nonspecific symptoms are common. Early symptoms of DCM can overlap those of carpal tunnel syndrome, peripheral neuropathy, arthritis, and general aging, among multiple other conditions. Further, it has been shown that nearly 80% of patients have neck pain at initial presentation often as their primary presenting symptom.[50] The clinical consequence of in adequate early detection tools is delayed diagnosis: patients with early myelopathy navigate an average of 5 physician visits and up to 46 months before receiving a correct diagnosis.[51]

The challenge of diagnosing DCM is compounded by the prevalence of spinal cord compression. Imaging studies show that disk degeneration of some degree is present in upwards of 80% of patients by the age of 50.[52] It is also estimated that nearly 1 in 5 adults has "asymptomatic spinal cord compression."[6,53] Thus, age-related compression is quite common.[54–56] However, there remain inconsistent clinical recommendations for these individuals. In a survey of 699 members of the AO Spine and CSRS societies, there was significant variability in how surgeons and health care providers chose to objectively assess and observe patients with mild DCM. Further, there was significant variability even in the clinical terminology, including "pre-symptomatic DCM," "cervical stenosis without myelopathy," and "non-myelopathic cervical spinal cord compression".[57]

The Prodromal Phase Concept

Given the prevalence of spinal cord compression and that a significant proportion of patients progress to myelopathy, it is possible that subtle early symptoms could be commonly missed. If this is the case, the commonly used term "asymptomatic spinal cord compression" could be a misnomer. Many neurological diseases have well-characterized prodromal phases that precede overt clinical symptoms. In Alzheimer disease, the concept of "Mild Cognitive Impairment" represents a stepwise decline to developing the disease, with imaging markers (medial temporal atrophy) and CSF markers (tau subtypes, amyloid-beta) identifying at-risk individuals.[58,59] In Parkinson disease, prodromal symptoms can predict later development, with decreased alpha-synuclein detectable from peripheral tissue biopsy in early disease.[60] In MS, Radiologically Isolated Syndrome (RIS) represents a prodromal state—early radiographic findings with mild or varied symptoms prior to formal diagnosis. This concept has proven so clinically useful that double-blinded, randomized treatment trials in RIS populations have been conducted.[61] The parallel to DCM is clear: patients with spinal cord compression who do not yet meet mJOA criteria may need to be evaluated for silent injury suggestive of the onset of early myelopathy.[56] Catching DCM early depends on developing reproducible techniques that can detect spinal cord distortion before overt clinical symptoms emerge. Reproducible and sensitive means of quantitative imaging may serve an important role here, as may outpatient neurologic tests that can detect injury prior to the development of clinical myelopathy.

OVERCOMING BARRIERS TO CLINICAL ADOPTION

Despite accumulating evidence, several barriers impede clinical translation of imaging biomarkers for the compressed spinal cord. These include variability in MRI acquisition parameters across vendors and sites, the prior dependence on labor-intensive manual region-of-interest analysis, the predominance of research-grade 3T scanners over widely available clinical 1.5T scanners, and limited disease-state datasets with normative data derived primarily from healthy controls.[57] Recent developments are directly addressing each of these barriers. The spine-generic protocol provides a standardized, open-access approach to acquisition that can be implemented across Siemens, GE, and Philips platforms.[3,10] Automated segmentation tools, such as the Spinal Cord Toolbox, eliminate manual analysis variability and have been validated across scanner types.[14] Importantly, multiple recent studies have demonstrated that automated morphometric and signal analysis techniques can be applied to clinical-grade scans at both 1.5T and 3T from multiple vendors, using both isotropic and anisotropic acquisitions.[8,36,34,47] The availability of open-source analysis code on platforms such as GitHub further lowers the barrier to adoption, enabling any research group or clinical center to implement these methods with minimal cost.[7,9,12,38]

SUMMARY

The evaluation of the compressed spinal cord has evolved substantially over the past 2 decades, transitioning from subjective, qualitative assessment to quantitative, automated, and increasingly standardized analysis (**Table 2**). Quantitative MRI techniques—particularly MTR—can detect microstructural injury in tissue that appears normal on conventional imaging, and these measures associate with clinical disability and predict surgical outcomes. Morphometric analysis derived from standard T2-weighted imaging provides complementary structural information that is accessible without research-grade sequences. Importantly, growing evidence supports the concept that "asymptomatic" spinal cord compression may in fact represent a prodromal state of early myelopathy, detectable through quantitative imaging and sensitive functional testing.

The path forward mirrors the translational arc demonstrated in MS research: from basic science observations that conventional imaging underestimates injury, through quantitative technique development, to clinical implementation as outcome measures and decision-making tools. With standardized acquisition protocols, automated analysis pipelines, and open-source tools now available, the field is poised to transform the early detection and management of DCM. The translation of these tools into routine clinical practice represents the next critical step in unlocking the silent injury of the compressed spinal cord.

CLINICS CARE POINTS

- Qualitative assessment of spinal cord compression on conventional MRI has limited sensitivity for detecting early myelopathy and correlates poorly with the degree of neurologic deficit.
- Quantitative MRI techniques DTI and MTR detect microstructural spinal cord injury before overt cord deformity is visible on conventional imaging; DTI FA decreases and ADC increase at the level of compression, while reduced MTR reflects demyelination and axonal loss; both measures correlate significantly with mJOA scores and surgical outcomes.
- Morphometric measures, including CSA and cord shape descriptors, can be derived from standard T2w imaging and associate with disease severity and surgical outcomes.
- Automated segmentation tools (eg, SCT) enable reproducible, operator-independent analysis applicable to scans from multiple MRI vendors.
- Patients with radiographic spinal cord compression who appear "asymptomatic" by conventional clinical scales may have measurable functional deficits and should be considered for longitudinal monitoring.
- Standardized MRI acquisition protocols are now available and should be considered for adoption to enable cross-site comparison and longitudinal assessment.

DISCLOSURES

The authors have nothing to disclose.

FUNDING

Presbyterian Health Foundation Team Science Grant.

REFERENCES

1. Sumi M, Miyamoto H, Suzuki T, et al. Prospective cohort study of mild cervical spondylotic myelopathy without surgical treatment. J Neurosurg Spine 2012;16(1):8–14.
2. Rhee JM, Shamji MF, Erwin WM, et al. Nonoperative management of cervical myelopathy: a systematic review. Spine 2013;38(22 Suppl 1):S55–67.
3. Cohen-Adad J, Alonso-Ortiz E, Abramovic M, et al. Open-access quantitative MRI data of the spinal cord and reproducibility across participants, sites and manufacturers. Sci Data 2021;8(1):219.
4. Martin AR, De Leener B, Cohen-Adad J, et al. Monitoring for myelopathic progression with multiparametric quantitative MRI. PLoS One 2018;13(4):e0195733. https://doi.org/10.1371/journal.pone.0195733.
5. Fehlings MG, Wilson JR, Kopjar B, et al. Efficacy and safety of surgical decompression in patients with cervical spondylotic myelopathy: results of the AOSpine North America prospective multi-center study. J Bone Joint Surg Am 2013;95(18):1651–8.
6. Fehlings MG, Tetreault LA, Riew KD, et al. A clinical practice guideline for the management of patients with degenerative cervical myelopathy: recommendations for patients with mild, moderate, and severe disease and nonmyelopathic patients with evidence of cord compression. Glob Spine J 2017;7(3 Suppl):70S–83S.
7. Muhammad F, Weber KA 2nd, et al. Semiautomated pipeline effectively assesses severity and monitor disease progression in compressed spinal cord of degenerative cervical myelopathy patients. Neurosurg Pract 2025;6(2):e00138.
8. Muhammad F, Weber KA, Bédard S, et al. Cervical spinal cord morphometrics in degenerative cervical myelopathy: quantification using semi-automated normalized technique and correlation with neurological dysfunctions. Spine J 2024;24(11):2045–57.
9. Naga Karthik E, Valošek J, Smith AC, et al. SCIseg: automatic segmentation of intramedullary lesions in

spinal cord injury on T2-weighted MRI scans. Radiol Artif Intell 2025;7(1):e240005. https://doi.org/10.1148/ryai.240005.
10. Cohen-Adad J, Alonso-Ortiz E, Abramovic M, et al. Generic acquisition protocol for quantitative MRI of the spinal cord. Nat Protoc 2021;16(10):4611–32.
11. Valošek J, Bédard S, Keřkovský M, et al. A database of the healthy human spinal cord morphometry in the PAM50 template space. Imaging Neurosci (Camb) 2024;2doi. https://doi.org/10.1162/imag_a_00075.
12. Valošek J, Cohen-Adad J. Reproducible spinal cord quantitative MRI analysis with the spinal cord toolbox. Magn Reson Med Sci 2024;23(3):307–15.
13. De Leener B, Fonov VS, Collins DL, et al. PAM50: unbiased multimodal template of the brainstem and spinal cord aligned with the ICBM152 space. Neuroimage 2018;165:170–9.
14. De Leener B, Levy S, Dupont SM, et al. SCT: spinal cord toolbox, an open-source software for processing spinal cord MRI data. Neuroimage 2017;145(Pt A):24–43.
15. Skotarczak M, Dzierżanowski J, Kaszubowski M, et al. Diagnostic value of diffusion tensor imaging in patients with clinical signs of cervical spondylotic myelopathy. Neurol Neurochir Pol 2022;56(4):341–8.
16. Mostafa NSA-A, Hasanin OAM, Al Yamani Moqbel EAH, et al. Diagnostic value of magnetic resonance diffusion tensor imaging in evaluation of cervical spondylotic myelopathy. Egypt J Radiol Nucl Med 2023/10/16 2023;54(1):175.
17. Dong F, Wu Y, Song P, et al. A preliminary study of 3.0-T magnetic resonance diffusion tensor imaging in cervical spondylotic myelopathy. Eur Spine J 2018;27(8):1839–45.
18. Ni M, Li S, Wen X, et al. A matched case-control study of early cervical spondylotic myelopathy based on diffusion magnetic resonance imaging. Insights Imaging 2024;15(1):25.
19. Maki S, Koda M, Kitamura M, et al. Diffusion tensor imaging can predict surgical outcomes of patients with cervical compression myelopathy. Eur Spine J 2017/09/01 2017;26(9):2459–66.
20. Grossman RI, Gomori JM, Ramer KN, et al. Magnetization transfer: theory and clinical applications in neuroradiology. Radiographics 1994;14(2):279–90.
21. Hartmann A, Noro F, Bahia PRV, et al. The clinical-radiological paradox in multiple sclerosis: myth or truth? Arq Neuropsiquiatr 2023;81(1):55–61. O paradoxo clínico radiológico na esclerose múltipla: mito ou verdade?
22. Barkhof F. MRI in multiple sclerosis: correlation with expanded disability status scale (EDSS). Mult Scler 1999;5(4):283–6.
23. Barkhof F. The clinico-radiological paradox in multiple sclerosis revisited. Curr Opin Neurol 2002;15(3):239–45.
24. Moccia M, van de Pavert S, Eshaghi A, et al. Pathologic correlates of the magnetization transfer ratio in multiple sclerosis. Neurology 2020;95(22):e2965–76.
25. Lee LE, Cohen-Adad J, Vavasour IM, et al. Cervical spinal cord magnetization transfer ratio and its relationship with clinical outcomes in multiple sclerosis. Ann Clin Transl Neurol 2025;12(9):1794–804.
26. Oh J, Chen M, Cybulsky K, et al. Five-year longitudinal changes in quantitative spinal cord MRI in multiple sclerosis. Mult Scler 2021;27(4):549–58.
27. Cloney MB, Smith ZA, Weber KA 2nd, et al. Quantitative magnetization transfer MRI measurements of the anterior spinal cord region are associated with clinical outcomes in cervical spondylotic myelopathy. Spine 2018;43(10):675–80.
28. Haynes G, Muhammad F, Weber KA 2nd, et al. Tract-specific magnetization transfer ratio provides insights into the severity of degenerative cervical myelopathy. Spinal Cord 2024;62(12):700–7.
29. Filimonova E, Abdaev M, Vasilenko I, et al. Evaluation of the structural integrity of different spinal cord tracts with magnetization transfer ratio in degenerative cervical myelopathy. Neuroradiology 2024;66(5):839–46.
30. Paliwal M, Weber KA 2nd, Hopkins BS, et al. Magnetization transfer ratio and morphometrics of the spinal cord associates with surgical recovery in patients with degenerative cervical myelopathy. World Neurosurg 2020;144:e939–47.
31. Lévy S, Benhamou M, Naaman C, et al. White matter atlas of the human spinal cord with estimation of partial volume effect. Neuroimage 2015;119:262–71.
32. Frostell A, Hakim R, Thelin EP, et al. A review of the segmental diameter of the healthy human spinal cord. Front Neurol 2016;7:238.
33. Grabher P, Mohammadi S, Trachsler A, et al. Voxel-based analysis of grey and white matter degeneration in cervical spondylotic myelopathy. Sci Rep 2016;6:24636.
34. Bédard S, Valošek J, Seif M, et al. Normalizing spinal cord compression measures in degenerative cervical myelopathy. Spine J 2025;25(9):1951–63.
35. Naga Karthik E, McGinnis J, Wurm R, et al. Automatic segmentation of spinal cord lesions in MS: A robust tool for axial T2-weighted MRI scans. Imaging Neurosci (Camb) 2025;3:IMAG.a.45.
36. Bédard S, Karthik EN, Tsagkas C, et al. Towards contrast-agnostic soft segmentation of the spinal cord. Med Image Anal 2025;101:103473. https://doi.org/10.1016/j.media.2025.103473.
37. Bédard S, Valošek J, Oliva V, et al. Rootlets-based registration to the PAM50 spinal cord template. Imaging Neurosci (Camb) 2025;3:IMAG.a.123.
38. Muhammad F, Weber Ii KA, Haynes G, et al. Magnetization transfer MRI (MT-MRI) detects white matter damage beyond the primary site of compression in

degenerative cervical myelopathy using a novel semi-automated analysis. Comput Biol Med 2025; 197(Pt B):111083. https://doi.org/10.1016/j.compbiomed.2025.111083.
39. Khan AF, Hameed S, Baha A, et al. Quantitative assessment of asymptomatic spinal cord compression using MRI: a multi-center study. GeroScience 2025;47(6):6749–64.
40. Yang S, Li J, Fei N, et al. A deep-learning-based diffusion tensor imaging pathological auto-analysis method for cervical spondylotic myelopathy. Bioengineering (Basel) 2025;12(8). https://doi.org/10.3390/bioengineering12080806.
41. Wang H, Wang K, Wang Y, et al. MRI-based machine learning and radiomics methods for assessing spinal cord function in patients with mild cervical spondylotic myelopathy. Bioengineering (Basel) 2025;12(6). https://doi.org/10.3390/bioengineering12060666.
42. Zhang Z, Li N, Ding Y, et al. Establishment and validation of a ResNet-based radiomics model for predicting prognosis in cervical spinal cord injury patients. Sci Rep 2025;15(1):9163.
43. Zhang Z, Li N, Ding Y, et al. An integrative nomogram based on MRI radiomics and clinical characteristics for prognosis prediction in cervical spinal cord injury. Eur Spine J 2025;34(3):1164–76.
44. Arnest RM, Koch MK, Budde MD, et al. Machine learning-based MRI radiomics identifies patients with degenerative cervical myelopathy and predicts baseline function. Eur Spine J 2026. https://doi.org/10.1007/s00586-026-10043-x.
45. Matsuda Y, Miyazaki K, Tada K, et al. Increased MR signal intensity due to cervical myelopathy. Analysis of 29 surgical cases. J Neurosurg 1991;74(6):887–92.
46. Morio Y, Yamamoto K, Kuranobu K, et al. Does increased signal intensity of the spinal cord on MR images due to cervical myelopathy predict prognosis? Arch Orthop Trauma Surg 1994;113(5):254–9.
47. Karthik EN, Valosek J, Smith AC, et al. SCIseg: automatic segmentation of T2-weighted intramedullary lesions in spinal cord injury. medRxiv 2024. https://doi.org/10.1101/2024.01.03.24300794.
48. Banerjee R, Kaptan M, Tinnermann A, et al. EPISeg: automated segmentation of the spinal cord on echo planar images using open-access multi-center data. Imaging Neurosci (Camb) 2025;3. https://doi.org/10.1162/IMAG.a.98.
49. Rhee JM, Heflin JA, Hamasaki T, et al. Prevalence of physical signs in cervical myelopathy: a prospective, controlled study. Spine 2009;34(9):890–5.
50. Schneider MM, Badhiwala JH, Alvi MA, et al. Prevalence of neck pain in patients with degenerative cervical myelopathy and short-term response after operative treatment: a cohort study of 664 patients from 26 global sites. Glob Spine J 2024;14(3):830–8.
51. Behrbalk E, Salame K, Regev GJ, et al. Delayed diagnosis of cervical spondylotic myelopathy by primary care physicians. Neurosurg Focus 2013; 35(1):E1.
52. Brinjikji W, Luetmer PH, Comstock B, et al. Systematic literature review of imaging features of spinal degeneration in asymptomatic populations. AJNR Am J Neuroradiol 2015;36(4):811–6.
53. Grodzinski B, Stubbs DJ, Davies BM. Most degenerative cervical myelopathy remains undiagnosed, particularly amongst the elderly: modelling the prevalence of degenerative cervical myelopathy in the United Kingdom. J Neurol 2023;270(1):311–9.
54. Yamaguchi S, Mitsuhara T, Abiko M, et al. Epidemiology and overview of the clinical spectrum of degenerative cervical myelopathy. Neurosurg Clin N Am 2018;29(1):1–12.
55. Smith SS, Stewart ME, Davies BM, et al. The prevalence of asymptomatic and symptomatic spinal cord compression on magnetic resonance imaging: a systematic review and meta-analysis. Glob Spine J 2021;11(4):597–607.
56. Hameed S, Muhammad F, Haynes G, et al. Early neurological changes in aging cervical spine: insights from PROMIS mobility assessment. GeroScience 2024;46(3):3123–34.
57. Brannigan JFM, Davies BM, Mowforth OD, et al. Management of mild degenerative cervical myelopathy and asymptomatic spinal cord compression: an international survey. Spinal Cord 2024;62(2):51–8.
58. Chandra A, Dervenoulas G, Politis M. Alzheimer's disease neuroimaging I. Magnetic resonance imaging in Alzheimer's disease and mild cognitive impairment. J Neurol 2019;266(6):1293–302.
59. Papaliagkas V, Kalinderi K, Vareltzis P, et al. CSF biomarkers in the early diagnosis of mild cognitive impairment and Alzheimer's Disease. Int J Mol Sci 2023;24(10). https://doi.org/10.3390/ijms24108976.
60. David A, Mechinaud F, Roze JC, et al. [A case of Cao-Gio. Possible confusion with abuse]. Arch Fr Pediatr 1986;43(2):147. Une observation de "Cao-Gio". Confusion possible avec des sevices.
61. Lebrun-Frenay C, Siva A, Sormani MP, et al. Teriflunomide and time to clinical multiple sclerosis in patients with radiologically isolated syndrome: the TERIS randomized clinical trial. JAMA Neurol 2023; 80(10):1080–8.

Neuroprotection of the Compressed Spine

A Systematized Narrative Review of Riluzole for Humans with Spinal Cord Injury

Teleale F. Gebeyehu, MD*, Ashmal S. Kabani, MD, Adam Leibold, MD, MSc, James S. Harrop, MD, MSHQS

KEYWORDS

• Riluzole • Neuroprotection • Compressed spine • Traumatic spinal cord injury • Neuroregeneration

KEY POINTS

- Riluzole has been studied as a neuroprotective agent for spinal cord injury, with evidence spanning mechanistic rationale, pharmacology, randomized trials, secondary analyses, and meta-analyses.
- Pharmacokinetic studies demonstrated acute spinal cord injury alters Riluzole disposition in a time-dependent manner, directly influencing drug exposure and underscoring the importance of optimized dosing.
- Pharmacodynamic analyses have linked Riluzole exposure to reductions in phosphorylated neurofilament heavy chain , providing biomarker-based evidence of axonal injury modulation in humans.
- Secondary and global statistical analyses have revealed treatment effects across neurologic, functional, and patient-reported outcomes that are not consistently captured by single primary endpoints.
- Other agents of interest include steroids, Nogo-A inhibitors, minocycline, and antirepulsive guidance molecule-a antibody, but their use is not conclusive.

INTRODUCTION

Traumatic spinal cord injury (tSCI) is associated with permanent disability, reduced quality of life, and substantial socioeconomic burden worldwide. Despite advances in surgical decompression, critical care, and rehabilitation, meaningful neurologic recovery following tSCI remains limited for many patients. This therapeutic gap reflects the complex pathophysiology of spinal cord injury (SCI), in which irreversible primary mechanical damage is followed by a prolonged and potentially modifiable secondary injury cascade that evolves over hours to days after the initial insult.[1,2]

Numerous pharmacologic agents have been evaluated for neuroprotection in tSCI; however, translation from promising preclinical findings to robust clinical benefit has proven challenging. Large randomized controlled trials (RCTs) investigating agents such as methylprednisolone, naloxone, gacyclidine, and gangliosides have not demonstrated consistent or clinically meaningful improvements, and concerns regarding adverse effects (AEs) have further limited widespread adoption.[3] Consequently, no universally accepted pharmacologic therapy directly targets the secondary injury cascade following tSCI, characterized

Department of Neurological Surgery, Thomas Jefferson University, 909 Walnut Street, 3rd Floor, Philadelphia, PA 19107, USA
* Corresponding author. 130 S. 9th Street, 12th Floor, Philadelphia, PA 19107.
E-mail address: tealealef.gebeyehu@jefferson.edu
Twitter: @AshmalSami; @LeiboldAdam

Neurosurg Clin N Am 37 (2026) 567–581
https://doi.org/10.1016/j.nec.2026.05.007

Abbreviations

ABEC	Area between Baseline and Effective Curve
AEs	Adverse Effects
AIS	American Spinal Injury Association (ASIA) Impairment Scale
ALS	Amyotrophic Lateral Sclerosis
ASIA	American Spinal Injury Association
AUCD0-D14	Area Under Curve of 14 days exposure
BL	Baseline
CL	Clearance
Cmax	maximum Concentration
Cmin	minimum Concentration
CSF	Cerebrospinal Fluid
DCM	Degenerative Cervical Myelopathy
EQ5D-HS	European Quality of Life 5-Dimension Health State
GTE	Global Treatment Effect
IQR	Inter Quartile Range
ISNCSCI	International Standards for Neurologic Classification of Spinal Cord Injury
MD	Mean Difference
mJOA	modified Japanese Orthopedic Association
MPSS	Methylprednisolone Sodium Succinate
NACTN	North American Clinical Trials Network
NASCIS-II	Second National Acute Spinal Cord Injury Study
NF	Neurofilament
NF-M	Neurofilament Medium Chain
NPRS	Numeric Pain Rating Scale
OR	Odds Ratio
PCS	Physical Component Score
PD	Pharmacodynamic
pNF-H	phosphorylated Neurofilament Heavy Chain
PK	Pharmacokinetic
RCTs	Randomized Controlled Trials
RGMa	Repulsive Guidance Molecule-a
RISCIS	Riluzole in Spinal Cord Injury Study
SCI	Spinal Cord Injury
SCIM	Spinal Cord Independence Measure
ΔTMS	Change in Total Motor Score
tSCI	traumatic Spinal Cord Injury
V	Volume of Distribution
VAS	Visual Analog Scale

by a convergence of pathologic mechanisms, including ischemia, disruption of ionic homeostasis, glutamate-mediated excitotoxicity, oxidative stress, inflammation, and apoptotic cell death.[1,4]

Riluzole, a benzothiazole compound approved by the US Food and Drug Administration to treat amyotrophic lateral sclerosis (ALS), has emerged as a leading candidate for neuroprotection in SCI. Its primary mechanisms of action include inhibition of voltage-gated sodium channels and modulation of glutamatergic neurotransmission, both of which are central to the pathophysiology of secondary SCI.[5,6] By stabilizing neuronal membranes, reducing sodium influx, and limiting calcium-mediated excitotoxicity, Riluzole has been shown in preclinical models to preserve white matter integrity, reduce lesion volume, and improve functional recovery.[5,6]

Beyond acute injury, converging evidence suggests that mechanisms underlying secondary injury, particularly excitotoxicity and ionic dysregulation, may persist in other forms of spinal cord pathology, further supporting investigation of Riluzole across spinal cord disorders.[6,7] Recent randomized trials and secondary analyses using global statistical approaches have demonstrated that Riluzole may improve motor function, pain, and health-related quality of life, reinforcing its relevance as a disease-modifying therapy rather than a narrowly targeted agent.[8]

Riluzole is among the most extensively studied neuroprotective agents in human SCI, with a uniquely strong foundation spanning mechanistic rationale, pharmacologic characterization, and randomized clinical investigation. Yet significant gaps remain in defining the precise clinical role of Riluzole. Variability in treatment response, uncertainty regarding optimal therapeutic windows, and the absence of validated biomarkers for patient stratification continue to limit definitive conclusions. Thus, the purpose of this narrative review is to compile the current evidence on Riluzole derived from RCTs, secondary analyses, and systematic evaluations, with a focus on pharmacologic mechanisms, pathophysiology of tSCI, effects on neurologic and functional outcome measures, and implications for future clinical translation.

MATERIALS AND METHODS OF STUDY SELECTION

This review includes human studies, human RCTs, and meta-analyses on Riluzole in compressed spine of humans, encompassing traumatic or degenerative spine causes. Articles cited within the results were also evaluated for inclusion. Animal studies were excluded because our purpose was to summarize evidence about Riluzole in human tSCI. On November 19, 2025, 16:50:52 PubMed was searched using the Medical Subject Headline "(Riluzole) AND (spinal cord injury)" and filters were applied for years 2015 to 2025 (Teleale F.

Gebeyehu). The search returned 82 articles, of which human studies, human RCTs, meta-analyses and secondary analyses of primary data were selected by title and abstract screening (TFG) leaving 10 studies[8–17] for full review. Two additional studies[18,19] were identified from citations that were deemed to be foundational, although published before 2015 (**Fig. 1**).[20] These were publications based on Phase I study of Riluzole in tSCI patients and contained significant preliminary findings relevant to this review. Of the 10 studies initially identified, one study included the rationale behind the need to study Riluzole for SCI.[12] Four studies[9,16,18,19] focused on pharmacokinetic, pharmacodynamic, safety, efficacy and clinical outcomes, as they were findings from Phase I and II/III studies as well as interim or various forms of analysis of the data from these phases of studies. Four other studies[10,11,14,15] were RCTs evaluating clinical effectiveness of Riluzole, 3[11,14,15] of which were on tSCI and one[10] on non-tSCI (degenerative cervical myelopathy). Two studies were a secondary data analysis of primary studies[8,13] and the final study was a meta-analysis.[17] All authors approved the final outline and article selection (Teleale F. Gebeyehu, Adam Leibold, Ashmal Sami Kabani, and James S. Harrop). Other references were added as needed to supplement the main findings of these studies. A brief discussion of other neuroprotective agents is also provided to inform readers about other current investigations in the areas of neuroprotection and neuroregeneration for tSCI.

DISCUSSION

Riluzole in Traumatic Spinal Cord Injury

Early animal investigations characterized the PK, safety, and preliminary efficacy of Riluzole in the acute postinjury setting.[21] Promising findings prompted a Phase I trial conducted in 6 North American Clinical Trials Network (NACTN) hospitals.[18,19] The prospective multicenter Phase I matched-comparison trial (n = 36) demonstrated that Riluzole administered within 12 hours of tSCI was well tolerated, with manageable transient elevations in liver enzymes and no serious drug-related AEs.[19] This study reported greater improvements in motor scores among Riluzole-treated patients compared with matched registry controls, particularly in cervical injuries, providing early clinical signals of efficacy.[19] Importantly, Riluzole's established clinical safety profile, oral bioavailability, and central nervous system penetration warranted large-scale evaluation in the acute trauma setting.

Rationale Behind Riluzole in Spinal Cord Injury Study

These findings informed the design of subsequent multicenter RCTs, notably the Riluzole in Spinal Cord Injury Study (RISCIS), a multicenter, randomized, placebo-controlled Phase IIb/III trial powered to detect clinically meaningful changes in motor outcomes when Riluzole was administered within 12 hours of injury.[11,12] Although challenges related to enrollment and study execution limited definitive conclusions, secondary analyses and complementary investigations have continued to elucidate Riluzole's therapeutic profile, including its PK variability and exposure–response relationships.[6,9,11,13] Collectively, these studies have highlighted the importance of timing, dosing, and patient selection in maximizing neuroprotective benefit. The trial's design has also influenced contemporary approaches to SCI clinical research,

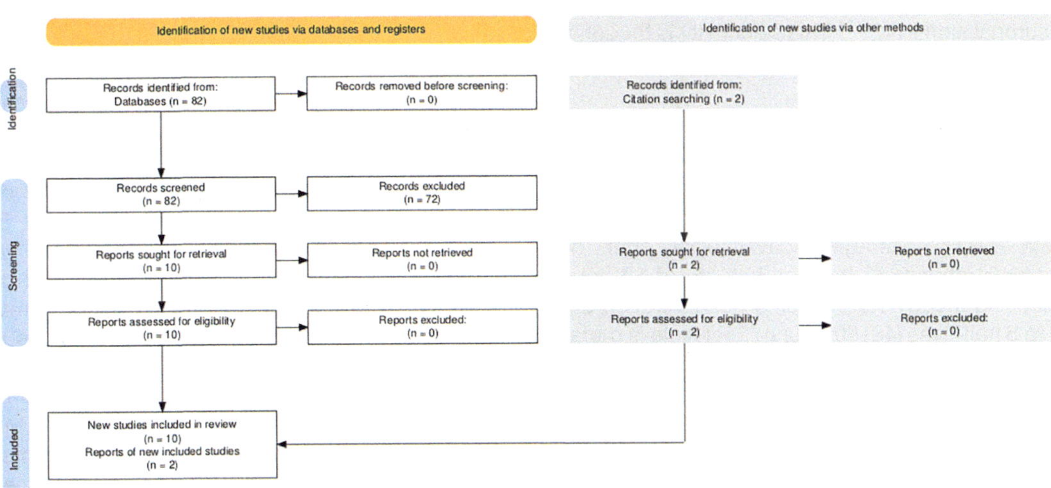

Fig. 1. Preferred reporting items for systematic reviews and meta-analyses (PRISMA) flow chart showing methods of study selection for reviewing Riluzole in humans with spinal cord injury. (Created using Shiny APP.)

emphasizing timing, biological plausibility, and patient-centered outcome metrics.

RISCIS represents a critical milestone in SCI therapeutics by establishing feasibility, safety, and the value of multidimensional outcome assessment beyond single primary endpoints.[9,11,13]

Neuroprotective Effect of Riluzole

PK investigations from RISCIS have further highlighted that acute SCI alters drug disposition, with time-dependent changes in clearance and volume of distribution influencing therapeutic exposure.[9,16] Importantly, Riluzole exposure has been linked to reductions in phosphorylated neurofilament heavy chain (pNF-H) levels, a biomarker of axonal injury, supporting a biologically meaningful neuroprotective effect in humans with SCI.[9] Thus, Riluzole's mechanism of action aligns closely with key drivers of secondary injury in SCI, offering a mechanistically targeted approach to mitigating excitotoxic and ionic-mediated neurodegeneration during the acute and subacute phases of injury.

Molecular Structure of Riluzole

Riluzole is a low-molecular-weight benzothiazole derivative with the chemical designation 2-amino-6-(trifluoromethoxy) benzothiazole.[5] Its benzothiazole core confers lipophilicity, facilitating efficient penetration across the blood–brain and blood–spinal cord barriers, a prerequisite for central neuroprotective activity.

The presence of a trifluoromethoxy substituent enhances metabolic stability and contributes to its affinity for voltage-gated sodium channels. Riluzole preferentially inhibits persistent sodium currents rather than transient physiologic channel activity, allowing it to attenuate pathologic depolarization without complete suppression of normal neuronal signaling.[5,16] This selectivity is thought to underlie its favorable safety profile in chronic neurologic conditions.

Pharmacokinetic Considerations

Previous studies have shown Riluzole is highly protein bound (96%) to albumin and lipoproteins with ~60% average bioavailability after oral administration.[22–24] It has a half-life of 12 hours, reaching steady state plasma concentration after 4 to 5 half-lives (48–60 hours).[18] Riluzole is metabolized by CYP 1A2, a subfamily of the CYP 450 family, leading to glucuronidation and urinary excretion. Only 2% of the dose is found in the urine unchanged.[22,25]

The PK and PD of Riluzole in humans with SCI were studied in both Phase I and II/III studies. In the Phase I study,[18] using human-equivalent dose and benefit-to-risk ratio reports based on previous studies, patients received PO/NG tube, tablet or crushed Riluzole 50 mg b.i.d for 14 days, starting at a mean time 8.7 $\pm$ 2.2 hours after injury. In Phase II/III, patients were given a 100 mg b.i.d dose for the first day and were maintained on 50 mg b.i.d for the remaining 13 days. For Phase I, sampling was 1 hour pre dose and 1 to 2 hours post dose on days 3 and 7. For Phase II/III, sampling was immediately before dose and approximately 3 hours after dose.

The Phase I and II/III studies[9,16,18] identified that median maximum concentration (Cmax), minimum concentration (Cmin), and Area Under Curve in 12 hours ($AUC_{0\text{-}12\ hours}$) were significantly higher on day 3 than day 14. These are due to lower hepatic blood flow causing low clearance (CL), hepatic gene expression, and smaller volume of distribution (V) on day 3 of SCI that increased by day 14 as these derangements subsided. In the Phase I study, extents of reduction were 68.6% and 56.5% for Cmax and Cmin, respectively, but half-life remained constant since both factors affecting it (CL and V) were offsetting each other with a comparable magnitude. Model for the time dependent PK of Riluzole is given in **Fig. 2** and explained in **Box 1**.

Pharmacodynamic Considerations

Change in total motor score

In Phase II/III,[9,11] compared to Phase I, a higher proportion of patients in the treatment group had higher gains in Total Motor Score (ΔTMS). Also, linear regression of the correlation of the ΔTMS with C_{peak} or C_{trough} (peak and minimum concentrations) of Riluzole did not result in an appreciable relationship. An initial attempt to correlate ΔTMS with Area Under Curve of 14 days Riluzole Exposure ([$AUC_{D0\text{-}D14}$] total exposure to Riluzole over 14 days) was performed (P = .028) but was inadequate to capture all subjects with high or low baseline (BL) TMS. Subsequently, ΔTMS in individual Riluzole-treated SCI patients at 6 months post-treatment was correlated with the $AUC_{D0\text{-}D14}$ and the BL TMS, showing the efficacy of the treatment was affected by both Riluzole exposure and the severity of the injury at BL. Based on this correlation, optimal outcomes were noted for exposure in the 16 to 48 mg*h/mL range at BL motor scores of 1 to 36. This finding established PK/PD correlation of ΔTMS with $AUC_{D0\text{-}D14}$ and BL TMS. Such formulation enables clinicians to project the optimal exposure range of Riluzole treatment ($AUC_{D0\text{-}D14}$) to achieve the intended clinical

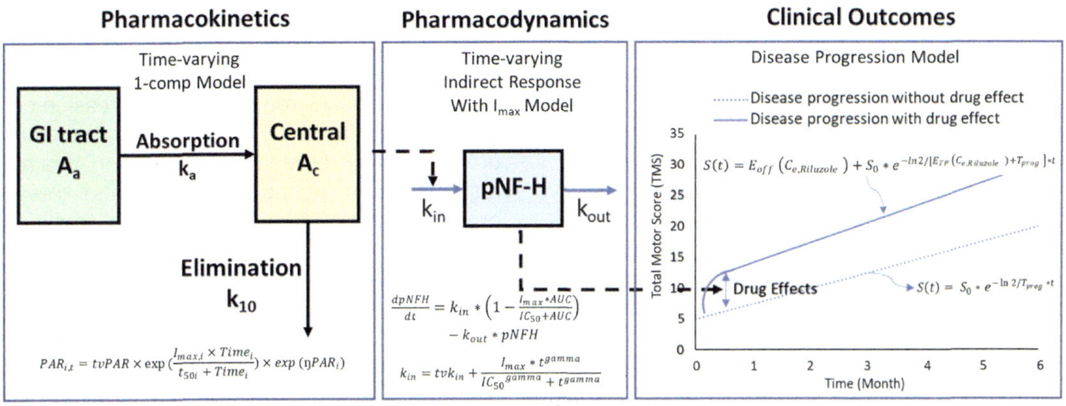

Fig. 2. Proposed model scheme of population PK, PD, pNF-H, and clinical outcome of Riluzole therapy in acute SCI population. (Chow DS, Nguyen A, Park J, et al. Riluzole in Spinal Cord Injury Study (RISCIS)-Pharmacokinetic (PK) Sub-Study: An Analysis of Pharmacokinetics, Pharmacodynamics, and Impact on Axonal Degradation of Riluzole in Patients with Traumatic Cervical Spinal Cord Injury Enrolled in the RISCIS Phase III Randomized Controlled Trial. J Neurotrauma. Sep 2023;40(17–18):1889–1906. Used by permission from Mary Ann Liebert Inc./Sage Publications.)

outcome (CO) in ΔTMS individually for patients (**Box 2**). Of note, correlations of changes in upper and lower-limb motor scores at 3 and 6 months did not result in apparent patterns.

Box 1
Model for time dependent pharmacokinetics of Riluzole

To explain the time-dependent change in PK parameters, one-compartment model incorporating empirical equations for time-varying clearance and volume of distribution (both normalized by bioavailability), using Phase I/II/III data, was established using Michaelis Menten Kinetics:

$$PAR_{i,t} = tvPAR \times exp\left(\frac{I_{max,i}.Time_i}{t50_i + Time_i}\right) \times exp(\eta PAR_i)$$

Where $PAR_{i,t}$ is the parameter value of individual í at time t; *tvPAR* is the typical value of PK parameters for the population; $I_{max,i}$ is the maximal fold-change of that parameter relative to baseline; $Time_i$ is the time after the first dose in individual í; $t50_i$ indicates the time at which 50% of I_{max} is reached; and ηPAR_i is interpatient variability in the parameter estimate for individual í. This model was checked by simulated datasets and prediction intervals at 95%, showing it captured the observed data, confirming the model.

Chow DS, Nguyen A, Park J, et al. Riluzole in Spinal Cord Injury Study (RISCIS)-Pharmacokinetic (PK) Sub-Study: An Analysis of Pharmacokinetics, Pharmacodynamics, and Impact on Axonal Degradation of Riluzole in Patients With Traumatic Cervical Spinal Cord Injury Enrolled in the RISCIS Phase III Randomized Controlled Trial. J Neurotrauma. Sep 2023;40(17–18):1889–1906. https://doi.org/10.1089/neu.2022.0499.

Effect of riluzole on phosphorylated neurofilament—heavy

Following neuronal damage, Neurofilaments (NF) are present in the bloodstream. The NF-H is the *heavy* or *high* subunit of the neurofilaments, belonging to a family of axonal proteins that form the neuronal cytoskeleton.[26] The protein NF-H, together with neurofilament medium chain (NF-M) and neurofilament light chain (NF-L), make

Box 2
Model of pharmacodynamics—clinical outcomes

It was possible to calculate the desired $AUC_{D0\text{-}D14}$, hence the desired dose and regime of Riluzole, using known baseline (BL) Total Motor Score (TMS) of an acute spinal cord injury patient and the desired, achievable clinical outcome goal of change (Δ) TMS at 6-month (6M), using the following equation:

$$\Delta TMS, 6M = -185.45 + 8.7 \times (BL) + 12.24 \times (AUC_{D0-D14}) - 0.13 \times (BL) \times (AUC_{D0-D14}) - 0.12 \times (BL)^2 - 0.15 \times (AUC_{D0-D14})^2$$

Chow DS, Nguyen A, Park J, et al. Riluzole in Spinal Cord Injury Study (RISCIS)-Pharmacokinetic (PK) Sub-Study: An Analysis of Pharmacokinetics, Pharmacodynamics, and Impact on Axonal Degradation of Riluzole in Patients With Traumatic Cervical Spinal Cord Injury Enrolled in the RISCIS Phase III Randomized Controlled Trial. J Neurotrauma. Sep 2023;40(17–18):1889–1906. doi:10.1089/neu.2022.0499.

up the neurofilament triplet.[26,27] Resistant to proteolytic enzymes, pNF-H is the ideal candidate out of the subunits for detection in human plasma and is shown to be elevated corresponding to the severity of SCI.[27,28]

Riluzole exerts its clinical impact indirectly through inhibition of axonal/neuronal degeneration; this is pharmacodynamically measured by the reduction of pNF-H production. The net drug effect will then be quantified by the difference between AUC showing concentration of pNF-H for treated and untreated patients during the treatment period, which is known as area between baseline and effective curve (ABEC). In patients treated with Riluzole, ΔTMS at 6 months is significantly correlated with this ABEC by multiple regression (**Fig. 2**).[9] This finding was proved to be accurate as treated patients had diminished progression of pNF-H, indicating drug efficacy. Model for time-dependent effect of Riluzole on pNF-H is explained in **Box 3**.

Box 3
Model for time dependent effect of riluzole on phosphorylated neurofilament—heavy

In the Phase II/III study, the time-dependent impact of Riluzole on pNF-H was quantified using Sigmoidal E max function with a multiplicative residual error model as follows,

$$\frac{\Delta pNFH}{\Delta t} = K_{in}\left(1 - \frac{I_{max} \times AUC}{IC_{50} + AUC}\right) - K_{out} \times pNFH_{nat}$$

Where–K_{in} and K_{out} define the rateconstants of production and loss of pNF-H, respectively. I_{max} represents maximum fractional inhibition by Riluzole, and IC_{50} indicates the AUC at which half I_{max} is reached, and $pNFH_{nat}$ is the progressive baseline pNF-H. Simply, the model depicts the change in pNF-H is described by subtracting the rate of elimination of pNF-H (K_{out}) from the blood stream corrected by natural time-dependent progression of pNF-H $(pNFH_{nat})$ from the rate of production of pNF-H (K_{in}) affected by the drug $\left(1 - \frac{I_{max} \times AUC}{IC_{50} + AUC}\right)$.

Chow DS, Nguyen A, Park J, et al. Riluzole in Spinal Cord Injury Study (RISCIS)-Pharmacokinetic (PK) Sub-Study: An Analysis of Pharmacokinetics, Pharmacodynamics, and Impact on Axonal Degradation of Riluzole in Patients With Traumatic Cervical Spinal Cord Injury Enrolled in the RISCIS Phase III Randomized Controlled Trial. J Neurotrauma. Sep 2023;40(17–18):1889–1906. doi:10.1089/neu.2022.0499.

Clinical outcome considerations

The final development of a clinical outcomes model for Riluzole considered disease-progression components that included BL clinical status, natural progression of disease over time, and treatment response in offsetting symptoms and disease-progression modification. In simple terms, the model defines clinical motor function status at a specific time by symptom-relieving effect of Riluzole, plus the initial motor function state as modified by time-dependent progression of motor function that is modified by Riluzole (**Box 4**). The net clinical benefit, therefore, is identified by the area difference between the curves for motor scores between placebo and Riluzole-treated patients (see **Fig. 2**).

TOXICOLOGY AND SIDE EFFECT CONSIDERATIONS

Comparison of severe AEs between the Riluzole group and cohort in the NACTN registry, both

Box 4
Model for final clinical outcome

The final PD impact model of Riluzole predicting clinical outcome in terms of motor function and symptom offset was defined by:

$$S(t) = E_{off}\left(C_{e,Riluzole}\right) + S_o \times e^{\frac{-ln\,2}{\left[E_{TP}\left(C_{e,Riluzole}\right) + T_{Prog}\right]} \times t}$$

Where $S(t)$ refers to motor status (clinical parameter) at time t, $E_{off}\left(C_{e,Riluzole}\right)$ refers to symptom offsetting by Riluzole, S_o refers to motor function status at BL, $E_{TP}\left(C_{e,Riluzole}\right)$ represents the time course of the effect of Riluzole concentrations at the effect site, and T_{Prog} refers to the half-life of natural SCI progression. In simple terms, the model defines clinical motor function status at a time (t) by symptom relieving effect of Riluzole, $\left[E_{off}\left(C_{e,Riluzole}\right)\right]$, plus the initial motor function state $[S_o]$ as modified by time-dependent progression $[T_{Prog}\ exponential\ (ln\ 2)]$ and further modified by Riluzole, $\left[E_{TP}\left(C_{e,Riluzole}\right)\right]$. The net clinical benefit, therefore, is identified by the area difference between the curves for motor scores between placebo and Riluzole-treated patients

Chow DS, Nguyen A, Park J, et al. Riluzole in Spinal Cord Injury Study (RISCIS)-Pharmacokinetic (PK) Sub-Study: An Analysis of Pharmacokinetics, Pharmacodynamics, and Impact on Axonal Degradation of Riluzole in Patients With Traumatic Cervical Spinal Cord Injury Enrolled in the RISCIS Phase III Randomized Controlled Trial. J Neurotrauma. Sep 2023; 40(17–18):1889–1906. doi:10.1089/neu.2022.0499.

matched and total reported in the registry, showed no significant difference.[9,18] No severe AEs or deaths were attributable to Riluzole, but there were mild-to-moderate elevations of bilirubin, alkaline phosphatase (ALP), alanine transaminase (ALT), aspartate transaminase (AST), and gamma-glutamyl transferase (GGT). There were 3 borderline severe elevations of ALT, AST, and GGT each in 3 different patients. The elevations were normalized mostly on the next day of testing, and the severely elevated enzymes were normal at 3 and 6 months' follow-up. Cmax of Riluzole and liver enzyme levels were found to be unrelated. In the Phase II/III study, no appreciable hepatic toxicity was reported.

Summary of molecular structure, PK, PD, and toxicity discussions are displayed in **Table 1**.

CLINICAL EFFICACY ANALYSIS

Preliminary Analysis of Efficacy from Phase I of Riluzole in Spinal Cord Injury Study

Motor score from Phase 1 Riluzole data[19] showed statistically significant improvement in motor score for all patients at 90 days after injury (+15.5 compared to registry patients, P = .021) but highest statistically significant benefit in American Spinal Injury Association Impairment Scale (AIS) B patients (+27.9 points compared to registry patients, P = .037). At 180 days, Riluzole showed a benefit in improving motor scores in those with AIS A, B, and cumulatively in all patients, but not to a statistically significant level when compared to registry patients. Pinprick, light touch, and AIS conversion were better for patients on Riluzole both at 90 and 180 days.

Phase II/III Analysis of Clinical Efficacy from Riluzole in Spinal Cord Injury Study

The RISCIS Phase II/III study[9] was prematurely terminated after enrolling 193 of the planned 351 patients (55%) due to the global corona virus disease 2019 (COVID-19) pandemic, limiting the study. However, important findings suggested benefits of Riluzole. At 180 days, the Riluzole-treated patients compared to placebo had an average of 1.8 points gained on upper extremity motor score, 1.45 points in lower extremity motor score, and 2.86 points higher ΔTMS, but none

Table 1
Summary of molecular structure, pharmacokinetic, pharmacodynamics, and toxicity considerations for Riluzole

Topic	Key Points
Riluzole Structure	2-amino-6-(trifluoromethoxy) benzothiazole Benzothiazole confers lipophilicity. Trifluoromethoxy confers metabolic stability and affinity for voltage-gated sodium channels.
Riluzole in Humans with SCI—Phase I study	Riluzole is well tolerated. Transient and manageable, mostly mild-to-moderate, liver enzyme elevation. No serious AE. Improvement in motor score among treated patients compared to previous patients (registry).
RISCIS - Phase IIb/III	
Pharmacokinetics	Riluzole administered within 12 hours of SCI. ~ 60% oral bioavailability. 96% albumin and lipoprotein bound. Half-life—12 hours. Maximum and trough concentrations—highest on day 3, normalize on day 14. Metabolized by CYP 1A2 - Glucuronidation and urinary excretion. 2% found in urine unchanged.
Pharmacodynamics	Effect on TMS depends on Riluzole exposure and baseline injury severity than maximum or minimum plasma concentrations. Optimal outcomes in TMS at 16–48 mg*h/ml and baseline motor score 1–36. Mechanism of effect is indirect - inhibits neurodegeneration. Effect is measured by reduction in phosphorylated neurofilament—heavy.
Toxicity	Generally safe, no death reported. No appreciable hepatic toxicity reported in Phase IIb/III study.

*Abbreviations:*AE, adverse effect; CYP 1A2, Cytochrome 1A2; mg*h/ml, milligram-hour per milliliter; TMS, total motor score.

were proved to be statistically significant, likely due to low power. At 180 days, gains were also higher in the Riluzole group in Spinal Cord Independence Measure (SCIM; 33.9 vs 27.8), neurologic levels (1.2 vs 0.4), SF-36 mental (−3.0 vs −5.2) and physical component (−23.5 vs −25.5), and European Quality of Life 5-dimension health state (EQ5D -HS) change (−14.9 vs −17.4). All were statistically insignificant.

In subgroup analysis of various outcomes at 180 days, patients with American Spinal Injury Association (ASIA) grades A and B who received Riluzole had certain outcomes that were close to being statistically significant by the *P*-value set in RISCIS (0.025). In AIS A cohort neurologic levels gained (0.5 vs 0.12, *P* = .077) were higher in the Riluzole group. In the AIS B cohort, the following were higher in the Riluzole-treated group: SCIM total score (45.3 vs 27.3, *P* = .036), SCIM respiratory management (18.9 vs 11.9, *P* = .041), SCIM self-care (10 vs 5.5, *P* = .032), SF36-MCS (1.6 vs −11.7, *P* = .012) and EQ5D HS (−12.1 vs −29.7, *P* = .031). For patients with AIS C, those who received Riluzole had higher chances of total and upper motor score changes (beta coefficients 13.8 and 7.96, p - values 0.011 and 0.016, respectively).

Assessment of neurologic recovery in tSCI relies heavily on standardized outcome measures, including the International Standards for Neurologic Classification of Spinal Cord Injury and associated motor and sensory scores.[29] While these metrics remain the cornerstone of clinical trials, their sensitivity to multidimensional recovery has been increasingly scrutinized. Considering these findings and the limitations observed in using single outcome measures and defining significance clinically, especially in the context of Riluzole's impact on the secondary injury cascade in SCI, the researchers suggested integrating functional outcomes, using biomarkers such as pNF-H and adding imaging in analyzing the benefits of Riluzole. Therefore, contemporary analyses emphasize the need to integrate neurologic, functional, and patient-reported outcomes to more comprehensively capture treatment effects, particularly for neuroprotective interventions expected to produce incremental but meaningful gains.[13] Observing the limitation of single primary endpoints to assess the effect of Riluzole, the same data from RISCIS trial, a multivariate nonparametric global statistical test (O'Brien's rank sum test), was used to assess the overall impact Riluzole has.[13] The analysis integrated ASIA, TMS, SCIM, and SF-36 PCS, and the respective rank sums for the values in these endpoints, with higher rank sums indicating better global (overall) patient outcomes. The results revealed that the Riluzole group exhibited a higher rank sum compared to placebo [median rank sum = 207 (Inter Quartile Range [IQR]: 166–246) in Riluzole versus 185 (IQR: 146–236) in placebo, *P* ≈ .04. Also, all patients receiving Riluzole had a 55% probability of having overall (Global) improvement compared to placebo (*P* = .04); AIS A patients had a 58% probability of overall improvement compared to placebo. The small sample size precluded statistical significance in AIS subgroups B and C, but positive treatment effects of Riluzole were observed for both subgroups. However, it should be underscored while global statistical approaches are innovative, they should be interpreted with caution and clearly framed as hypothesis-generating rather than confirmatory.

Other Randomized Controlled Trials of Clinical Efficacy and Safety

Kumarsamay and colleagues[14] performed an RCT in a tertiary institute in India to examine the safety, efficacy, implications, and benefits of Riluzole for incomplete cervical SCI. The study was conducted in a small cohort containing treatment group (n = 23) and control group (n = 20) with final analysis done on 21 of the treated and 17 of the control patients due to patient deaths in each group. The treatment dose was comparable to RISCIS. The study assessed change in motor, sensory, SCIM, Numeric Pain Rating Scale (NPRS) and AISA conversion at 6 weeks and 3, 6, and 12 months. Both groups showed similar and a statistically significant improvement in the outcome measures as time progressed when compared to the BL values. However, comparing the groups revealed no significant differences in all the variables at all times. When calculated, the net gains from the mean values in the published study showed a very small difference in the scores of the variables at 6 months and 1 year. Net gain at 1 year for Riluzole versus control, respectively, was 43.7 versus 44.8 for motor score, 59.6 versus 67.3 for sensory score, 78.2 versus 74.3 for SCIM III, and −7.9 versus −7.8 for NPRS. There were no Riluzole-associated AEs reported. However, this study had a very small number of patients, excluded AISA A patients up to 72 hours interval from injury to Riluzole administration, and depended on clinical rather than biological or radiological markers to measure the effect of Riluzole treatment. It would also have benefitted from calculating the global treatment effect (GTE) combining various outcomes.

The other RCT studying Riluzole was conducted in Iran by Meshkini and colleagues.[15] The study included 60 patients transferred to a university hospital after SCI with 30 patients in the Riluzole group. Although the inclusion criteria were similar to the RISCIS, the measure of neurologic impairment was Frankel grade. Patients with Frankel grades A–C and injury levels C4–L2 were included. The exact timing of Riluzole administration and surgical intervention after injury was not specified, and Riluzole was administered at a dose of 50 mg every 12 hr for 8 weeks. No International Standards for Neurologic Classification of Spinal Cord Injury (ISNCSCI) motor and sensory scores were reported before and after treatment. The study reported patients benefitted from Riluzole at 6 months in the areas of motor and sensory scores based on Frankel score changes, but it reported no benefit for pain measured in visual analog scale (VAS). Despite the details of motor and sensory benefits being not clearly quantified, the average VAS score was shown to be better for the control group by 0.2 points. There were no Riluzole-associated AEs reported. The small number of patients limited the study findings, as well as the design, execution, and reporting. Therefore, it is challenging to make a quantitative estimation or comment on the net benefit of Riluzole based on this published report.

Insight from a Meta-Analysis

Weisbrod and colleagues[17] conducted a systematic review with meta-analyses to evaluate the safety and efficacy of Riluzole compared with placebo or standard of care in adults with acute tSCI. The meta-analyses used 5 of the studies we reviewed in this article.[9,11,14,15,19] Using a data from 378 patients, of whom 187 received Riluzole and 191 served as controls, the study demonstrated that Riluzole treatment was associated with higher ASIA motor scores at both 3 months (mean difference [MD] 0.26; 95% CI −0.10–0.61; I^2 = 0%) and 6 months (MD 0.21; 95% CI −0.17–0.60; I^2 = 0%) compared with controls; however, these differences did not reach statistical significance. Similarly, Riluzole was associated with increased odds of AIS grade improvement at 3 months (odds ratio [OR] 0.59; 95% CI −0.12–1.30; I^2 = 0%) and 6 months (OR 0.28; 95% CI −0.50–1.06; I^2 = 0%), though again without statistical significance.

Regarding safety outcomes, Riluzole was not associated with an increased incidence of AEs compared with controls (OR 0.12; 95% CI −1.59–1.35; I^2 = 0%). No AEs were directly attributed to Riluzole, and transient liver enzyme elevations were reported without clinically significant sequelae. Mortality was numerically lower in the Riluzole group (OR 0.20; 95% CI −1.03–0.63; I^2 = 0%), though this difference was not statistically significant.

Overall, the meta-analysis demonstrated that Riluzole administration in acute tSCI is safe and associated with consistent trends toward improved neurologic outcomes, although pooled effects did not achieve statistical significance. It also demonstrated consistent trends toward improved neurologic outcomes without increased AEs. Although pooled analyses did not achieve statistical significance for ASIA motor score improvement or AIS grade conversion at 3 or 6 months, the directionality of effect consistently favored Riluzole. It also confirmed Riluzole's favorable safety profile, with no significant increase in AEs or mortality compared with controls. These findings support the biological plausibility and clinical tolerability observed in individual trials, including RISCIS, and emphasize the impact of limited sample size and heterogeneity on statistical power rather than absence of therapeutic signal.

RILUZOLE IN DEGENERATIVE CERVICAL MYELOPATHY—EFFECT ON CLINICAL, FUNCTIONAL, AND PATIENT-REPORTED OUTCOMES

Clinical evaluation of Riluzole in degenerative cervical myelopathy (DCM) has provided important insights into its multidimensional effects beyond traditional neurologic scoring systems. The primary CSM-PROTECT trial demonstrated no significant difference in improvement in modified Japanese Orthopedic Association (mJOA) scores at 6 months between Riluzole and placebo when assessed as a single endpoint.[10] However, subsequent secondary and global analyses revealed a more nuanced therapeutic profile.

Using a global statistical test integrating multiple outcome domains, including ASIA motor score, Nurick grade, SF-36 Physical Component Score (PCS), and pain measures, Riluzole was associated with a significantly greater probability of overall clinical improvement at 1 year.[8] This composite approach captured benefits that were not fully reflected by mJOA alone, highlighting limitations of unidimensional outcome measures in DCM.

Riluzole-treated patients demonstrated favorable trends or significant improvements across motor and sensory scores, grip strength, and functional independence metrics. Patient-reported outcomes, including neck and arm pain assessed by Numeric Rating Scales, showed meaningful reductions, aligning with observed improvements in quality-of-life indices such as SF-36 PCS and EQ-5D.[8,10] Improvements in dysphagia severity, measured by the Bazaz scale, and reductions in arm and shoulder pain further suggest a broader symptomatic benefit.

Notably, Riluzole's GTE analysis indicated a greater than 50% probability of achieving superior outcomes compared with placebo, underscoring its potential role as an adjunctive therapy in surgically managed DCM.[8] These findings reinforce the importance of multidimensional assessment frameworks when evaluating neuroprotective agents in chronic compressive myelopathy. Summary of the clinical effects of Riluzole discussed is given in **Table 2**.

OTHER AGENTS OF INTEREST

Methylprednisolone Sodium Succinate

Steroids, especially methylprednisolone sodium succinate (MPSS), commonly methylprednisolone, have been highly investigated as neuroprotective agents in tSCI.[30–32] Steroids in general reduce inflammation and theoretically would be expected to mitigate the secondary cascade of SCI that ensues.[30–32] Yet they have also been one of the most contended drugs in the tSCI setting, with references to minimal clinical benefit and associated systemic AEs.[33–38] After a long period of questioning their use according to Second National Acute Spinal Cord Injury Study (NASCIS-II) protocol, the AO spine gave recommendations on the use of steroids, suggesting a 24-hour infusion of high-dose MPSS for patients presenting within 8 hours of injury but not for injuries presenting after 8 hours (weak recommendation based on a moderate evidence).[39] In addition, 48 hours of high-dose MPSS was not recommended (weak recommendation; no studies included).[39] Recent meta-analyses and systematic reviews overall suggest against their use in SCI.[36–38] However, by using a combined dataset from the North American Clinical Trials Network SCI registry, Surgical Timing in

Table 2
Summary of the clinical effects of Riluzole

Topic	Key Points
Clinical Efficacy	
RISCIS - Phase IIb/III	Limited by termination of study due to global COVID-19 pandemic. Primary end points were not met. *All Patients* Treatment arm had slightly higher average in UEMS, LEMS and ΔTMS at 180 days - statistically insignificant. Treatment arm had higher neurologic levels, SCIM, SF-36 MCS and PCS, and EQ5D - HS change - satistically insignificant. Treatment arm had 55% probability of global improvement (combining AIS, TMS, SCIM and SF-36 PCS) using GTE analysis - statistically significant. *AIS - A* Nuerological level gained is higher and almost significant for treatment arm. Treatment arm had 58% probability of global improvement using GTE analysis. *AIS - B* SCIM (total, respiratory management and slef-care) and EQ5D -HS was higher and amost significant, $0.05 > P > .025$, in treatment arm. SF36-MCS is higher and significant in treatment arm. *AIS - C* Treatment arm had statistically significant higher odds of changes in TMS and UEMS.
Meta-Analysis	Riluzole treated individuals had higher ASIA motor scores at 3 and 6 months - statistically insignificant. Riluzole treated individuals had higher odds of AIS improvement at 3 and 6 months - statistically insignificant. No increased incidence of AE.
CSM-Protect Trial	No significant difference in mJOA scores between treatment and placebo. Treatment arm had >50% probability of superior global outcomes using GTE analysis.

Abbreviations: AIS, American Spinal Injury Association (ASIA) Impairment Score; COVID-19, Corona Virus Disease 2019, CSM, Cervical Spondylotic Myelopathy; EQ5D - HS, European Quality of Life 5 Dimensions - Health State; GTE, global treatment effect; LEMS, lower extremity motor score; MCS, mental component score; mJOA, modified Japanese Orthopaedic Association; PCS, physical component score; SCIM, spinal cord independence measure; SF-36, short form 36; TMS, total motor score; UEMS, upper extremity motor score; ΔTMS, change in total motor score;

Acute Spinal Cord Injury Study, and the NASCIS-II, a newer study by Mimura and colleagues[40] showed MPSS was associated with improved lower extremity motor score in AIS A cervical SCI and fewer cardiopulmonary, gastrointestinal, and genitourinary AEs, indicating a potential subgroup of patients can benefit from it. Despite these controversies, their use in acute tSCI is still reported among some physicians in major SCI centers, although the majority report not using them.[41] Steroids remain a focus of research for tSCI.[42,43]

Nogo-A Inhibitors

Nogo-A is a membrane protein prevalent in myelin and is known to prevent neurite growth after SCI.[44] Therefore, it has been a target of neutralization to prevent neural growth inhibition. A recent Phase 2b trial in multiple European centers was conducted by Weidner and colleagues.[45] Patients received multiple bolus doses of the investigational intrathecal medication (ATI355 - antibody that inhibits Nogo-A). The medication was proved to be safe and feasible to administer with no significant difference in AEs or severe AEs between treatment and placebo arms. However, the treatment arm failed to meet the expected primary end point, which is a clinically significant recovery of upper extremity motor score (UEMS). Secondary end points were also not met. Notably, in a subgroup of patients with motor incomplete injury, there was a statistically significant but clinically insignificant improvement of UEMS and favorable SCIM self-care in the treatment arm. The favorable SCIM self-care was explained as a possibility due to a better UEMS recovery shown. These findings suggest that certain groups of SCI patients with spared neuronal bridge after trauma have a potentially favorable pathology that can be redirected toward recovery. This was also indirectly indicated in the study as the median (IQR) extent of preserved neural tissue within the cord of patients with motor incomplete injury was 1.9 mm (1.2–2.8) versus 0.85 mm (0–2.2) for motor complete injury on MRI, although overall findings in this study may not fully support this concept since multiple endpoints were not met.

It should be noted, however, that the study was mainly on neuro-regeneration rather than neuroprotection, where intervention took place days after tSCI occurred. In addition, CSF analysis for medication concentration showed potentially effect-compromising "dosing holiday" hours between doses, wherein the trough CSF concentration of the medication was below 10 μg/mL, the minimum required concentration for in vitro neurite outgrowth on a spinal cord extract substrate. Therefore, future studies that potentially adjust for these gaps may reveal its benefits.

Minocycline

Minocycline, a second-generation tetracycline antibiotic, has demonstrated neuroprotective potential through its pleiotropic anti-inflammatory and anti-apoptotic properties. Studies have consistently shown that minocycline attenuates microglial activation, reduces pro-inflammatory cytokine release, and inhibits caspase-dependent neuronal apoptosis. Shultz and Zhong[46] highlighted that minocycline targets multiple secondary injury pathways, including suppression of matrix metalloproteinases and reduction of oxidative stress, thereby preserving blood–spinal cord barrier integrity and limiting lesion expansion. These mechanisms are particularly relevant in the acute phase of tSCI, where secondary injury significantly contributes to neuronal loss.

Clinical applications of these findings have been encouraging but remain evolving. A recent study by Omair and colleagues[47] reported that minocycline administration in acute tSCI was associated with improved motor recovery trends, particularly in cervical injuries, although statistical significance varied across subgroups and functional significance was not established. Subtherapeutic central nervous system penetration was a noted challenge. Similarly, systematic analyses have supported minocycline's therapeutic promise. Hu and colleagues[48] through meta-analysis and network pharmacology, demonstrated that minocycline exerts multi-target effects involving inflammatory signaling pathways such as Nuclear Factor – Kappa B and mitogen-activated protein kinase, reinforcing its role as a broad-spectrum modulator of secondary injury. Despite these promising findings, variability in dosing regimens, timing of administration, and study design continues to limit definitive conclusions regarding its clinical efficacy. As noted by Sherrod and colleagues,[49] minocycline remains a compelling candidate for adjunctive therapy, though larger randomized trials are necessary to establish standardized protocols and confirm long-term benefits.

Repulsive Guidance Molecule-a Monoclonal Antibody

Repulsive guidance molecule-a (RGMa) has also been identified as a key inhibitory factor following central nervous system injury. After SCI, RGMa is upregulated and interacts with its receptor, neogenin, which activates intracellular pathways that inhibit axonal growth and limit plasticity. In experimental models, blocking this pathway not only enhances axonal sprouting but also preserves neural tissue and improves functional recovery. Notably, Jacobson and colleagues[50] demonstrated in a nonhuman primate model that treatment with elezanumab promoted corticospinal tract integrity and functional improvement, supporting the idea that RGMa inhibition may have a dual role of reducing secondary injury while facilitating repair.

Early-phase clinical trials of RGMa antibodies in humans have primarily focused on safety and PK. In a phase 1 study, Kalluri and colleagues[51] demonstrated elezanumab was well tolerated in both healthy participants and individuals with multiple sclerosis, with no statistically significant AEs. The drug had a cerebrospinal fluid (CSF) penetration of 0.1% to 0.4% with levels of free RGMa reduced by greater than 40% with maximal effect at 1800 mg IV. A subsequent study by Kalluri and colleagues[52] confirmed consistent safety and PK profiles across diverse populations, further supporting its clinical feasibility. In a randomized, placebo-controlled trial, Cree and colleagues[53] found that while elezanumab remained well tolerated, it did not produce significant improvement in clinical outcomes when added to standard therapy for multiple sclerosis. These results imply that while RGMa inhibition is biologically active and safe, its neuroprotective effects in humans may be limited or may require more precise timing, dosing, in combination with other therapies. Overall, RGMa is still a crucial target binding factor; however, recent human evidence suggests that its function in SCI is probably supportive rather than novel.

LIMITATIONS

There are certain limitations to this study. As this is a systematized narrative review, potential study selection bias can be present. Another limitation is the existing clinical evidence for Riluzole in SCI and DCM is constrained by underpowered trials, heterogeneity in injury severity, and reliance on single primary endpoints that may inadequately capture multidimensional recovery. Premature termination of RISCIS limited definitive conclusions regarding efficacy. It is also evident that primary endpoints in major RCTs (eg, RISCIS, CSM-PROTECT) were not met, and that evidence remains suggestive rather than definitive despite encouraging subgroup and GTE analyses.[11,13] However, GTE interpretation should be limited due to the hypothesis-generating rather than definitive nature of the analysis. Additionally, from the studies conducted to date, it is hard to conclude whether Riluzole is ready for routine use or if it should remain investigational. Yet these conclusions are severely limited due to multiple *unknowns*. Further, because phase II/III study was terminated prematurely, the developed models are not fully proven. Further data is needed to validate and enhance the power of PK/PD/CO models.

FUTURE DIRECTIONS

Future studies should prioritize adaptive trial designs, biomarker-guided dosing strategies, and CO measures integrating neurologic, functional, and patient-reported domains. PK-PD modeling may further optimize therapeutic exposure in the evolving physiologic milieu of acute SCI. Collectively, these strategies may better define Riluzole's role within a precision-based neuroprotective framework for SCI. Questions regarding routine use of Riluzole should also be addressed. Looking at the mechanism of action and the complex pathology of SCI, perhaps attaining the expected primary end points requires a technique that restores the damaged neural tissue within the cord. Riluzole may not be the agent for neuro-regenerative purposes, although it might have spared a substantial amount of neural tissue that could have been permanently damaged without its use. Therefore, considering its safety profile and suggested benefits, routine off-label use may be beneficial for patients as well as future studies, especially in situations where conducting RCTs presents logistical challenges.

SUMMARY

Across RCTs, secondary analyses, and systematic reviews, Riluzole has demonstrated a consistent pattern of safety and tolerability, with no significant increase in AEs compared with standard care or placebo. Although primary efficacy endpoints were not uniformly met, multiple studies have reported favorable trends toward improved neurologic, functional, and patient-reported outcomes. Emerging evidence suggests that traditional unidimensional outcome measures may underestimate the therapeutic impact of Riluzole, whereas multidimensional approaches are better suited to capture clinically meaningful benefits.

PK and PD analyses further underscore the importance of optimized dosing strategies and individualized exposure in the evolving physiologic environment of acute SCI. Together, these findings highlight Riluzole's potential role as a disease-modifying adjunct rather than a stand-alone therapy.

Future research should focus on adequately powered trials, biomarker-informed patient stratification, and outcome frameworks that reflect the multidimensional nature of recovery after SCI. Within this context, Riluzole continues to serve as a critical reference compound in the ongoing pursuit of effective neuroprotective therapies for SCI.

CLINICS CARE POINTS

- RISCIS showed that in SCI patients (ASIA A-C) presenting within 12 hours of injury may stand to benefit from a Riluzole use.
- Patients can be given 100mg BID Riluzole for the first 24 hours, followed by 50mg BID for 13 days.
- Patients on Riluzole should have their liver enzymes monitored for potential liver injury as the primary side effect, as well as monitored for respiratory complications and neutropenia, though, none of these side effects occurred at higher rates compared with placebo in the trial.

ACKNOWLEDGMENT

A special thanks to Pamela Walter at Thomas Jefferson University library for meticulously editing this article.

DISCLOSURE

Funding—The authors did not receive any funding for this work. Conflict of Interest—None.

REFERENCES

1. Ahuja CS, Nori S, Tetreault L, et al. Traumatic spinal cord injury-repair and regeneration. Neurosurgery 2017;80(3s):S9–22.
2. Hawryluk GW, Rowland J, Kwon BK, et al. Protection and repair of the injured spinal cord: a review of completed, ongoing, and planned clinical trials for acute spinal cord injury. Neurosurg Focus 2008; 25(5):E14.
3. An KD, Noh CY, Jang J, et al. Potential pharmacologic treatments in spinal cord injury: a narrative review. Korean J Neurotrauma 2025;21(4):237–54.
4. Ahuja CS, Fehlings M. Concise review: bridging the gap: novel neuroregenerative and neuroprotective strategies in spinal cord injury. Stem Cells Transl Med 2016;5(7):914–24.
5. Nagoshi N, Nakashima H, Fehlings MG. Riluzole as a neuroprotective drug for spinal cord injury: from bench to bedside. Molecules 2015;20(5): 7775–89.
6. Pedro KM, Alvi MA, Goulart GR, et al. Riluzole as a pharmacological therapy for spinal cord injury: where does this therapy stand? Curr Opin Neurol 2025;38(6):625–34.
7. Kalsi-Ryan S, Karadimas SK, Fehlings MG. Cervical spondylotic myelopathy: the clinical phenomenon and the current pathobiology of an increasingly prevalent and devastating disorder. Neuroscientist 2013;19(4):409–21.
8. Fehlings MG, Pedro KM, Alvi MA, et al. Riluzole for degenerative cervical myelopathy: a secondary analysis of the CSM-PROTECT trial. JAMA Netw Open 2024;7(6):e2415643.
9. Chow DS, Nguyen A, Park J, et al. Riluzole in spinal cord injury Study (RISCIS)-Pharmacokinetic (PK) Sub-Study: an analysis of pharmacokinetics, pharmacodynamics, and impact on axonal degradation of riluzole in patients with traumatic cervical spinal cord injury enrolled in the RISCIS phase III randomized controlled trial. J Neurotrauma 2023;40(17–18): 1889–906.
10. Fehlings MG, Badhiwala JH, Ahn H, et al. Safety and efficacy of riluzole in patients undergoing decompressive surgery for degenerative cervical myelopathy (CSM-Protect): a multicentre, double-blind, placebo-controlled, randomised, phase 3 trial. Lancet Neurol 2021;20(2):98–106.
11. Fehlings MG, Moghaddamjou A, Harrop JS, et al. Safety and efficacy of Riluzole in acute spinal cord injury Study (RISCIS): a Multi-Center, randomized, Placebo-Controlled, double-blinded trial. J Neurotrauma 2023; 40(17–18):1878–88.
12. Fehlings MG, Nakashima H, Nagoshi N, et al. Rationale, design and critical end points for the Riluzole in Acute Spinal Cord Injury Study (RISCIS): a randomized, double-blinded, placebo-controlled parallel multi-center trial. Spinal Cord 2016;54(1): 8–15.
13. Fehlings MG, Pedro KM, Alvi MA, et al. The sodium-glutamate antagonist riluzole improves outcome after acute spinal cord injury: results from the RISCIS randomised controlled trial analysed using a global statistical analytic technique. EBioMedicine 2025; 118:105863.
14. Kumarasamy D, Viswanathan VK, Shetty AP, et al. The role of riluzole in acute traumatic cervical spinal cord injury with incomplete neurological deficit: a prospective, randomised controlled study. Indian J Orthop 2022;56(12):2160–8.
15. Meshkini A, Salehpour F, Aghazadeh J, et al. Riluzole can improve sensory and motor function in patients with acute spinal cord injury. Asian J Neurosurg 2018;13(3):656–9.

16. Nguyen A, Chow DS, Wu L, et al. Longitudinal impact of acute spinal cord injury on clinical pharmacokinetics of riluzole, a potential neuroprotective agent. J Clin Pharmacol 2021;61(9):1232–42.
17. Weisbrod LJ, Nilles-Melchert TT, Bergjord JR, et al. Safety and efficacy of Riluzole in traumatic Spinal Cord injury: a systematic review with meta-analyses. Neurotrauma Rep 2024;5(1):117–27.
18. Chow DS, Teng Y, Toups EG, et al. Pharmacology of riluzole in acute spinal cord injury. J Neurosurg Spine 2012;17(1 Suppl):129–40.
19. Grossman RG, Fehlings MG, Frankowski RF, et al. A prospective, multicenter, phase I matched-comparison group trial of safety, pharmacokinetics, and preliminary efficacy of riluzole in patients with traumatic spinal cord injury. J Neurotrauma 2014;31(3):239–55.
20. Haddaway NR, Page MJ, Pritchard CC, et al. PRISMA2020: an R package and shiny app for producing PRISMA 2020-compliant flow diagrams, with interactivity for optimised digital transparency and open synthesis. Campbell Syst Rev 2022;18(2):e1230.
21. Tetreault LA, Zhu MP, Wilson JR, et al. The impact of riluzole on neurobehavioral outcomes in preclinical models of traumatic and nontraumatic spinal cord injury: results from a systematic review of the literature. Glob Spine J 2020;10(2):216–29.
22. Bryson HM, Fulton B, Benfield P. Riluzole. A review of its pharmacodynamic and pharmacokinetic properties and therapeutic potential in amyotrophic lateral sclerosis. Drugs 1996;52(4):549–63.
23. Le Liboux A, Cachia JP, Kirkesseli S, et al. A comparison of the pharmacokinetics and tolerability of riluzole after repeat dose administration in healthy elderly and young volunteers. J Clin Pharmacol 1999;39(5):480–6.
24. Le Liboux A, Lefebvre P, Le Roux Y, et al. Single- and multiple-dose pharmacokinetics of riluzole in white subjects. J Clin Pharmacol 1997;37(9):820–7.
25. Rorer R-P. Riluzole prescribing information. Collegeville (PA). 1996.
26. Hoffman PN, Lasek RJ. Axonal transport of the cytoskeleton in regenerating motor neurons: constancy and change. Brain Res 1980;202(2):317–33.
27. Shaw G, Yang C, Ellis R, et al. Hyperphosphorylated neurofilament NF-H is a serum biomarker of axonal injury. Biochem Biophys Res Commun 2005;336(4):1268–77.
28. Hayakawa K, Okazaki R, Ishii K, et al. Phosphorylated neurofilament subunit NF-H as a biomarker for evaluating the severity of spinal cord injury patients, a pilot study. Spinal Cord 2012;50(7):493–6.
29. Kalsi-Ryan S, Wilson J, Yang JM, et al. Neurological grading in traumatic spinal cord injury. World Neurosurg 2014;82(3–4):509–18.
30. Bracken MB, Collins WF, Freeman DF, et al. Efficacy of methylprednisolone in acute spinal cord injury. JAMA 1984;251(1):45–52.
31. Bracken MB, Shepard MJ, Collins WF, et al. A randomized, controlled trial of methylprednisolone or naloxone in the treatment of acute spinal-cord injury. Results of the Second National Acute Spinal Cord Injury Study. N Engl J Med 1990;322(20):1405–11.
32. Bracken MB, Shepard MJ, Holford TR, et al. Administration of methylprednisolone for 24 or 48 hours or tirilazad mesylate for 48 hours in the treatment of acute spinal cord injury. Results of the Third National Acute Spinal Cord Injury Randomized Controlled Trial. National Acute Spinal Cord Injury Study. JAMA 1997;277(20):1597–604.
33. Hurlbert RJ. Methylprednisolone for acute spinal cord injury: an inappropriate standard of care. J Neurosurg 2000;93(1 Suppl):1–7.
34. Hurlbert RJ, Hadley MN, Walters BC, et al. Pharmacological therapy for acute spinal cord injury. Neurosurgery 2013;72(Suppl 2):93–105.
35. Hurlbert RJ, Hamilton MG. Methylprednisolone for acute spinal cord injury: 5-year practice reversal. Can J Neurol Sci 2008;35(1):41–5.
36. Liu Z, Yang Y, He L, et al. High-dose methylprednisolone for acute traumatic spinal cord injury: a meta-analysis. Neurology 2019;93(9):e841–50.
37. Sultan I, Lamba N, Liew A, et al. The safety and efficacy of steroid treatment for acute spinal cord injury: a systematic review and meta-analysis. Heliyon 2020;6(2):e03414.
38. Sunshine JE, Dagal A, Burns SP, et al. Methylprednisolone therapy in acute traumatic Spinal Cord injury: analysis of a regional Spinal Cord model systems database. Anesth Analg 2017;124(4):1200–5.
39. Fehlings MG, Wilson JR, Tetreault LA, et al. A Clinical Practice Guideline for the management of patients with acute spinal cord injury: recommendations on the use of methylprednisolone sodium succinate. Glob Spine J 2017;7(3 Suppl) 203s–11s.
40. Mimura T, Moghaddamjou A, Badhiwala JH, et al. Effect of methylprednisolone in cervical spinal cord injury stratified by injury severity: analysis in 908 patients. Spinal Cord 2026;64(2):177–85.
41. Gebeyehu TF, Sokol Z, Guest JD, et al. Variations in managing acute spinal cord injury in the north American clinical trials network and partner institutes. Glob Spine J 202621925682261421192. https://doi.org/10.1177/21925682261421192.
42. Lin Y, Li C, Li J, et al. NEP(1-40)-modified human serum albumin nanoparticles enhance the therapeutic effect of methylprednisolone against spinal cord injury. J Nanobiotechnology 2019 17(1):12.
43. Qi L, Jiang H, Cui X, et al. Synthesis of methylprednisolone loaded ibuprofen modified dextran based

nanoparticles and their application for drug delivery in acute spinal cord injury. Oncotarget 2017;8(59): 99666–80.

44. Kucher K, Johns D, Maier D, et al. First-in-Man intrathecal application of neurite growth-promoting Anti-Nogo-A antibodies in acute spinal cord injury. Neurorehabil Neural Repair 2018;32(6–7):578–89.
45. Weidner N, Abel R, Maier D, et al. Safety and efficacy of intrathecal antibodies to Nogo-A in patients with acute cervical spinal cord injury: a randomised, double-blind, multicentre, placebo-controlled, phase 2b trial. Lancet Neurol 2025;24(1):42–53.
46. Shultz RB, Zhong Y. Minocycline targets multiple secondary injury mechanisms in traumatic spinal cord injury. Neural Regen Res 2017;12(5): 702–13.
47. Omair J, Sheth A, Elsamadicy AA, et al. Efficacy of minocycline in acute traumatic spinal cord injury. J Neurotrauma 20268977151261432165. https://doi.org/10.1177/08977151261432165.
48. Hu CW, Li ZY, Zhu K, et al. Exploring the effectiveness and potential pharmacological mechanism of minocycline for spinal cord injury through meta-analysis and network pharmacology. Curr Neuropharmacol 2025;23(9):1060–80.
49. Sherrod BA, Porche K, Condie CK, et al. Pharmacologic therapy for spinal cord injury. Clin Spine Surg 2024;37(9):433–9.
50. Jacobson PB, Goody R, Lawrence M, et al. Elezanumab, a human anti-RGMa monoclonal antibody, promotes neuroprotection, neuroplasticity, and neurorecovery following a thoracic hemicompression spinal cord injury in non-human Primates. Neurobiol Dis 2021;155:105385.
51. Kalluri HV, Rosebraugh MR, Misko TP, et al. Phase 1 evaluation of elezanumab (Anti-Repulsive guidance molecule A monoclonal antibody) in healthy and multiple sclerosis participants. Ann Neurol 2023;93(2): 285–96.
52. Kalluri HV, Rosebraugh MR, Boehm N, et al. Comparability of Elezanumab safety, tolerability, and pharmacokinetics in healthy Japanese, Chinese, and white participants. Clin Pharmacol Drug Dev 2024; 13(2):180–9.
53. Cree BAC, Freedman MS, Gold M, et al. Randomized, double-blind, placebo-controlled, multiple-dose studies to assess the safety and efficacy of elezanumab when added to standard of care in relapsing and progressive forms of multiple sclerosis. Ann Neurol 2025;98(3):590–602.

Optimizing Surgical Cord Decompression in Traumatic Spinal Cord Injury and Degenerative Cervical Myelopathy

Bizhan Aarabi, MD[a,*], Timothy Chryssikos, MD, PhD[a], Carl M. Zipser, MD[b], Youssef Chedid, MD, MBBS, BSc (hons)[c,d], Noori Akhtar-Danesh, PhD[e], Benjamin M. Davies, BSC, MPhil, MRCS[c], Mark R. Kotter, MD, MPhil, PhD[c]

KEYWORDS

- Spinal cord injury • Intramedullary lesion length • Laminectomy • Decompression
- Degenerative cervical myelopathy

KEY POINTS

- Intramedullary lesion length is a key biomarker associated with severity of spinal cord injury (SCI) and plays a central role in planning decompression surgery.
- Spinal cord compression in the setting of SCI can result from either an extrinsic (boney/disco-ligamentous complex) or an intrinsic (dura) cause.
- Laminectomy and its extent are key surgical techniques for optimal spinal cord decompression.
- Intraoperative ultrasonography can be used during surgery for both cervical myelopathy and SCI to verify the extent of decompression and may play a role in selection of patients for expansion duraplasty in addition to laminectomy.
- Optimal decompression in DCM should be defined by effective restoration of space around the spinal cord rather than by canal realignment alone; what constitutes *adequate* physiologic decompression remains incompletely defined.

TRAUMATIC SPINAL CORD INJURY

Traumatic spinal cord injury (tSCI) remains a formidable challenge in modern medicine, with a global incidence of between 1 and 4 per 100,000.[1–3] Nearly half of these patients suffer complete injuries, and approximately one-third remain permanently quadriplegic.[1,4,5] To date, medical management strategies have yielded inconclusive results[6–9]; even the benefits of mean arterial pressure (MAP) augmentation remain under debate.[10] While early and complete surgical decompression appears neuroprotective—potentially facilitating neurologic recovery as measured by American Spinal Injury Association Impairment Scale (AIS) grade conversion[11–13]—the precise definition and methodology of *optimal* surgical decompression remain incompletely defined. In the landmark STASCIS prospective multicenter study, decompression methodology was left to

[a] Department of Neurosurgery, University of Maryland School of Medicine, Baltimore City, MD, USA; [b] Department of Neurology and Neurophysiology, Balgrist University, Zurich; [c] Division of Neurosurgery, Department of Clinical Neurosciences, University of Cambridge, Cambridge, UK; [d] Department of Clinical Neurosciences, Cambridge University Hospitals NHS Foundation Trust; [e] Faculty of Health Sciences, McMaster University, Hamilton, Ontario, Canada
* Corresponding author. 22 South Greene Street, Baltimore, MD, 21201.
E-mail address: baarabi@som.umaryland.edu

Neurosurg Clin N Am 37 (2026) 583–596
https://doi.org/10.1016/j.nec.2026.05.008

neurosurgery.theclinics.com

Abbreviations

AIS	American Spinal Injury Association Impairment Scale
BSCB	blood–spinal cord barrier
CSF	cerebrospinal fluid
DCM	degenerative cervical myelopathy
IMLL	intramedullary lesion length
IOUS	intraoperative ultrasound
ISP	intraspinal pressure
MAP	mean arterial pressure
NDI	Neck Disability Index
SCPP	spinal cord perfusion pressure
TSCI	traumatic spinal cord injury

surgeon discretion, with no requirement to confirm results via postoperative MRI.[14] However, subsequent clinical studies suggest that incorporating intramedullary lesion length (IMLL) into preoperative planning and evaluating the extent of decompression on postoperative MRI are critical variables for recovery.[15–17] Furthermore, intraoperative ultrasound (IOUS) has been increasingly used to assess and verify adequacy of spinal cord decompression during surgical decompression for tSCI. This modality provides the opportunity to perform additional bony decompression (laminectomy) should IOUS reveal persistent compression at the rostral and/or caudal ends of the laminectomy bed and could be used to select candidates for expansion duraplasty if severe intradural swelling with obliteration of the subarachnoid space is demonstrated despite adequate bony decompression. Collectively, preoperative MRI, IOUS, and postoperative MRI continue to guide the decision-making process for surgical decompression in tSCI and together offer a standardized approach to tSCI intervention.[18,19]

Preclinical studies have established that early decompression of the spinal cord following tSCI improves motor and functional outcomes.[20] Similarly, translational investigations in humans have confirmed that early decompression may be neuroprotective and can facilitate AIS grade conversion.[11,13,14,20–25]

However, the optimal surgical methodology and the definitive *proof of decompression* remain significant gaps in current knowledge.[15,18] While evidence suggests that the extent of decompression may correlate with improved neurologic recovery, MRI remains the gold standard for postoperative verification of decompression extent.[15,19] This highlights a critical need to refine management protocols and intraoperative planning to consistently achieve—and verify—adequate spinal cord decompression.

MRI AND PREOPERATIVE INTRAMEDULLARY LESION LENGTH IN TRAUMATIC SPINAL CORD INJURY

Evaluation of the admission IMLL is fundamental to preoperative planning and is a critical step in achieving optimal spinal cord decompression and AIS grade conversion.[16,26,27] As an imaging biomarker, IMLL has been shown to correlate strongly with injury severity.[26,28–31] While injury morphology (**Fig. 1**) and gender have negligible effects on IMLL, there is a significant inverse correlation with the ASIA motor score: as the score drops, the IMLL increases (**Fig. 2**).[17,27] Consequently, IMLL is notably larger in complete (AIS grade A) versus incomplete spinal cord injuries (AIS grades B, C, and D) (**Fig. 3**).[27,31]

The expansion of intramedullary lesions is most rapid immediately following trauma. For example the patient in **Fig. 4**, evaluated 5.5 hours postaccident, exhibited an IMLL of 69.2 mm—an expansion rate of 12.6 mm/hour. By contrast, the expansion rate between admission and postoperative MRI also increases but at a significantly slower rate, averaging 0.9 mm in motor-complete patients and 0.3 mm in motor-incomplete patients.[27] Research indicates that IMLL is the strongest predictor of AIS grade conversion at 6-month follow-up. Specifically, the predictive model suggests that for every 1-mm and 10-mm increase in IMLL, the odds of AIS grade conversion decrease by 4% and 40%, respectively (**Fig. 5**).[16]

DECOMPRESSION BASED ON INJURY MORPHOLOGY IN TRAUMATIC SPINAL CORD INJURY

The traditional approach to spinal cord decompression was primarily rooted in preoperative injury morphology as seen on computed tomography (CT) scans.[14,32–35] Today, we continue to come across a definition of *decompression* as synonymous with successful anatomic realignment and internal fixation. Even in the landmark prospective multicenter STASCIS study, the methodology remained surgeon-dependent rather than following a standardized algorithm; notably, postoperative MRIs were performed only if complications arose.[14] However, recent evidence has shifted this paradigm toward MRI-verified outcomes.[11,35] A 2017 investigation demonstrated that for patients with AIS grades A–C, the probability of AIS grade conversion at a 6-month follow-up was 58.9% with complete decompression, compared with only 18.5% when decompression was incomplete (see **Fig. 5**).[16] In this context, *complete decompression* was strictly defined as the presence of cerebrospinal fluid

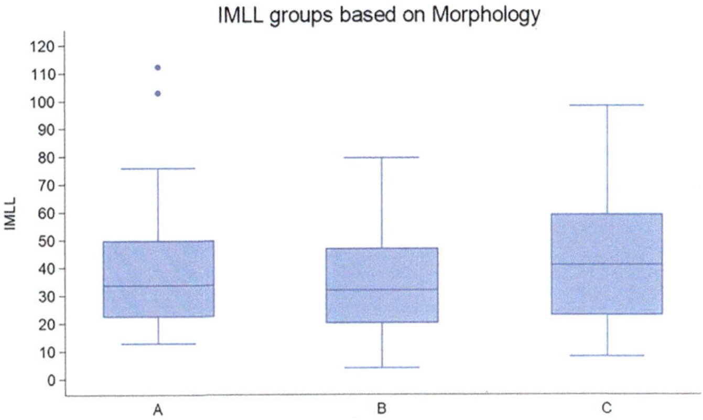

Fig. 1. Lack of significant statistical relationship between IMLL and AO-Spine Injury Morphology Classes A, B, and C.

(CSF) surrounding the injured cord segment on postoperative MRI.[15,18] Subsequent research in 2019 further quantified this, finding that the success of decompression in motor-complete patients directly correlated with selection and extent of the decompression procedure.[15] Regardless of whether a discectomy or corpectomy was performed, laminectomy proved essential: a five-level laminectomy was associated with complete decompression in nearly 100% of patients (**Fig. 6**).

CONTRIBUTION OF INTRAOPERATIVE ULTRASOUND IN OPTIMIZATION OF CORD DECOMPRESSION AND EXPANSIVE DURAPLASTY IN TRAUMATIC SPINAL CORD INJURY

Evidence indicates that when preoperative planning disregards IMLL—relying instead on non-standardized algorithms with emphasis on anatomic alignment and internal fixation alone—spinal cord decompression is often suboptimal. In a cohort of 184 consecutive patients where IMLL was not considered, adequate decompression rates varied significantly by procedure: 46.8% for discectomy, 58.6% for corpectomy, 71.7% for discectomy with laminectomy, 73.1% for corpectomy with laminectomy, and 86.2% for laminectomy alone.[15] In contrast, when IMLL was integrated into preoperative planning—specifically by performing one level of laminectomy for every 15 mm of IMLL, regardless of anterior surgery—more than 90% of patients (AIS grades A-C) achieved adequate decompression on postoperative MRI.

IOUS has also emerged as a useful supplement to verify the extent of decompression at the time of surgery. In a 2023 study of patients who underwent laminectomy including both IOUS and postoperative evaluation of decompression with MRI and CT myelography, 9.8% of these patients had additional laminectomy performed based on persistent spinal cord compression as revealed by IOUS. Patients who were found to have inadequate decompression in 15.69% despite surgeon judgment of adequate decompression using IOUS at the time of the operation had significantly larger IMLL and more severe clinical injuries,

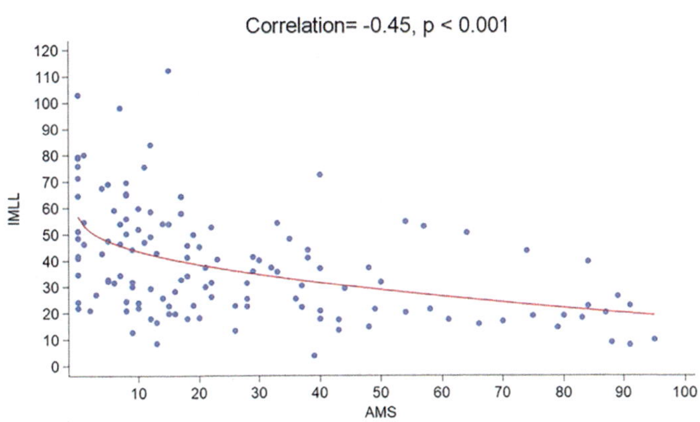

Fig. 2. Significant statistical relationship between IMLL and ASIA motor score.

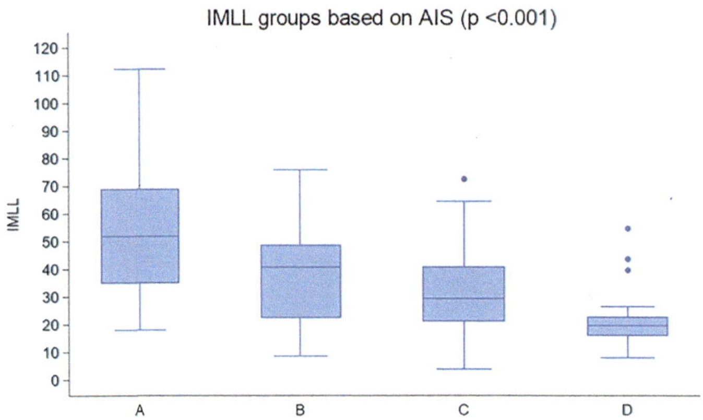

Fig. 3. Significant statistical relationship between IMLL and ASIA Impairment Scale grades A–D.

suggesting a potential additional role for IOUS in selecting patients for expansion duraplasty.[18] By providing additional verification of decompression with IOUS as a supplement to the laminectomy algorithm (based on IMLL), patients are more likely to have successful, de facto decompression of the injured spinal cord. Additional experience, further refinement in IOUS technology, and establishment of objective IOUS parameters will further define the role of this promising imaging modality in the management of tSCI (**Figs. 7** and **8**).

In summary, primary tSCI results in dynamic volumetric progression of the initial contusion and is typically associated with spinal cord swelling. By the time a patient is resuscitated and has undergone an MRI, the presence and length of the intramedullary lesion can be determined. IMLL not only provides prognostic information but is also critical for surgical planning. Optimal decompression relies on both anatomic alignment and internal fixation, but for severe tSCI it also typically requires adequate laminectomy based on the IMLL. Specifically, we have proposed that one level of laminectomy be performed for every 15 mm of IMLL to optimize decompression (successful in nearly 90% of patients). Furthermore, IOUS can provide real-time assessment of the extent of bony decompression and intradural swelling and may indicate additional bony decompression or expansion duraplasty in select patients (e.g., severe tSCI)

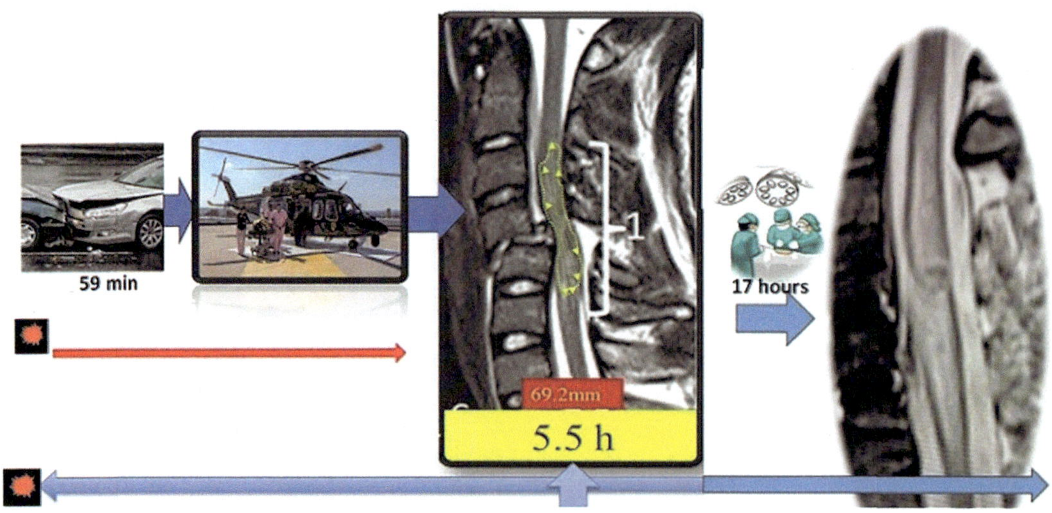

Fig. 4. Timeline delay from the moment of accident until the compressed cord was visualized preoperatively, and immediately following decompression by MRI. In the preoperative MRI, obtained 5.5 hours after trauma, the IMLL in this AIS grade A patient measured 69.2 mm. Surgical decompression was completed 17 hours after trauma; the postoperative MRI indicated an IMLL measuring 102 mm.

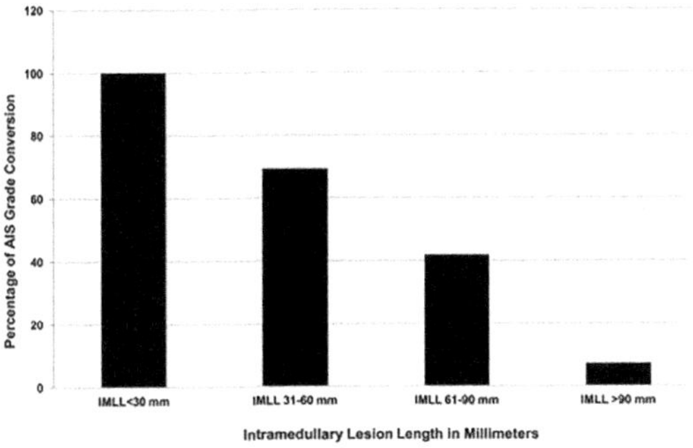

Fig. 5. Significant relationship between IMLL and AIS grade conversion at 6 months in cervical tSCI. A longer IMLL correlates with a lower likelihood of AIS grade conversion ($P<.001$). (*Adapted from*[16])

SPINAL CORD COMPRESSION IN DEGENERATIVE CERVICAL MYELOPATHY

Degenerative cervical myelopathy (DCM) is the most common cause of spinal cord dysfunction world-wide.[36,37] It is classically conceptualized as chronic disorder in which sustained mechanical compression leads to progressive axonal injury, demyelination, and neuronal loss, ultimately resulting in intramedullary myelomalacia and spinal cord atrophy. This paradigm is supported by histopathological studies demonstrating irreversible parenchymal damage in advanced disease and has strongly influenced both diagnostic interpretation and surgical timing.[38,39]

The temporal evolution of SCI in DCM differs fundamentally from that observed after traumatic injury yet shares important biological features. Whereas tSCI is characterized by abrupt onset and rapid progression over hours, DCM typically evolves over timespans ranging from weeks to sometimes many months. Despite clear differences in etiology and temporal evolution, the intramedullary response observed in DCM shares key features with posttraumatic spinal cord swelling.

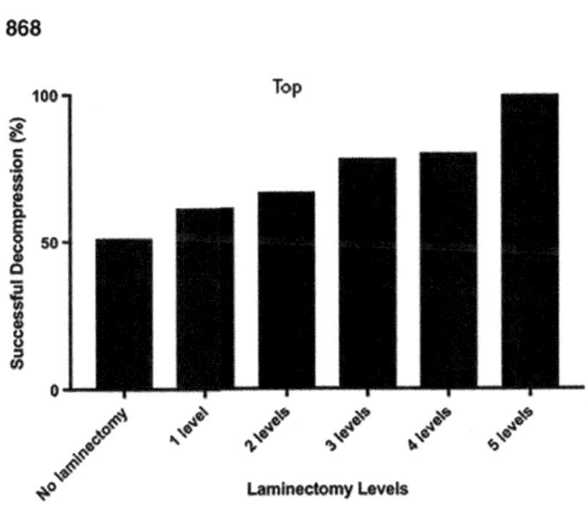

Fig. 6. The relationship between the number of laminectomy levels and the probability of decompression. (*Adapted from*[15])

DYNAMIC MICROTRAUMA

Although tSCI and DCM differ fundamentally in their initiating insults, both conditions involve mechanical factors that amplify intramedullary injury over time. In tSCI, a single catastrophic event produces immediate tissue deformation and vascular disruption. In DCM, repetitive subthreshold injury at the area of cervical compression, exacerbated by spinal cord motion, instability, and dynamic compression, with associated transient intradural pressure changes, is likely to exert cumulative effects on spinal cord parenchyma and microvasculature.[40,41]

Despite these differences, both scenarios converge on similar downstream biology: blood–spinal cord barrier (BSCB) failure, edema, ischemia, and longitudinal lesion propagation. Dynamic microtrauma therefore serves as a unifying amplifier that links acute and chronic SCI within a shared mechanistic framework (**Fig. 9**). A central mechanism underlying tSCI and DCM is disruption of the BSCB. In tSCI, mechanical deformation of the spinal cord produces immediate endothelial injury, followed by ischemia–reperfusion, oxidative stress, and inflammatory activation, all of which contribute to loss of barrier integrity and extravasation of plasma proteins into the interstitial space.[39,42,43] The resulting vasogenic edema is a major contributor to early spinal cord swelling and secondary injury progression.

In DCM, BSCB disruption appears to occur through a different but convergent pathway. Chronic mechanical compression, repetitive microtrauma, and sustained microvascular compromise have been shown to impair spinal cord blood flow and endothelial function, leading to increased vascular permeability and interstitial edema.[40,44,45] The presence of intramedullary gadolinium enhancement in a subset of DCM provides in vivo evidence of BSCB dysfunction, analogous to that observed in acute traumatic injury.[46]

Ischemia represents a second unifying mechanism linking spinal cord swelling across traumatic and degenerative etiologies. In tSCI, primary vascular disruption and systemic hypotension are compounded by rising intraspinal pressure (ISP) as the swollen cord expands within the confines of the dura. Experimental and clinical studies demonstrate that increasing ISP reduces spinal cord perfusion pressure (SCPP), creating a state in which perfusion becomes pressure-dependent

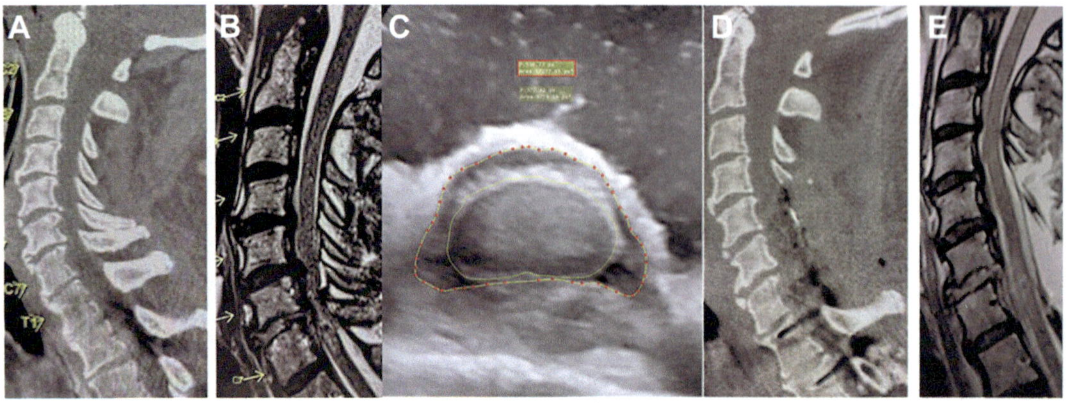

Fig. 7. Preoperative and postoperative midsagittal CT and MRI (*A* and *B*) of a 62-year-old male patient involved in a motor vehicle accident. Admission AIS grade was A, and ASIA motor score was 3. The IMLL at admission (6 hours posttrauma) measured 27.1 mm (*B*). Ten hours after trauma, the patient underwent a 3.5-level laminectomy (*D*). IOUS at the injury epicenter (*C*) demonstrated adequate decompression, confirmed by postoperative MRI 27 hours after trauma (*E*).

and highly vulnerable to small additional increases in cord volume.[47–49]

In DCM, ischemia develops more insidiously but follows a similar physiologic logic. Chronic compression is associated with microvascular compromise, potentially mediated by endothelial dysfunction, leading to further impairment of perfusion.[40,44] In the case of a compressed spinal cord there is little reserve capacity, and even modest fluctuations in cord or systemic blood pressure may therefore result in episodic hypoperfusion, aggravating the injury.

In both conditions, this interaction between intramedullary pathology and a noncompliant external canal may create a compartment-like state in which ischemia and edema reinforce one another. Importantly, this physiology explains why neurologic deterioration may continue despite

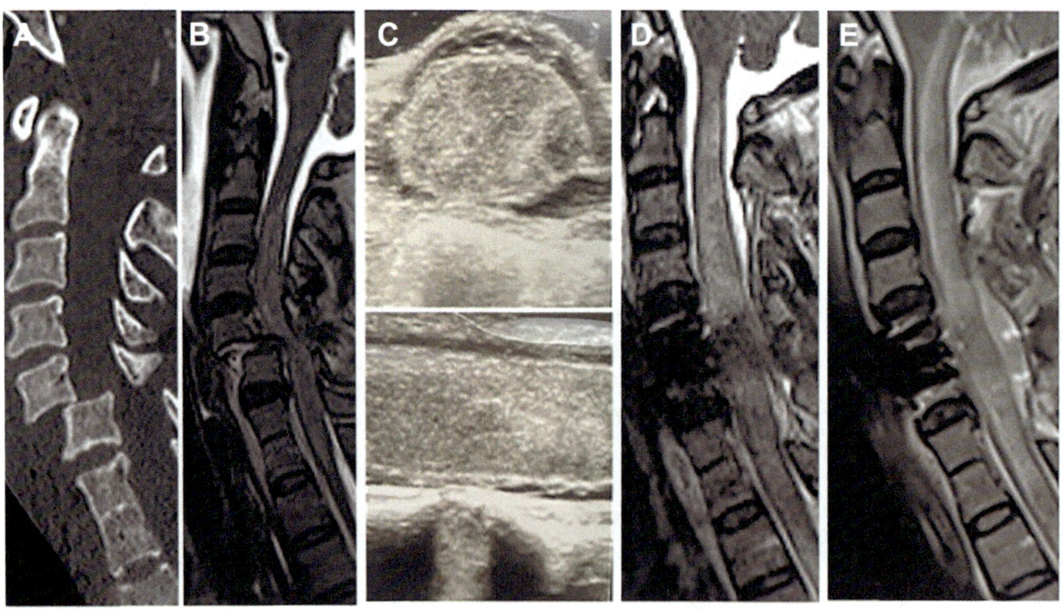

Fig. 8. Preoperative and postoperative midsagittal CT and MRI (*A* and *B*) of a 37-year-old female patient who sustained a ground-level fall and C5/6 bilateral locked facets (*A*). The admission IMLL was 98.1 mm (*B*). The dislocation was initially reduced, followed by C5/6 ACDF. Postoperative MRI 78 hours after trauma revealed an IMLL of 165 mm and inadequate decompression (*D*). Following a reoperation for 5-level laminectomies, intraoperative MRI showed continued dural compression (*C*). An expansion duraplasty was then performed (*E*).

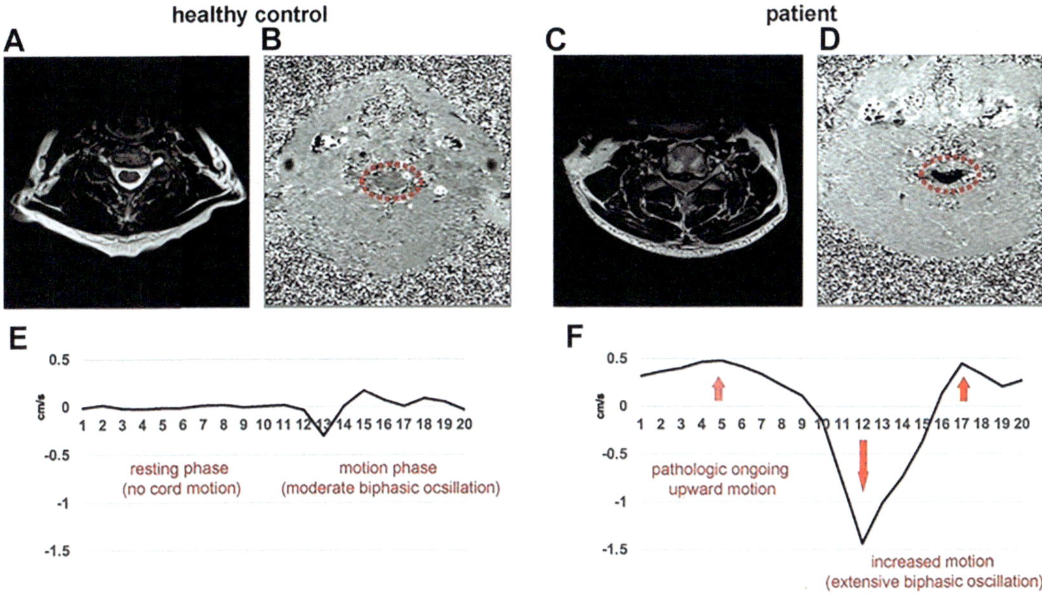

Fig. 9. (*A-F*) Dynamic mechanical stress resulting from exaggerated spinal cord motion at the level of compression, visualized with specialized MRI sequences.

stabilization of the spinal column and why decompression strategies that fail to adequately relieve intradural constraint may be insufficient to interrupt secondary injury.

Disruption of CSF dynamics constitutes another common mechanism linking spinal cord swelling in tSCI and DCM. In acute trauma, cord expansion and subarachnoid hemorrhage can obstruct CSF pathways, contributing to pressure gradients across the injured segment that further compromise perfusion.[48] Indeed, perioperative intradural pressure monitoring via lumbar drainage in individuals with DCM provides direct, real-time insight into the intradural compartment.[48] Under physiologic conditions, CSF freely communicates across the whole craniospinal compartment—intraspinal and intrathecal (CSF-) pressure measurements can be reliably measured with different techniques. Generally, CSF pressure metrics of interest are mean pressure, cardiac-related CSF pulsations (or CSF pulsation), and CSF pressure response to jugular vein compression (Queckenstedt's test) (**Fig. 10**). In DCM, canal stenosis may function as a chronic CSF *dam*, impairing normal pulsatile flow and promoting interstitial fluid accumulation within the spinal cord. This mechanism is reminiscent of the *resyrinx* state in Chiari's syndrome, which precedes cavitation and syrinx formation if compression is not relieved.[50,51] Current data, including unpublished observations from the authors, suggest that patients commonly exhibit attenuated CSF pulse amplitude distal to the site of compression, consistent with reduced intradural compliance. In the prospective monocentric COMP-CORD study, it was demonstrated that CSF pulsatility significantly increased following surgical decompression, while other intraoperative events such as CSF leakage could be discerned.

These findings support the concept of a compartmentalized intradural space in DCM that may contribute to spinal cord injury, analogous to the pressure–perfusion derangements observed in acute tSCI when the swollen cord is constrained within a noncompliant dural compartment.[47,48] Altered pulsatile pressure transmission across a focal stenosis may contribute to repetitive mechanical stress on the cord, a concept similar to that proposed in Chiari malformations, in which CSF flow obstruction and pressure gradients at the foramen magnum are implicated in syrinx formation and cord injury.[50,51]

Intraoperative and bedside CSF pressure findings in tSCI have shown a more severely attenuated situation as compared to DCM, with non-pulsatile CSF not being uncommon. However, as in patients with DCM, improved pressure metrics are found following surgical decompression. Notably, a study in tSCI with parallel assessment of intraspinal pressure at the level of injury and lumbar intrathecal pressure revealed site-dependent differences that warrant further investigation.

Noteworthy, most studies have evaluated lumbar intrathecal pressure metrics in a predecompressio, to postdecompression fashion, instead

CSF pressure in a spine-healthy cohort

	Mean CSFP	CSFPp	QT rise	Max CSFPp	RPPC-Q	P0-Q	VM rise
Young (N=14)	6.9 – 18.5	0.3 – 2	5.4 – 30.7	0.6 – 5.8	0.04 – 0.26	-8.0 – 8.4	7.3 – 43.7
Old (N=14)	8.2 – 20.3	0.4 – 2.1	5.3 – 34.1	1.5 – 8.8	0.1 – 0.44	-0.1 – 15.1	27.4 – 60.8

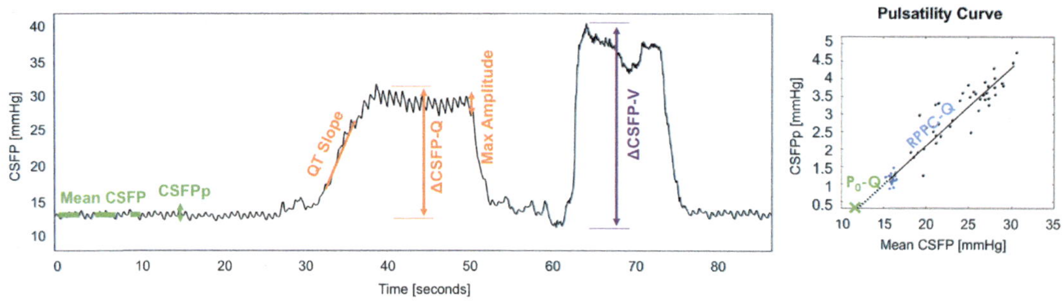

Fig. 10. CSF pressure metrics of interest for determining CSF space patency. Reference age-dependent values are from patients without cord compression, according to Kheram and colleagues (2025). CSFP, CSF pressure; CSFPp, cardiac-related CSF pulsations; QT, Queckenstedt's test; P0-Q, pressure at infinite compliance obtained using QT; VM, Valsalva maneuver. (*Data from* Kheram N, Boraschi A, Rasenack M, et al. Age-Dependence of Cerebrospinal Fluid Pressure Metrics During Queckenstedt's Test. Chauhan A, ed. Acta Neurologica Scandinavica. 2025;2025(1) doi:https://doi.org/10.1155/ane/2761843)

of comparing them to reference ranges. This represents a pragmatic approach, partly owing to the lack of reference ranges from sedated and ventilated patients without cord compression, who have distinct patterns as compared to awake patients. Another explanation is the generally wide range of CSF pressure. Future research is required to determine thresholds for clinically relevant perioperative changes in CSF pressure.

In summary, across tSCI and DCM, impaired CSF flow may therefore interact with edema, ischemia, to exacerbate intramedullary pressure and tissue injury, reinforcing the concept that secondary injury mechanisms in the spinal cord form a multifactorial and self-sustaining process.

IMPLICATIONS FOR DECOMPRESSION STRATEGY: EXTENDING PRINCIPLES ACROSS DISEASES

It follows that a constellation of interacting mechanisms common to both traumatic and degenerative injury, including BSCB disruption, ischemia and perfusion failure, venous congestion, impaired CSF dynamics, and mechanical amplification converge to produce injury. While the initiating insults and temporal profiles differ, the downstream biological consequences are strikingly similar. This shared mechanistic substrate provides the foundation for considering tSCI and DCM within a unified framework, which in turn underpins the rationale for decompression strategies that prioritize restoration of a permissive intradural environment for the injured spinal cord.

This shared biological framework necessitates a reassessment of how spinal cord decompression is conceptualized and evaluated. The optimal surgical methodology and the definitive "proof of decompression" remain significant gaps in current knowledge, particularly in the management of severe tSCI.[11,16] The traditional approaches have largely focused on restoration of spinal alignment and canal dimensions, yet these criteria do not directly address the intramedullary consequences of spinal cord swelling.

The traditional approach to spinal cord decompression was primarily rooted in preoperative injury morphology as seen on computed tomography, with the implicit assumption that correction of osseous displacement and stabilization of the spinal column would adequately relieve neural compression. However, MRI-based analyses demonstrate that anatomy-centric strategies frequently fail to account for the longitudinal and intradural nature of secondary injury in tSCI, particularly in patients with extensive intramedullary edema.[16] When spinal cord swelling is recognized as the dominant biological driver of ongoing injury, decompression must be evaluated at the level of the cord rather than the canal.

CONCEPTUAL EXTENSION AND SURGICAL APPROACHES TO DEGENERATIVE CERVICAL MYELOPATHY

Although the evidence supporting these decompression principles is strongest in tSCI, the shared biology of secondary injury mechanisms suggests potential relevance to selected cases of degenerative cervical myelopathy. In patients with DCM, bony decompression of the most compressed segments may not fully relieve intradural constraint. A substantive body of work has sought to address the question of whether a specific surgical approach leads to better outcomes and whether anterior or posterior surgery is more effective in DCM. The recent CSM Surgery trial provided robust evidence that in patients where there is equipoise with regards to the approach, the outcomes are equivalent, if the spinal cord is *adequately* decompressed.[52] However, what constitutes *adequate* is yet to be defined. At present, there is insufficient evidence to define decompression algorithms for DCM. Another important question is whether posterior approaches consisting of a decompression alone in the form of a laminectomy enable optimal recovery, or whether additional instrumentation and fusion is required. This question is currently being addressed via both registry studies[53,54] and controlled RCTs,[55] including our Polyfix DCM trial (**Figs. 11** and **12**).[56]

Surgeon judgment alone is insufficient to reliably determine the adequacy of spinal cord decompression, particularly in the presence of extensive intramedullary swelling.[11] In tSCI,IOUS has demonstrated that residual intradural compression frequently persists despite surgeon-perceived adequate decompression, and that IOUS-guided extension of decompression improves postoperative MRI-verified outcomes.[11] IOUS therefore emerges as a potential tool to guide surgical decompression.

Index Case: Sixty-seven-year-old female with past medical history (PMH) including hypertension (HTN) and chronic obstructive pulmonary disease (COPD) and prior C3-4, C4-5, C5-6 anterior cervical discectomy and fusion (ACDF) at outside facility presents with neck pain, progressive difficulty walking, difficulty with dexterity and "frostbite" sensation in her hands, with shooting pain down the triceps to the wrist. Her mJOA was 10. She did not benefit from a trial of physical therapy before evaluation. On neurologic examination she had mild weakness of her grips and hip flexors (4/5). There was bilateral sustained clonus in the lower extremities. MRI indicated evidence of previous surgery and stenosis at C6/C7 level. There was a faint high signal intensity change at C6/C7 (**Fig. 13**A, B). She underwent C6/C7 posterior laminectomy and fusion. Real-time intraoperative ultrasound indicated complete decompression of the spinal cord (see **Fig. 13**C). Two months postoperatively her mJOA score was 14 with Visual Analogue Scale score of 2/10 for neck pain and 3/10 for arm pain (see **Fig. 13**D).

Index Case: This 73-year-old man with history of hypertension, prostate cancer, and diabetes mellitus referred to the clinic with neck pain, hand numbness and left lower extremity weakness and worsening gait instability. At the time of admission his mJOA score was 11 and her Neck Disability Index (NDI) 48%. Neurologically he was intact except for the decreased sensation in both hands

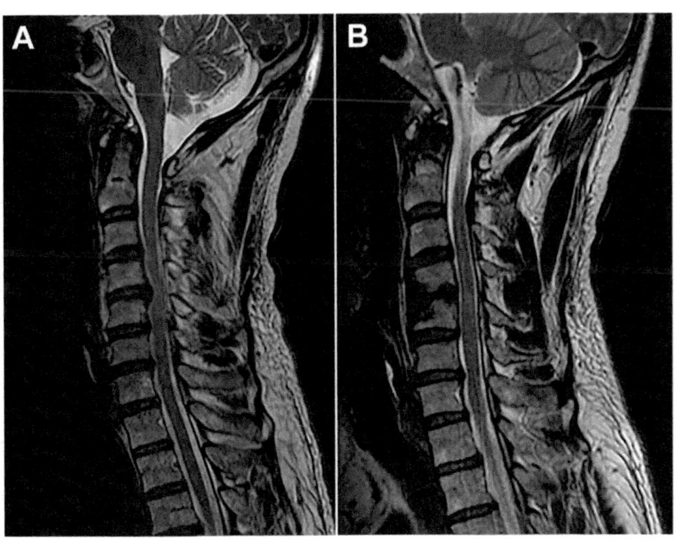

Fig. 11. (*A, B*) Preoperative and postoperative midsagittal T2WI MRI following a single-level ACDF, showing resolution of compression at C4-5.

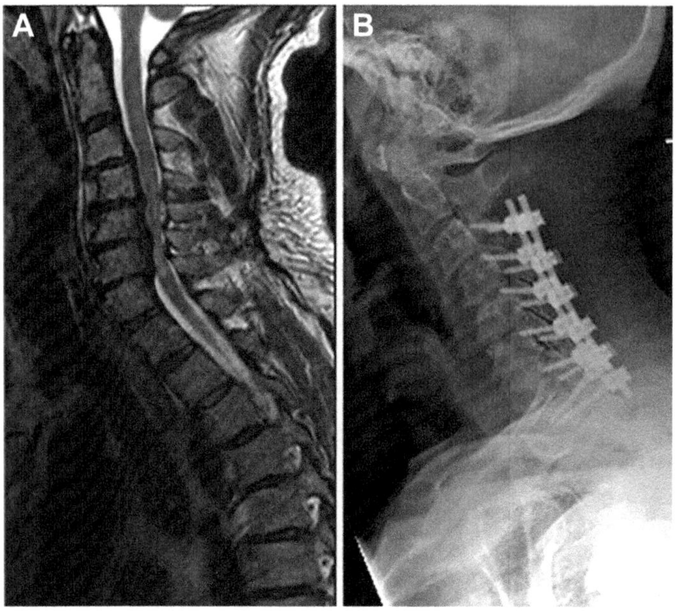

Fig. 12. (*A, B*) Preoperative midsagittal T2WI MRI demonstrating multilevel stenosis with cord compression and hyperintense signal; postoperative X-ray demonstrating a C3-6 laminectomy and C3-T1 instrumented fusion.

and legs. There was no Hoffman and reflexes 1+. CT scan indicated spinal stenosis and T2WMRI indicated a mild high signal change at C3/4 and C4/5 (**Fig. 14**A, B). He underwent C3-C5 laminectomy and posterior spina fusion (see **Fig. 14**C). Real-time intraoperative ultrasonsography and postoperative MRI indicated complete decompression of the spinal cord (see **Fig. 14**D, E). Six weeks after surgery her mJOA was 14 and he was neurologically intact.

Another physiologic correlation is the change in pressure waves that are regularly observed following decompression of the spinal cord during surgery. In the author's experience, intraoperative intradural pressure monitoring is able to detect changes in pressure wave amplitude even in cases where compressions on MRI images are subtle. Therefore, intraoperative pressure monitoring may serve as another potential indicator that can address the unresolved question of what constitutes *adequate* decompression of the spinal cord.

At this time, intraoperative physiologic verification remains inconsistently applied and lacks

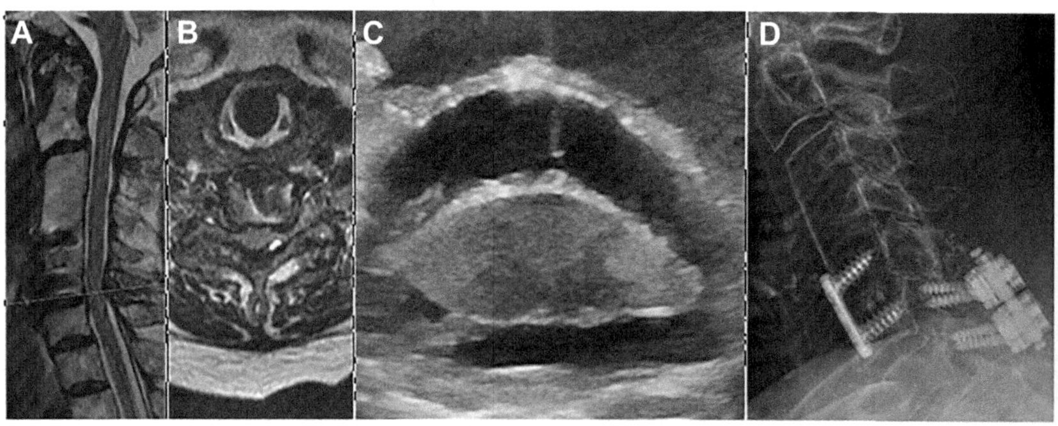

Fig. 13. Preoperative midsagittal T2W MRI (*A*) and axial image (*B*) of the cervical spine, indicating focal pressure on the spinal cord at the C6/C7 level and high signal intensity. Real-time intraoperative ultrasound indicates complete decompression of the spinal cord and an echogenic shadow at the level of the corticospinal tracts (*C*) Midsagittal postoperative X-ray (*D*) shows evidence of previous anterior and recent posterior surgical intervention and fusion.

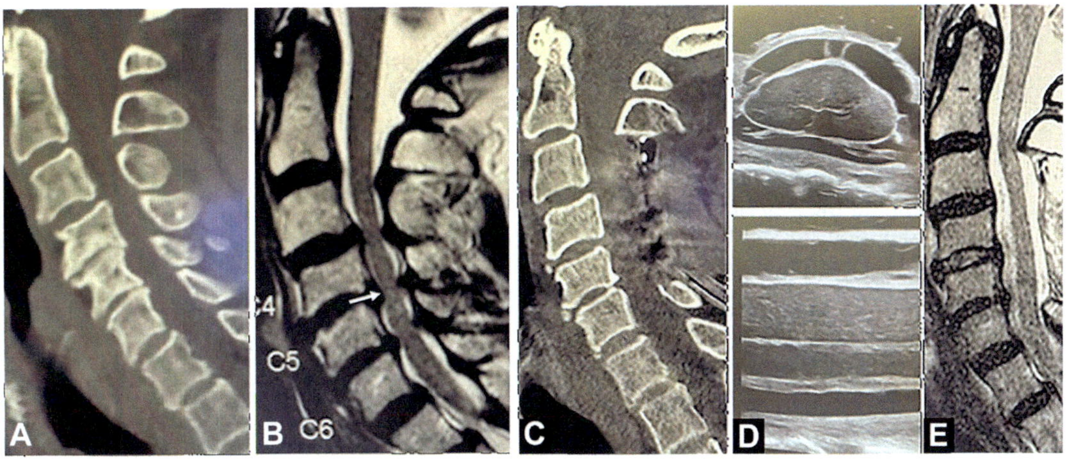

Fig. 14. Preoperative midsagittal CT scan (*A*) and preoperative midsagittal T2WI-MRI (*B*) of the cervical spine, indicating spinal stenosis and high signal intensity at the C4/C5 segment. Midsagittal CT of the cervical spine indicating C3-C5 laminectomy and fusion (*C*). Axial and midsagittal sections of real-time intraoperative ultrasound and midsagittal MRI indicating complete spinal cord decompression of the spinal cord (*D, E*).

standardized criteria. Beyond trauma, there is little guidance on how to assess decompression adequacy intraoperatively in chronic or degenerative conditions. The absence of objective, reproducible intraoperative metrics to confirm restoration of a permissive intradural environment represents an important unmet need, particularly if decompression principles are to be translated beyond acute injury.

Taken together, these findings establish that optimal decompression is not necessarily synonymous with anatomic realignment or canal enlargement. Adequate decompression may require restoration of CSF space around the injured spinal cord and relief of intradural constraint, goals that can only be reliably assessed using MRI and/or intraoperative techniques, such as ultrasound or intradural pressure recordings. In traumatic injury, this biology-informed approach is associated with improved neurologic outcomes. The convergence of mechanisms between traumatic and degenerative spinal cord injury suggests that these principles may have broader relevance, providing a coherent foundation for interpreting outcomes and guiding future translational work.

IMPLICATIONS FOR DECOMPRESSION STRATEGY: EXTENDING PRINCIPLES ACROSS DISEASES

The shared biological framework outlined above necessitates a reassessment of how spinal cord decompression is conceptualized and evaluated. The optimal surgical methodology and the definitive *proof of decompression* remain significant gaps in current knowledge. Traditional approaches have largely focused on restoration of spinal alignment and canal dimensions, yet these criteria do not directly address the intramedullary consequences of spinal cord swelling in tSCI. In DCM the evidence base is still lacking; however, given the similarities in injury mechanisms, one can expect similar principles to apply.

The optimal surgical methodology and the definitive *proof of decompression* remain significant gaps in current knowledge, particularly when decompression is judged solely by anatomic realignment or canal enlargement. The data synthesized here demonstrate that effective decompression should be defined physiologically, by restoration of cerebrospinal fluid space, relief of intradural constraint, and improvement of spinal cord perfusion.

CLINICS CARE POINTS

- Mechanisms of Injury: In traumatic spinal cord injury (tSCI) correctly identify the *primary injury* as the mechanical event (fracture/dislocation) occurring in milliseconds. This emphasizes the urgency of decompressing and stabilizing the spine to prevent *secondary injury* (ischemia, inflammation, and edema). In degenerative cervical myelopathy (DCM) the *primary injury* is chronic mechanical compression and dynamic microtrauma rather than a single catastrophic event. However, secondary injury mechanisms—microvascular compromise, ischemia, and interstitial edema—

may drive ongoing neurologic decline. This emphasizes the importance of timely decompression to interrupt progressive intramedullary injury.

- Neurologic Baseline: Use the International Standards for Neurologic Classification of Spinal Cord Injury examination as the gold standard for defining the ASIA Impairment Scale grade at admission. In DCM careful clinical characterization using standardized functional scales (eg, mJOA) is critical to define baseline impairment and monitor progression. Neurologic deterioration in DCM may be gradual or stepwise, and objective documentation of decline is central to surgical decision-making.
- MRI Metrics: In tSCI defining intramedullary Lesion Length (IMLL) via admission MRI is a sophisticated prognostic indicator. Hemorrhagic contusions generally suggest a more severe injury than does edema alone. In DCM intramedullary T2 signal change reflects underlying cord pathology but represents a spectrum ranging from potentially reversible edema to established myelomalacia. The longitudinal extent of signal abnormality, presence of T1 hypointensity, and enhancement patterns provide important prognostic information and should inform urgency and expectations of recovery
- Surgical Precision: The most critical takeaway here is the 15-mm rule. Linking the length of the laminectomy directly to the IMLL (1 level per 15 mm) ensures that decompression accounts for the internal longitudinal spread of the injury, not just the bony fracture site. Decompression in DCM should not be conceptualized solely as anatomic canal widening. The goal is restoration of adequate space around the spinal cord and normalization of its physiologic environment. Selection of anterior versus posterior approaches should prioritize achieving effective cord decompression rather than adherence to a fixed morphologic paradigm.
- Intraoperative Validation: Using real-time ultrasound (intraoperative ultrasound) is an excellent care point. It allows the surgeon to visualize the *thecal sac refill* and CSF flow, providing objective data on whether a standard decompression is sufficient or if the pressure requires an expansive duraplasty. In DCM although less standardized than in tSCI, intraoperative adjuncts such as ultrasound or assessment of dural pulsatility may help verify restoration of CSF space and decompression adequacy. Objective physiologic verification represents an important translational opportunity in DCM surgery.

DISCLOSURE

No disclosures.

REFERENCES

1. Barbiellini Amidei C, Salmaso L, Bellio S, et al. Epidemiology of traumatic spinal cord injury: a large population-based study. Spinal Cord 2022;60(9): 812–9.
2. Furlan JC, Sakakibara BM, Miller WC, et al. Global incidence and prevalence of traumatic spinal cord injury. Can J Neurol Sci 2013;40(4):456–64.
3. Rahimi-Movaghar V, Sayyah MK, Akbari H, et al. Epidemiology of traumatic spinal cord injury in developing countries: a systematic review. Neuroepidemiology 2013;41(2):65–85.
4. Zariffa J, Curt A, Steeves JD, et al. Functional motor preservation below the level of injury in subjects with American Spinal Injury Association Impairment Scale grade A spinal cord injuries. Arch Phys Med Rehabil 2012;93(5):905–7.
5. DeVivo MJ, Chen Y. Trends in new injuries, prevalent cases, and aging with spinal cord injury. Arch Phys Med Rehabil 2011;92(3):332–8.
6. Bracken MB, Shepard MJ, Collins WF, et al. A randomized, controlled trial of methylprednisolone or naloxone in the treatment of acute spinal-cord injury. Results of the Second National Acute Spinal Cord Injury Study. N Engl J Med 1990;322(20): 1405–11.
7. Fehlings MG, Moghaddamjou A, Harrop JS, et al. Safety and efficacy of Riluzole in acute spinal cord injury study (RISCIS): a Multi-Center, randomized, Placebo-Controlled, double-blinded trial. J Neurotrauma 2023 40(17–18):1878–88.
8. Fehlings MG, Pedro KM, Alvi MA, et al. The sodium-glutamate antagonist riluzole improves outcome after acute spinal cord injury: results from the RISCIS randomised controlled trial analysed using a global statistical analytic technique. EBioMedicine 2025; 118:105863.
9. Pedro KM, Alvi MA, Goulart GR, et al. Riluzole as a pharmacological therapy for spinal cord injury: where does this therapy stand? Curr Opin Neurol 2025;38(6):625–34.
10. Sajdeya R, Yanez ND, Kampp M, et al. Early blood pressure targets in acute spinal cord injury: a randomized clinical trial. JAMA Netw Open 2025;8(9): e2525364.
11. Aarabi B, Akhtar-Danesh N, Chryssikos T, et al. Efficacy of ultra-early (< 12 h), early (12-24 h), and late (>24-138.5 h) surgery with magnetic resonance imaging-confirmed decompression in American spinal injury Association impairment Scale grades A, B and C cervical spinal cord injury. J Neurotrauma 2020;37(3):448–57.

12. Badhiwala JH, Wilson JR, Kulkarni AV, et al. A novel method to classify cervical incomplete spinal cord injury based on potential for recovery: a group-based trajectory analysis. J Neurotrauma 2022; 39(23–24):1654–64.
13. Badhiwala JH, Wilson JR, Witiw CD, et al. The influence of timing of surgical decompression for acute spinal cord injury: a pooled analysis of individual patient data. Lancet Neurol 2021;20:117–26.
14. Fehlings MG, Vaccaro A, Wilson JR, et al. Early versus delayed decompression for traumatic cervical spinal cord injury: results of the Surgical Timing in Acute Spinal Cord Injury Study (STASCIS). PLoS One 2012;7(2):e32037.
15. Aarabi B, Olexa J, Chryssikos T, et al. Extent of spinal cord decompression in motor complete (American spinal injury Association impairment Scale grades A and B) traumatic spinal cord injury patients: Post-Operative magnetic resonance imaging analysis of standard operative approaches. J Neurotrauma 2019;36(6):862–76.
16. Aarabi B, Sansur CA, Ibrahimi DM, et al. Intramedullary lesion length on postoperative magnetic resonance imaging is a strong predictor of ASIA impairment scale grade conversion following decompressive surgery in cervical spinal cord injury. Neurosurgery 2017;80(4):610–20.
17. Aarabi B, Simard JM, Kufera JA, et al. Intramedullary lesion expansion on magnetic resonance imaging in patients with motor complete cervical spinal cord injury. J Neurosurg Spine 2012;17(3): 243–50.
18. Aarabi B, Chixiang C, Simard JM, et al. Proposal of a management algorithm to predict the need for expansion duraplasty in American spinal injury Association impairment Scale grades A-C traumatic cervical spinal cord injury patients. J Neurotrauma 2022;39(23–24):1716–26.
19. Chryssikos T, Stokum JA, Ahmed AK, et al. Surgical decompression of traumatic cervical spinal cord injury: a pilot Study comparing real-time intraoperative ultrasound after laminectomy with postoperative MRI and CT myelography. Neurosurgery 2023;92(2): 353–62.
20. Furlan JC, Noonan V, Cadotte DW, et al. Timing of decompressive surgery of spinal cord after traumatic spinal cord injury: an evidence-based examination of pre-clinical and clinical studies. J Neurotrauma 2011;28(8):1371–99.
21. Godzik J, Dalton J, Hemphill C, et al. Early surgical intervention among patients with acute central cord syndrome is not associated with higher mortality and morbidity. J Spine Surg 2019;5(4):466–74.
22. Jug M, Kejzar N, Vesel M, et al. Neurological recovery after traumatic cervical spinal cord injury is superior if surgical decompression and instrumented fusion are performed within 8 hours versus 8 to 24 hours after injury: a single Center experience. J Neurotrauma 2015;32(18):1385–92.
23. Stokum JA, Serra R, Gorny N, et al. Mechanisms of traumatic spinal cord injury AIS grade conversion. Neurotrauma Rep 2025;6(1):506–24.
24. van Middendorp JJ. Letter to the editor regarding: "early versus delayed decompression for traumatic cervical spinal cord injury: results of the Surgical Timing in Acute Spinal Cord Injury Study (STASCIS)". Spine J 2012;12(6):540 [author reply: 541–2].
25. Wilson JR, Arnold PM, Singh A, et al. Clinical prediction model for acute inpatient complications after traumatic cervical spinal cord injury: a subanalysis from the Surgical Timing in Acute Spinal Cord Injury Study. J Neurosurg Spine 2012;17(1 Suppl):46–51.
26. Miyanji F, Furlan JC, Aarabi B, et al. Acute cervical traumatic spinal cord injury: MR imaging findings correlated with neurologic outcome–prospective study with 100 consecutive patients. Radiology 2007;243: 820–7.
27. Le E, Aarabi B, Hersh DS, et al. Predictors of intramedullary lesion expansion rate on MR images of patients with subaxial spinal cord injury. J Neurosurg Spine 2015;1–11. https://doi.org/10.3171/2014.10.spine14576.
28. Aarabi B, Oner C, Vaccaro AR, et al. Application of AOSpine subaxial cervical spine injury classification in simple and complex cases. J Orthop Trauma 2017;31(Suppl 4):S24–32.
29. Flanders AE, Schaefer DM, Doan HT, et al. Acute cervical spine trauma: correlation of MR imaging findings with degree of neurologic deficit. Radiology 1990;177:25–33. NOT IN FILE.
30. Mushlin H, Kole MJ, Chryssikos T, et al. AOSpine subaxial cervical spine injury classification system: the relationship between injury morphology, admission injury severity, and long-term neurologic outcome. World Neurosurg 2019;130:e368–74.
31. Boldin C, Raith J, Fankhauser F, et al. Predicting neurologic recovery in cervical spinal cord injury with postoperative MR imaging. Spine (Phila Pa 1976) 2006;31(5):554–9.
32. Vaccaro AR, Daugherty RJ, Sheehan TP, et al. Neurologic outcome of early versus late surgery for cervical spinal cord injury. Spine (Phila Pa 1976) 1997;22(22):2609–13.
33. Levi L, Wolf A, Rigamonti D, et al. Anterior decompression in cervical spine trauma: does the timing of surgery affect the outcome? Neurosurgery 1991; 29(2):216–22.
34. Vale FL, Burns J, Jackson AB, et al. Combined medical and surgical treatment after acute spinal cord injury: results of a prospective pilot study to assess the merits of aggressive medical resuscitation and blood pressure management. J Neurosurg 1997; 87(2):239–46.

35. Aarabi B, Alexander M, Mirvis SE, et al. Predictors of outcome in acute traumatic central cord syndrome due to spinal stenosis. J Neurosurg Spine 2011;14:122–30. NOT IN FILE.
36. Davies BM, Munro C, Khan DZ, et al. Outcomes of degenerative cervical myelopathy from the perspective of persons living with the condition: findings of a semistructured interview process with partnered internet survey. Glob Spine J 2022;12(3):432–40.
37. Smith SS, Stewart ME, Davies BM, et al. The prevalence of asymptomatic and symptomatic spinal cord compression on magnetic resonance imaging: a systematic review and meta-analysis. Glob Spine J 2021;11(4):597–607.
38. Kameyama T, Hashizume Y, Ando T, et al. Spinal cord morphology and pathology in ossification of the posterior longitudinal ligament. Brain 1995;118(Pt 1):263–78.
39. Tator CH, Fehlings MG. Review of the secondary injury theory of acute spinal cord trauma with emphasis on vascular mechanisms. J Neurosurg 1991;75(1):15–26.
40. Morio Y, Teshima R, Nagashima H, et al. Correlation between operative outcomes of cervical compression myelopathy and mri of the spinal cord. Spine (Phila Pa 1976) 2001;26(11):1238–45.
41. Penning L. Some aspects of plain radiography of the cervical spine in chronic myelopathy. Neurology 1962;12:513–9.
42. Popovich PG, Horner PJ, Mullin BB, et al. A quantitative spatial analysis of the blood-spinal cord barrier. I. Permeability changes after experimental spinal contusion injury. Exp Neurol 1996;142(2):258–75.
43. Figley SA, Khosravi R, Legasto JM, et al. Characterization of vascular disruption and blood-spinal cord barrier permeability following traumatic spinal cord injury. J Neurotrauma 2014;31(6):541–52.
44. Takahashi M, Sakamoto Y, Miyawaki M, et al. Increased MR signal intensity secondary to chronic cervical cord compression. Neuroradiology 1987;29(6):550–6.
45. Uchida K, Nakajima H, Takeura N, et al. Prognostic value of changes in spinal cord signal intensity on magnetic resonance imaging in patients with cervical compressive myelopathy. Spine J 2014;14(8):1601–10.
46. Pessini Ferreira LM, Auger C, Kortazar Zubizarreta I, et al. MRI findings in cervical spondylotic myelopathy with gadolinium enhancement: review of seven cases. BJR Case Rep 2021;7(2):20200133.
47. Kwon BK, Curt A, Belanger LM, et al. Intrathecal pressure monitoring and cerebrospinal fluid drainage in acute spinal cord injury: a prospective randomized trial. J Neurosurg Spine 2009;10(3):181–93.
48. Saadoun S, Chen S, Papadopoulos MC. Intraspinal pressure and spinal cord perfusion pressure predict neurological outcome after traumatic spinal cord injury. J Neurol Neurosurg Psychiatry 2017;88(5):452–3.
49. Werndle MC, Saadoun S, Phang I, et al. Monitoring of spinal cord perfusion pressure in acute spinal cord injury: initial findings of the injured spinal cord pressure evaluation study. Crit Care Med 2014;42(3):646–55.
50. Fischbein NJ, Dillon WP, Cobbs C, et al. The "presyrinx" state: a reversible myelopathic condition that may precede syringomyelia. AJNR Am J Neuroradiol 1999;20(1):7–20.
51. Levine DN. The pathogenesis of syringomyelia associated with lesions at the foramen magnum: a critical review of existing theories and proposal of a new hypothesis. J Neurol Sci 2004;220(1–2):3–21.
52. Fehlings MG, Barry S, Kopjar B, et al. Anterior versus posterior surgical approaches to treat cervical spondylotic myelopathy: outcomes of the prospective multicenter AOSpine North America CSM study in 264 patients. Spine (Phila Pa 1976) 2013;38(26):2247–52.
53. de Dios E, Heary RF, Lindhagen L, et al. Laminectomy alone versus laminectomy with fusion for degenerative cervical myelopathy: a long-term study of a national cohort. Eur Spine J 2022;31(2):334–45.
54. Revesz DF, Charalampidis A, Gerdhem P. Effectiveness of laminectomy with fusion and laminectomy alone in degenerative cervical myelopathy. Eur Spine J 2022;31(5):1300–8.
55. Ghogawala Z, Terrin N, Dunbar MR, et al. Effect of ventral vs dorsal spinal surgery on patient-reported physical functioning in patients with cervical spondylotic myelopathy: a randomized clinical trial. JAMA 2021;325(10):942–51.
56. Yordanov S. Does laminectomy alone or laminectomy with fusion lead to better recovery in patients undergoing surgery for degenerative cervical myelopathy from the back. 2025;doi:10.1186/ISRCTN12638817.

Optimizing Spinal Cord Perfusion in Traumatic and Non-traumatic Spinal Cord Injury

Mark Jun Shah-Ostrowski, BM, BCh[a], Yaw Antwi-Yeboah, MBBS, BSc, FRCS[a],
Lara Prisco, MD, MSc, MPH[b,c],
Michael G. Fehlings, MD, PhD, FRCSC, FRSC, FCAHS[d],
Mario Ganau, MD, PhD, MBA, LLM, FEBNS, FRCSEd, FFSTEd[a,c,e,*]

KEYWORDS

• Spinal cord injury • Spinal cord perfusion • Trauma • Degenerative cervical myelopathy
• Hemodynamic management

KEY POINTS

- The pathophysiology of traumatic and non-traumatic spinal cord injury (SCI) differs substantially in terms of mechanism of injury and shares only some commonalities in the secondary cascade of damage.
- The recent AO Spine/Praxis guideline indicates that in patients with traumatic SCI mean arterial pressure, targets should range between 75 and 80 mm Hg as a lower limit and 90 and 95 mm Hg as an upper limit for 3 to 7 days following injury.
- Non-traumatic SCI patients will also benefit from optimized hemodynamic management to ensure adequate perfusion pressure, however consensus is lacking regarding the most appropriate targets range.

INTRODUCTION

Spinal cord injury (SCI) remains one of the most challenging conditions encountered in neurosurgical practice. Despite advances in operative techniques, imaging, and neurocritical care, neurological recovery following SCI is often limited and long-term disability remains common. Secondary injury mechanisms that may be amenable to intervention have therefore garnered increasing attention. Among these, impairments of spinal cord perfusion have emerged as central modifiable determinants of outcome in traumatic and non-traumatic SCI through prompt surgical decompression, medical optimization, and adequate monitoring. This review examines the pathophysiology of SCI and the evidence supporting use of perfusion-guided strategies in neurosurgical practice.

Overview of Spinal Cord Injury Epidemiology and Burden

SCI is a potentially devastating neurological condition associated with substantial morbidity,

[a] Department of Neurosurgery, Oxford University Hospitals NHS Foundation Trust, Oxford, UK; [b] Neuro-Anaesthesia and Intensive Care Medicine, Department of Anaesthesia, Oxford University Hospitals NHS Foundation Trust, Oxford, UK; [c] Nuffield Department of Clinical Neurosciences, University of Oxford, Oxford, UK; [d] Department of Neurosurgery, University of Toronto, Toronto, Canada; [e] BAU International University Batumi, Batumi, Georgia
* Corresponding author. John Radcliffe Hospital, Neurosciences Offices, West Wing, Headley Way, Oxford OX3 9DU, UK.
E-mail address: Mario.Ganau@alumni.harvard.edu

Neurosurg Clin N Am 37 (2026) 597–607
https://doi.org/10.1016/j.nec.2026.05.009

Abbreviations

ASA	anterior spinal artery
CEUS	contrast-enhanced ultrasound
CSF	cerebrospinal fluid
DCM	degenerative cervical myelopathy
ISP	intraspinal pressure
ITP	intrathecal pressure
MAP	mean arterial pressure
NIRS	near-infrared spectroscopy
OSP	opposing spinal pressure
SCI	spinal cord injury
SCPP	spinal cord perfusion pressure
TAAA	thoracoabdominal aortic aneurysm
WCS	White Cord Syndrome

mortality and socioeconomic burden worldwide. The global incidence of SCI is estimated between 700,000 and 1.2 million new cases annually.[1] Absolute burden has increased substantially over the last 3 decades and is projected to rise further with an aging population and improved survival following injury.[2] Marked regional variation is observed in SCI incidence and prevalence, reflecting disparities in socioeconomic status, injury prevention strategies, access to specialist care and data collection infrastructure.[3]

Traumatic mechanisms, mainly falls and road injuries, account for most new cases of SCI globally.[1] Non-traumatic mechanisms including neoplasms, vascular disorders and degenerative myelopathies increasingly contribute to overall disease burden particularly in higher-income, aging populations.[1] SCI disproportionately affects males and older adults, and is associated with lifelong disability, reduced quality of life and a substantial economic strain on health care systems.[1,2]

From a neurosurgical perspective, the burden of SCI extends beyond immediate neurological deficits. Patients are susceptible to a spectrum of secondary complications that vary according to the level and extent of injury. These may include cardiovascular instability, respiratory compromise, bladder and bowel dysfunction, sexual dysfunction, chronic pain syndromes, and increased susceptibility to pressure injuries and infection.[4] Collectively, these sequelae impose a profound economic impact driven by acute surgical and critical care, prolonged rehabilitation, long-term medical support and need for assistive technology.

Pathophysiology: Primary and Secondary Mechanisms of Injury

SCI pathophysiology is often conceptualized as a biphasic process comprising primary and secondary injury. Primary injury refers to the immediate mechanical insult to the spinal cord, such as contusion, compression, distraction or transection, which irreversibly disrupts neurons, glia and microvasculature.[5] This initial event causes direct tissue destruction, hemorrhage and disruption of spinal cord blood flow, establishing the conditions for further secondary injury.

Secondary injury evolves over minutes to weeks following the initial insult, encompassing a cascade of biochemical, cellular and vascular processes that amplify tissue damage beyond the original lesion. Central components include ischemia and impaired spinal cord perfusion, which act as initiators and perpetuators of further downstream molecular cascades including inflammation, edema, glutamate excitotoxicity, and oxidative stress.[5–7] Cumulatively these lead to progressive neuronal and glial loss, demyelination and formation of a hostile microenvironment that impedes regeneration and functional recovery.[8]

For neurosurgeons, secondary injury represents a principal therapeutic target. Many of the driving mechanisms, particularly impaired perfusion and mechanical compression, are potentially modifiable through timely surgical and perioperative intervention.

Rationale for Optimizing Perfusion

Optimizing spinal cord perfusion represents a key clinically actionable strategy for mitigating secondary injury following SCI. Unlike many molecular pathways involved in secondary injury, spinal cord perfusion can be modified in real time through hemodynamic manipulation, cerebrospinal fluid (CSF) drainage, and timely surgical decompression. The American Association of Neurological Surgeons and Congress of Neurological Surgeons emphasize that hemodynamic management and urgent decompression are among the few interventions supported by clinical and experimental evidence for reducing secondary damage and improving recovery in traumatic and non-traumatic SCI.[9]

PATHOPHYSIOLOGY OF SPINAL CORD PERFUSION AND ISCHEMIA

Vascular Anatomy and Autoregulation of the Spinal Cord

Spinal cord vascular anatomy (**Fig. 1**) consists of 3 longitudinal arterial trunks reinforced through segmental inflow, which makes it vulnerable to ischemia. The anterior spinal artery (ASA) arises from the vertebral arteries and runs along the ventral midline of the spinal cord. It approximately supplies the anterior two-thirds of the cord including the anterior horns, corticospinal, and spinothalamic tracts. A paired set of posterior spinal

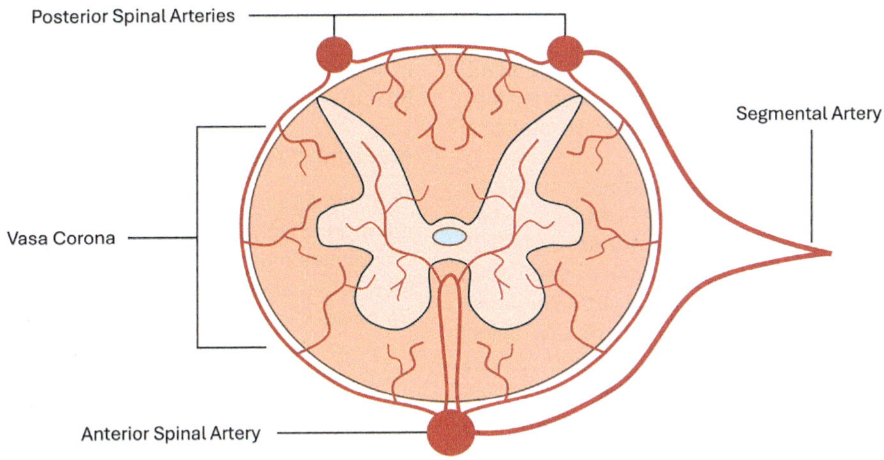

Fig. 1. Spinal cord vascular anatomy.

arteries course dorsolaterally supplying the dorsal columns and posterior horns. This vascular network is interconnected by the vasa corona, a delicate pial arterial plexus which wraps around the cord.[10]

The vertebral arteries themselves only perfuse the upper cervical cord; our longitudinal blood supply therefore relies on numerous radiculomedullary and segmental arteries for reinforcement. In most individuals, the lower thoracic and lumbar ASA is supplied by the artery of Adamkiewicz which is typically left sided and originates between T9 and L2.[11] The segmental, almost discontinuous nature of arterial supply to the cord can therefore predispose regions to hypoperfusion and ischemia in the context of traumatic and non-traumatic SCI.[12]

Under physiological conditions, blood flow to the spinal cord is tightly regulated to maintain stable perfusion despite variation in mean arterial pressure (MAP). Spinal cord autoregulation is an evolving research field, with experimental studies suggesting roles for sympathetic drive, metabolic coupling to neuronal activity and myogenic responses of arteriolar smooth muscle[13] in generating a plateau on the Lassen curve of spinal cord blood flow between MAPs of 50 to 150 mm Hg.[14]

Pathophysiology in Traumatic Spinal Cord Injury

Depending on the level and severity of injury, SCI has the potential to profoundly disrupt autoregulation. Traumatic SCI causes immediate mechanical disruption of neural and vascular structures leading to focal hemorrhage and ischemia at the site of injury. Vasospasm, endothelial damage, microthrombosis, and loss of sympathetic tone are some proposed mechanisms by which autoregulation can begin to fail within hours of injury,[15] effectively making blood flow to affected areas of the spinal cord MAP-dependent. As a result, even brief periods of hypotension may risk ischemia,[16] while excessive hypertension potentially contributes to edema, bleeding and reperfusion injury.[17]

Microvascular failure is amplified further through inflammatory processes which further impair capillary perfusion.[13] Data from animal models suggests that calcium dysregulation promotes cytotoxic injury, while oxidative stress and mitochondrial dysfunction accelerate neuronal apoptosis.[15] These synergistic processes create a vicious cycle, in which impaired perfusion drives further edema, metabolic failure and thus progressive ischemia in potentially salvageable tissue. Loss of autoregulation is a central mechanism underpinning secondary injury, supporting the rationale for strict hemodynamic control in acute phases of traumatic SCI.

Pathophysiology in Non-traumatic Spinal Cord Injury

Non-traumatic SCI describes a spectrum of diseases with distinct but overlapping mechanisms contributing to spinal cord ischemia. The temporal profile of ischemia in such cases is often subacute or chronic, with hypoxia and impaired autoregulation leading to poor perfusion and subsequent neurological deterioration.[13,18] Compressive lesions, including tumors and degenerative stenosis, progressively increase pressure on neural tissue, collapsing microvasculature and venous outflow. Over time, this chronic hypoperfusion leads to reduced capillary density, impaired autoregulation and subsequent metabolic failure.[13]

Inflammatory lesions like transverse myelitis and epidural abscesses have the potential to further disrupt autoregulation through cytokine-mediated endovascular injury. Together these mechanisms result in demyelination and progressive neuronal loss at affected levels.

Iatrogenic injury during thoracoabdominal aortic aneurysm (TAAA) surgery is a well-described, clinically significant cause of non-traumatic SCI. Aortic cross-clamping, interruption of segmental arteries supplying the cord, and intra-operative systemic hypotension can critically reduce spinal cord blood flow, especially in watershed regions with limited collateralization.[19] Reperfusion injury following clamp release may further exacerbate neural damage. Multimodal perioperative protocols including staging of procedures (aimed to preserve collateral supply to the cord), selective CSF drainage and permissive hypertension are employed to mitigate these risks, however permanent neurological deficits remain a significant concern.[20]

DETERMINANTS OF SPINAL CORD PERFUSION PRESSURE

Spinal cord perfusion pressure (SCPP) represents the primary driving force for spinal cord blood flow and oxygen delivery. It is defined as the difference between MAP and opposing pressure within the spinal canal, which we will define as opposing spinal pressure (OSP).[21]

Reductions in MAP, elevations in OSP or both can compromise perfusion and exacerbate ischemic injury (**Fig. 2**). MAP provides continuous assessment of systemic perfusion and is usually measured through arterial catheterization.[22] Measurement of OSP, and therefore calculation of SCPP, is more complex and depends on the technique employed.[23] SCPP has attracted increasing interest in perioperative management of SCI. Observational data suggest that utilizing SCPP targets of 60-65 mm Hg may be a better predictor of enhanced neurological recovery compared with MAP alone,[24] with exposure to SCPP below 50 mm Hg conferring poorer prognosis.[21]

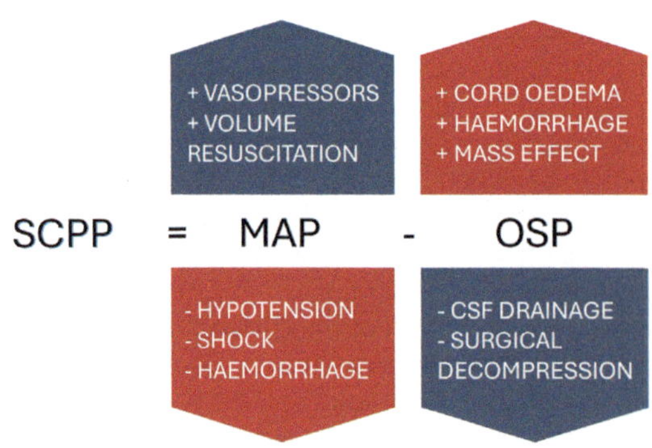

Fig. 2. Determinants of SPCC. SCPP, spinal cord perfusion pressure.

Measuring Pressure Within the Spinal Cord

The terminology surrounding pressure measurement in SCI requires clarification, as different techniques measure distinct physiologic compartments. Saadoun and colleagues have proposed a framework analogous to the Monroe-Kellie doctrine: following SCI, the injured cord swells and displaces surrounding CSF to mitigate local rises in pressure. Once this compensatory reserve is exhausted, the cord becomes compressed against the inflexible theca. Alongside external compression (which depends on the mechanism of SCI), this leads to an increase in pressure at the site of injury.[23]

Intraspinal pressure (ISP) refers to pressure directly measured from within the subdural space at the site of SCI, typically using a fiberoptic pressure probe (eg, Codman microsensors) placed on the surface of the swollen cord following laminectomy and durotomy. Pioneered by the Injured Spinal Cord Pressure Evaluation study,[25] this technique provides direct measurement of pressure exerted by the swelling cord against the dura and correlates more closely with neurological outcomes.[26] Direct ISP measurement has important limitations; intradural probe placement risks additional cord injury and increases the risk of pseudomeningocoele and CSF leak. Probes must be placed under direct microscopic guidance intraoperatively and can become displaced.[27]

Intrathecal pressure (ITP) refers to CSF pressure measured remotely from the injury site, typically via a lumbar drain catheter. These are widely available and technically straightforward; they can be inserted in an intensive care setting and can be used to drain CSF to directly reduce ITP, potentially increasing SCPP.[21] The rationale for monitoring ITP arises from vascular TAAA surgery in which the technique is deployed to monitor and reduce CSF pressure to mitigate ischemia in an otherwise undamaged spinal cord.[20] In the context of focal SCI, however, lumbar ITP correlates poorly with ISP at the site of injury, with lumbar CSF drainage having a limited impact on focally reducing ISP.[28]

Clinical Implications for Spinal Cord Perfusion Pressure Optimization

These distinctions have important implications when translated to clinical practice. SCPP calculated through lumbar ITP, while safer and more straightforward, may not accurately reflect perfusion conditions at the injury site. SCPP derived from injury-site ISP appears to be a stronger predictor of neurological recovery, but remains experimental and highly specialist.

As SCPP integrates the effects of MAP and OSP, it serves as a useful physiological endpoint for optimization through surgical decompression. Evidence suggests that laminectomy alone is ineffective at reducing ISP at the site of injury due to ongoing dural compression of the swollen cord. Laminectomy combined with duroplasty or durotomy is more effective at increasing SCPP compared with laminectomy alone.[29,30] If MAP is not concurrently supported, the resulting increase in SCPP achieved through decompression alone may be insufficient to restore adequate perfusion to the cord,[31,32] highlighting the need for coordinated surgical and hemodynamic management.

Despite promising data, SCPP monitoring is not yet standard practice. While most contemporary systematic reviews conclude that SCPP optimization appears associated with improved neurological recovery, they highlight that current literature is insufficient to generate strong clinical recommendations.[9,32–34] Furthermore, a growing body of evidence supports the idea that "optimal SCPP" can differ substantially on a patient-by-patient basis and can vary over time. This supports the rationale for the use of personalized, real-time monitoring strategies rather than fixed hemodynamic targets in the future.[33,34] MAP has therefore remained the primary hemodynamic target in routine clinical practice.

EVIDENCE FOR OPTIMIZING PERFUSION IN TRAUMATIC SPINAL CORD INJURY

Hemodynamic Targets

Maintenance of elevated MAP in the acute phases of traumatic SCI is a cornerstone of perioperative management. Current AO Spine/Praxis clinical practice guidelines suggest targeting MAP between 75 and 80 mm Hg as a lower limit and 90 and 95 mm Hg as an upper limit for 3 to 7 days following injury.[9,33,34] This strategy aims to support microcirculation, counteract ischemia and stabilize the injured cord during the period of maximal vulnerability to secondary injury.

MAP has historically been our primary hemodynamic target due to its simplicity and reproducibility across clinical environments. Arterial catheterization is widely available, and MAP can be monitored continuously in theater and in any intensive care setting without specialized equipment or expertise.[9,31] The overall evidence base underpinning MAP threshold recommendations remains highly heterogenous, with prospective cohort data (n = 92) indicating adherence to MAP goals of 80 to 85 mm Hg is associated with neurological improvement at 6 months.[21] Meanwhile, retrospective cohort data (n = 105) do not demonstrate a correlation between increased frequency of hypotensive episodes and worse neurological outcomes at discharge.[35] 2024 AO Spine/Praxis guidelines therefore rate the quality of evidence underpinning MAP guidelines as "very low".[9]

Achieving Hemodynamic Targets

Vasopressor selection plays an important role in optimizing perfusion and is highly patient specific; choice depends on comorbidities, level of injury and cardiopulmonary function (**Table 1**). Norepinephrine (noradrenaline) is often favored as a first-line therapy due to its balanced α-adrenergic vasoconstrictive and modest β-adrenergic inotropic effects that raise MAP while preserving cardiac output and maintaining chronotropic support.[17] Phenylephrine, a pure α-agonist, is also commonly used although it lacks the chronotropic support which may confer benefit in bradycardic patients with high cervical or thoracic injuries. Animal studies indicate that norepinephrine may promote improved restoration of spinal cord blood flow and oxygenation compared with phenylephrine.[36] Dopamine is associated with higher rates of cardiovascular complications particularly in older patient populations and has been demonstrated to cause MAP-dependent increases in ITP thus reducing SCPP.[9,37] Patients with pre-existing cardiac conditions or SCI-induced myocardial dysfunction may benefit from inotropic agents such as dobutamine.[38]

Unfortunately, no randomized trials have compared vasopressors head-to-head for neurological outcomes in SCI, and current AO Spine/Praxis guidelines leave vasopressor choice at the discretion of attending physicians.[9] A 2025 retrospective cohort study (n = 3,636) found that phenylephrine was most used (57%) with norepinephrine selected in more severely injured patients; while norepinephrine was associated with worse outcomes overall, this likely reflects indication bias.[39]

The risks of vasopressor therapy must be weighed against perfusion benefits. Key complications include arrhythmia, myocardial strain, acute kidney injury and tissue necrosis secondary to extravastation.[17] Central venous access is often required for prolonged administration; enteral agents such as midodrine may facilitate weaning from intravenous therapy once clinically appropriate.[40] Volume resuscitation with balanced

Table 1
Vasopressors commonly used in spinal cord injury management

Vasopressor	Mechanism of Action	SCI Clinical Indication	Adverse Effects	Central Line Required
Norepinephrine	α_1-adrenergic vasoconstriction (predominant); β_1-adrenergic inotropy and chronotropy	First-line agent for MAP augmentation; preferred in high cervical/thoracic injuries with bradycardia; balanced effect on peripheral resistance and cardiac output	Arrhythmias, myocardial strain, acute kidney injury, tissue necrosis (extravasation)	Yes
Phenylephrine	Pure α_1-adrenergic vasoconstriction	MAP augmentation; commonly used (57% of patients in large cohort); suitable when chronotropic support not required	Reflex bradycardia, reduced cardiac output, tissue necrosis (extravasation)	Yes
Dopamine	Dose-dependent: D_1 (low), β_1 (moderate), α_1 (high dose)	Alternative agent; historically common but declining use	Higher rates of arrhythmia (sinus/ventricular tachycardia), troponin elevation, atrial fibrillation; MAP-dependent increase in ITP (reduces SCPP); increased complications in elderly	Yes
Dobutamine	β_1-adrenergic inotropy (predominant); mild β_2 vasodilation	Patients with SCI-induced cardiac dysfunction; cardio-centric hemodynamic management	Tachycardia, arrhythmias, hypotension (via β_2 vasodilation)	Only required with prolonged use at high doses
Midodrine	Oral α_1-adrenergic agonist	Enteral agent for weaning from IV vasopressors; facilitates ICU discharge	Supine hypertension, urinary retention, piloerection	No

crystalloids should precede initiation of vasopressors in most cases, though excessive fluid risks exacerbating edema and elevating ITP.[40]

PERFUSION MANAGEMENT IN NON-TRAUMATIC SPINAL CORD INJURY

In non-traumatic SCI arising from compressive lesions perfusion impairment arises from elevated tissue pressure, venous outflow obstruction, and reduced arteriovenous pressure gradients. Surgical decompression is the primary intervention to restore perfusion in these contexts.

Degenerative Cervical Myelopathy

Degenerative cervical myelopathy (DCM) is the most common cause of non-traumatic spinal cord dysfunction worldwide. Unlike acute traumatic mechanisms, DCM involves chronic, progressive cord compression leading to reduced capillary density, impaired autoregulation, and subsequent metabolic failure.[41] MRI perfusion studies indicate reduced spinal cord blood flow at the site of compression correlates proportionally to severity of stenosis and subsequent neurological impairment.[42] Surgical decompression is the cornerstone of DCM management, with the goal of halting neurological deterioration and improving function.

Intra-operative hemodynamic management

General perioperative guidance from the American Heart Association suggests maintaining MAP above 60 to 70 mm Hg to prevent end-organ injury during non-cardiac surgery. Given the impaired autoregulatory capacity present in chronic cord compression, some authors advocate higher thresholds in DCM patients, though this remains an area of active investigation.[43]

Intra-operative hypotension is common during cervical decompression surgery, occurring in up to 43% of patients.[44] risk factors include prone positioning,[45] pre-existing systemic hypertension, treatment of upper cervical levels, and multilevel disease.[44] Patients who develop intra-operative hypotension experience higher rates of acute kidney injury, greater need for intensive care admission, and longer hospital stays.[44] Very few data are available directly comparing MAP targets with neurological outcomes in DCM, with most currently accepted hemodynamic targets extrapolated from traumatic SCI literature.[9]

A small recent randomized controlled trial (n = 60) investigated links between higher MAP targets ($\geq$85 mm Hg) and neurological outcomes in DCM surgery.[43] While the trial suggested a trend toward improved recovery with higher MAP targets, the small sample size precludes definitive conclusions. Further investigation is urgently needed to establish evidence-based hemodynamic targets specific to DCM.

White Cord Syndrome

White Cord Syndrome (WCS) is a rare but dangerous cause of acute neurological deterioration following spinal cord decompression. It is characterized by new T2 hyperintensity on post-operative MRI correlated with a sudden motor deficit below the level of surgery. Pathophysiology remains controversial and is thought to involve ischemia-reperfusion injury in the context of chronic hypoperfusion.[46] A 2025 systematic review of 27 reported cases identified several key risk factors for WCS: advanced age (mean 54 years), extensive surgery, posterior surgical approach (70% of cases), and presence of ossification of the posterior longitudinal ligament (33% of cases). Common comorbidities included hypertension (30%), diabetes mellitus (20%), and previous cervical surgery (8%).[47]

The current management strategies for WCS are underpinned by limited and poor-quality evidence, primarily consisting of case reports and small case series rather than prospective trials or high-level studies. Treatment recommendations—such as high-dose intravenous steroids, maintaining MAP above 85 mm Hg, additional decompression, and rehabilitation—are based on expert opinion and anecdotal experience rather than controlled studies.[47] The pathophysiological basis for interventions, including MAP augmentation and steroids, is extrapolated from broader SCI literature and not validated in WCS-specific populations - current strategies should therefore be interpreted with caution.

Metastatic Spinal Cord Compression and Inflammatory Myelopathies

Metastatic spinal cord compression is an oncological emergency affecting up to 10% of patients with spinal metastases. Back pain precedes neurological deterioration in up to 95% of cases, and pretreatment ambulatory status is the strongest predictor of post-treatment function, underscoring the importance of early recognition.[48]

Corticosteroids should be initiated immediately upon clinical suspicion, even before imaging confirmation. A standard regimen of 10 mg intravenously, followed by 4 mg every 6 hours is commonly used, although dosing strategies vary and should be individualized according to comorbidity and oncological context.[48] Surgical decompression followed by radiotherapy is supported by Category 1 evidence for selected patients. The Patchell trial demonstrated that surgery followed by radiotherapy resulted in significantly better ambulatory outcomes than radiotherapy alone (84% vs 57%), with patients in the surgical arm maintaining ambulation for a median of 122 days compared with 13 days. Surgery is particularly indicated for patients with spinal instability, radioresistant tumors, single-site compression, or rapid neurological deterioration, and is generally reserved for those with life expectancy greater than or equal to 3 months and paraplegia for less than 24 hours.[49]

Inflammatory myelopathies

For inflammatory myelopathies such as transverse myelitis and epidural abscess, perfusion impairment arises through cytokine-mediated endothelial injury and vasogenic edema. High-dose intravenous corticosteroids are the standard first-line treatment for transverse myelitis. For epidural abscess, urgent surgical drainage combined with appropriate antimicrobial therapy is essential to relieve compression and restore perfusion before irreversible cord injury occurs.[50]

Aortic and Vascular Surgery

Spinal cord ischemia is an important complication of TAAA repair, with an incidence of up to 10%

depending on aneurysm extent, comorbidities, procedural urgency, and institutional experience. Patients who develop SCI have a poor prognosis, with mortality rates reaching 75% within the first year.[20] Contemporary spinal cord protection protocols are multimodal. CSF drainage targeting ITP less than or equal to 10 mm Hg is recommended in high-risk patients undergoing open TAAA repair based on randomized clinical trial evidence, which demonstrates significant reductions in both temporary and permanent neurological deficits.[51,52] Most centers target MAP greater than or equal to 90 mm Hg and hemoglobin greater than or equal to 10 g/dL perioperatively, with additional adjuncts including targeted revascularization, staged repair, mild permissive hypothermia (32–34°C) and neuromonitoring.[20] Delayed SCI may occur up to 2 weeks post-operatively and requires aggressive management including CSF drain re-insertion and MAP augmentation.

EMERGING TECHNIQUES

Emerging technologies have the potential to refine perfusion-guided care by moving beyond surrogate markers such as MAP toward direct assessment of spinal cord blood flow and oxygenation.

Near-infrared spectroscopy (NIRS) has been initially proposed in traumatic brain injury as an addition to multimodality monitoring for its ability to provide real-time, non-invasive estimates of tissue oxygenation by measuring changes in oxygenated and deoxygenated hemoglobin.[53] Data from animal models demonstrate high sensitivity and specificity for detecting changes also in spinal cord oxygenation during hypoxic episodes and MAP alterations.[54] Animal studies on collateral network NIRS, which monitors paraspinous muscle oxygenation as a surrogate for spinal cord perfusion, have promisingly demonstrated correlation with neurological outcomes in the context of thoracoabdominal aortic surgery.[55] In human studies, NIRS has been used intra-operatively to assess spinal cord perfusion and auto-regulation.[56,57] Further clinical validation and standardization are needed before routine implementation in neurosurgical practice.[56]

Intra-operative contrast-enhanced ultrasound (CEUS) has emerged as a promising modality for real-time assessment of cord perfusion.[58] In both traumatic and non-traumatic SCI models, CEUS can identify perfusion deficits and calculate spinal perfusion indices which correlate injury severity and predict long-term functional outcomes in both animal and human studies.[59,60] In the context of DCM, CEUS studies have demonstrated that greater increases in spinal cord blood flow immediately after decompression are associated with superior neurological recovery.[61] Fascinatingly, rodent studies have demonstrated the efficacy of transcutaneous CEUS for non-invasive, post-operative monitoring of cord perfusion via laminectomy windows.[62] With further large-scale human validation, CEUS may provide an excellent tool to guide intra-operative and post-operative decision making based on real time assessment of perfusion deficits.

All the above underscores once again the efforts to ensure critically important holistic care to the full spectrum of SCI patients, from pediatric to adult cases, by leveraging on the increased understanding of the pathologic mechanisms surrounding the secondary cascade of damage ensuing in the context of SCI.[63–65]

SUMMARY

Impaired spinal cord perfusion is a central and potentially modifiable driver of secondary injury across both traumatic and non-traumatic SCI. Experimental and clinical evidence support the role of timely perfusion optimization through coordinated surgical decompression, hemodynamic management, and CSF control in limiting ischemic injury and improving neurological outcomes. While MAP remains the most practical and widely used surrogate for perfusion in current practice, its limitations are increasingly recognized. SCPP may represent a more physiologically relevant target moving forward. A growing body of evidence suggests that uniform hemodynamic thresholds are likely not optimal, reinforcing the need for personalized strategies guided by real-time physiology. Emerging monitoring techniques, including NIRS and CEUS, offer promising avenues for real-time assessment of cord perfusion although further validation is urgently needed. Until such approaches are established, meticulous avoidance of hypotension, timely decompression, and an informed understanding of spinal cord perfusion physiology remain among the most effective neuroprotective interventions available to the neurosurgeon.

CLINICS CARE POINTS

- Optimizing spinal cord perfusion via careful control of MAP can remarkably increase chances of neurological recovery following traumatic and non-traumatic SCI.

DISCLOSURE

No COI or other disclosure.

REFERENCES

1. GBD Spinal Cord Injuries Collaborators. Global, regional, and national burden of spinal cord injury, 1990-2019: a systematic analysis for the global burden of disease study 2019. Lancet Neurol 2023; 22(11):1026–47. https://doi.org/10.1016/S1474-4422(23)00287-9.
2. Liu Y, Yang X, He Z, et al. Spinal cord injury: global burden from 1990 to 2019 and projections up to 2030 using Bayesian age-period-cohort analysis. Front Neurol 2023;14:1304153.
3.. Wang S, Chen S, Fan W, et al. Global inequalities in the burden of traumatic spinal cord linjury from 1990 to 2021: findings from the Global Burden of Disease Study 2021. Neuroepidemiology 2025; 1–19.
4. Adegeest CY, van Gent JAN, Stolwijk-Swüste JM, et al. Influence of severity and level of injury on the occurrence of complications during the subacute and chronic stage of traumatic spinal cord injury: a systematic review. J Neurosurg Spine 2021;36(4): 632–52.
5. Mortazavi MM, Verma K, Harmon OA, et al. The microanatomy of spinal cord injury: a review. Clin Anat 2015;28(1):27–36.
6. Hellenbrand DJ, Quinn CM, Piper ZJ, et al. Inflammation after spinal cord injury: a review of the critical timeline of signaling cues and cellular infiltration. J Neuroinflammation 2021;18(1):284.
7. Lima R, Monteiro A, Salgado AJ, et al. Pathophysiology and therapeutic approaches for spinal cord injury. Int J Mol Sci 2022;23(22):13833.
8. Ahuja CS, Wilson JR, Nori S, et al. Traumatic spinal cord injury. Nat Rev Dis Primers 2017;3:17018.
9. Kwon BK, Tetreault LA, Martin AR, et al. A clinical practice guideline for the management of patients with acute spinal cord injury: recommendations on hemodynamic management. Glob Spine J 2024; 14(3_suppl):187S–211S.
10. Bosmia AN, Hogan E, Loukas M, et al. Blood supply to the human spinal cord: part I. Anatomy and hemodynamics. Clin Anat 2015;28(1):52–64.
11. Taterra D, Skinningsrud B, Pękala PA, et al. Artery of adamkiewicz: a meta-analysis of anatomical characteristics. Neuroradiology 2019;61(8):869–80.
12. Gailloud P, Gregg L, Galan P, et al. Periconal arterial anastomotic circle and posterior lumbosacral watershed zone of the spinal cord. J Neurointerv Surg 2015;7(11):848–53.
13.. Routkevitch D, Jiang K, Weber-Levine C, et al. Spinal cord vascular autoregulation: key concepts and opportunities to improve management. Spinal Cord 2026;64(1):14–28.
14. Kobrine AI, Doyle TF, Martins AN. Autoregulation of spinal cord blood flow. Clin Neurosurg 1975;22: 573–81.
15. Senter HJ, Venes JL. Loss of autoregulation and posttraumatic ischemia following experimental spinal cord trauma. J Neurosurg 1979;50(2):198–206.
16. Tanvir A, Rizk AA, Wang W, et al. Effect of blood pressure threshold on adverse outcomes in patients with acute spinal cord injury: a systematic review and meta-analysis. Crit Care 2025;29(1):308.
17. Taman M, Abdulrazeq H, Chuck C, et al. Vasopressor use in acute spinal cord injury: current evidence and clinical implications. J Clin Med 2025; 14(3):902.
18. Hernandez-Gerez E, Fleming IN, Parson SH. A role for spinal cord hypoxia in neurodegeneration. Cell Death Dis 2019;10(11):861.
19. Awad H, Lowes S, Gigax B, et al. MRI patterns in ischemic spinal cord injury after thoracoabdominal aorta repair: narrative review with illustrative case series. J Stroke Cerebrovasc Dis 2025;34(12): 108479.
20. Lella SK, Waller HD, Pendleton A, et al. A systematic review of spinal cord ischemia prevention and management after open and endovascular aortic repair. J Vasc Surg 2022;75(3):1091–106.
21. Squair JW, Bélanger LM, Tsang A, et al. Spinal cord perfusion pressure predicts neurologic recovery in acute spinal cord injury. Neurology 2017;89(16): 1660–7.
22. Chen S, Smielewski P, Czosnyka M, et al. Continuous monitoring and visualization of optimum spinal cord perfusion pressure in patients with acute cord injury. J Neurotrauma 2017;34(21):2941–9.
23. Saadoun S, Asif H, Papadopoulos MC. The concepts of Intra Spinal Pressure (ISP), Intra Thecal Pressure (ITP), and Spinal Cord Perfusion Pressure (SCPP) in acute, severe traumatic spinal cord injury: narrative review. Brain Spine 2024;4:103919.
24. Squair JW, Bélanger LM, Tsang A, et al. Empirical targets for acute hemodynamic management of individuals with spinal cord injury. Neurology 2019;93-(12):e1205–11.
25. Werndle MC, Saadoun S, Phang I, et al. Monitoring of spinal cord perfusion pressure in acute spinal cord injury: initial findings of the injured spinal cord pressure evaluation study. Crit Care Med 2014; 42(3):646–55.
26. Hogg FRA, Kearney S, Zoumprouli A, et al. Acute spinal cord injury: correlations and causal relations between intraspinal pressure, spinal cord perfusion pressure, lactate-to-pyruvate ratio, and limb power. Neurocrit Care 2021;34(1):121–9.
27. Phang I, Zoumprouli A, Saadoun S, et al. Safety profile and probe placement accuracy of intraspinal pressure monitoring for traumatic spinal cord injury: injured Spinal Cord Pressure Evaluation study. J Neurosurg Spine 2016;25(3):398–405.
28. Hogg FRA, Gallagher MJ, Kearney S, et al. Acute spinal cord injury: monitoring lumbar cerebrospinal

fluid provides limited information about the injury site. J Neurotrauma 2020;37(9):1156–64.
29. Tykocki T, Poniatowski Ł, Czyż M, et al. Intraspinal pressure monitoring and extensive duroplasty in the acute phase of traumatic spinal cord injury: a systematic review. World Neurosurg 2017;105:145–52.
30. Phang I, Werndle MC, Saadoun S, et al. Expansion duroplasty improves intraspinal pressure, spinal cord perfusion pressure, and vascular pressure reactivity index in patients with traumatic spinal cord injury: injured spinal cord pressure evaluation study. J Neurotrauma 2015;32(12):865–74.
31. Weber-Levine C, Judy BF, Hersh AM, et al. Multimodal interventions to optimize spinal cord perfusion in patients with acute traumatic spinal cord injuries: a systematic review. J Neurosurg Spine 2022;37(5):729–39.
32. Hovis GEA, Sherrod B, Agarwal N, et al. Optimization of spinal cord perfusion pressure for improvement of neurological outcome in traumatic spinal cord injury: a systematic review and meta-analysis. Neurotrauma Rep 2025;6(1):813–23.
33. Evaniew N, Davies B, Farahbakhsh F, et al. Interventions to optimize spinal cord perfusion in patients with acute traumatic spinal cord injury: an updated systematic review. Glob Spine J 2024;14(3_suppl):58S–79S.
34. Hubertus V, Badhiwala JH, Hejrati N, et al. AO spine clinical practice recommendations for the surgical management of acute traumatic spinal cord injury: contemporary concepts. Glob Spine J 2025;15(8):3572–9.
35. Martin ND, Kepler C, Zubair M, et al. Increased mean arterial pressure goals after spinal cord injury and functional outcome. J Emerg Trauma Shock 2015;8(2):94–8.
36. Streijger F, So K, Manouchehri N, et al. A direct comparison between norepinephrine and phenylephrine for augmenting spinal cord perfusion in a porcine model of spinal cord injury. J Neurotrauma 2018;35-(12):1345–57.
37. Altaf F, Griesdale DE, Belanger L, et al. The differential effects of norepinephrine and dopamine on cerebrospinal fluid pressure and spinal cord perfusion pressure after acute human spinal cord injury. Spinal Cord 2017;55(1):33–8.
38. Williams AM, Manouchehri N, Erskine E, et al. Cardiocentric hemodynamic management improves spinal cord oxygenation and mitigates hemorrhage in acute spinal cord injury. Nat Commun 2020;11(1):5209.
39. Hashemaghaie M, Ohnuma T, Sajdeya R, et al. Early vasopressor utilization in critically ill patients with acute traumatic spinal cord injury: a retrospective cohort study. Crit Care Med 2025;53(10):e1952–62.
40. Iovine JA, Villanueva RD, Werth CM, et al. Contemporary hemodynamic management of acute spinal cord injuries with intravenous and enteral vasoactive agents: a narrative review. Am J Health Syst Pharm 2022;79(18):1521–30.
41. Fehlings MG, Evaniew N, Ter Wengel PV, et al. AO spine clinical practice recommendations for diagnosis and management of degenerative cervical myelopathy: evidence based decision making - a review of cutting edge recent literature related to degenerative cervical myelopathy. Glob Spine J 2025;15(5):2585–93.
42. Ellingson BM, Woodworth DC, Leu K, et al. Spinal cord perfusion MR imaging implicates both ischemia and hypoxia in the pathogenesis of cervical spondylosis. World Neurosurg 2019;128:e773–81.
43. Sharma A, Jaiswal A, Marathe N, et al. Does elevated mean-arterial pressure lead to better outcomes in degenerative cervical Myelopathy?- A prospective, pilot randomized control trial. Glob Spine J 2025;15(3):1653–61.
44. Chiang TY, Wang YK, Huang WC, et al. Intraoperative hypotension in non-emergency decompression surgery for cervical spondylosis: the role of chronic arterial hypertension. Front Med (Lausanne) 2022;9:943596.
45. Manohar N, Ramesh VJ, Radhakrishnan M, et al. Haemodynamic changes during prone positioning in anaesthetised chronic cervical myelopathy patients. Indian J Anaesth 2019;63(3):212–7.
46. So JS, Kim YJ, Chung J. White cord syndrome: a reperfusion injury following spinal decompression surgery. Korean J Neurotrauma 2022;18(2):380–6.
47. Bagherzadeh S, Rostami M, Jafari M, et al. "White Cord Syndrome" as clinical manifestation of the spinal cord reperfusion syndrome: a systematic review of risk factors, treatments, and outcome. Eur Spine J 2025;34(1):50–63.
48.. Vega Moreno DA, Reyes Soto G, Lopez-Valdes JC et al. Comprehensive guide to the diagnosis, management, and treatment of metastatic spinal cord compression syndrome. Surg Oncol 2026;64:102341.
49. Patchell RA, Tibbs PA, Regine WF, et al. Direct decompressive surgical resection in the treatment of spinal cord compression caused by metastatic cancer: a randomised trial. Lancet 2005;366(9486):643–8.
50. Molinares DM, Gater DR, Daniel S, et al. Nontraumatic spinal cord injury: epidemiology, etiology, and management. J Pers Med 2022;12(11):1872.
51. Svensson LG, Hess KR, D'Agostino RS, et al. Reduction of neurologic injury after high-risk thoracoabdominal aortic operation. Ann Thorac Surg 1998;66(1):132–8.
52. Coselli JS, LeMaire SA, Köksoy C, et al. Cerebrospinal fluid drainage reduces paraplegia after thoracoabdominal aortic aneurysm repair: results of a

randomized clinical trial. J Vasc Surg 2002;35(4): 631–9.
53. Forcione M, Ganau M, Prisco L, et al. Mismatch between tissue partial oxygen pressure and near-infrared spectroscopy neuromonitoring of tissue respiration in acute brain trauma: the rationale for implementing a multimodal monitoring strategy. Int J Mol Sci 2021;22(3):1122.
54. Cheung A, Tu L, Manouchehri N, et al. Continuous optical monitoring of spinal cord oxygenation and hemodynamics during the first seven days post-injury in a porcine model of acute spinal cord injury. J Neurotrauma 2020;37(21):2292–301.
55. von Aspern K, Haunschild J, Ziemann M, et al. Evaluation of collateral network near-infrared spectroscopy during and after segmental artery occlusion in a chronic large animal model. J Thorac Cardiovasc Surg 2019;158(1):155–64.e5.
56. Amiri AR, Lee CH, Leung TS, et al. Intraoperative assessment of human spinal cord perfusion using near infrared spectroscopy with indocyanine green tracer technique. Spine J 2013;13(12):1818–25.
57. Rashnavadi T, Macnab A, Cheung A, et al. Monitoring spinal cord hemodynamics and tissue oxygenation: a review of the literature with special focus on the near-infrared spectroscopy technique. Spinal Cord 2019;57(8):617–25.
58. Ganau M, Syrmos N, Martin AR, et al. Intraoperative ultrasound in spine surgery: history, current applications, future developments. Quant Imaging Med Surg 2018;8(3):261–7.
59. Khaing ZZ, Leyendecker J, Harmon JN, et al. Perfusion imaging metrics after acute traumatic spinal cord injury are associated with injury severity in rats and humans. Sci Transl Med 2024;16(765): eadn4970.
60.. Saway BF, Routkevitch D, Suresh R, et al. Contrast-enhanced ultrasound perfusion imaging of the spinal cord before and after surgical decompression for cervical spondylotic myelopathy. Neurosurgery 2026;98:688–97.
61.. Wei X, Song Q, Huang L, et al. Intraoperative ultrafast ultrasound doppler imaging of degenerative cervical myelopathy helps predict neurological recovery. J Ultrasound Med 2026;45(3):639–51.
62. Khaing ZZ, Cates LN, Hyde JE, et al. Transcutaneous contrast-enhanced ultrasound imaging of the posttraumatic spinal cord. Spinal Cord 2020; 58(6):695–704.
63. Eraifej J, Nnadi C, Ganau M. Early and ultra-early surgical decompression for acute spinal cord injury: bracing for the winds of change. Eur Spine J 2022; 31(7):1691–2.
64. Hachem LD, Zhu M, Aarabi B, et al. A practical classification system for acute cervical spinal cord injury based on a three-phased modified Delphi process from the AOSpine spinal cord injury knowledge forum. Glob Spine J 2024;14(2):535–45.
65. Ganau M, Fehlings MG. Clinical and health policy-related challenges of pediatric spinal cord injuries. Neurol India 2017;65(3):475–6.

Delayed C5 Palsy after Cervical Spine Surgery

Laura Ganau[a], So Kato, MD, PhD[b], Zheqing Zhang, BA[c], Gianfranco K.I. Ligarotti, MD[d],
Michael G. Fehlings, MD, PhD, FRCSC, FRSC, FCAHS[e],
Mario Ganau, MD, PhD, MBA, LLM, FEBNS, FRCSEd, FFSTEd[c,f,g,*]

KEYWORDS

- Degenerative cervical myelopathy • Anterior cervical discectomy and fusion • Cervical laminectomy
- Postoperative C5 palsy

KEY POINTS

- Various mechanistic theories have been proposed for C5 nerve palsy (C5NP): such plethora of theories suggests a multifactorial etiology for this postoperative complication.
- Optimizing prevention strategies and adopting Early Recovery after Surgery (ERAS) protocols represent meaningful approaches to minimize the risk of C5NP.
- Promising pharmacologic strategies, such as riluzole, currently under assessment in international randomized clinical trials could become game changer for the treatment of C5NP.

INTRODUCTION

Postoperative C5 nerve palsy (C5NP) is a well-recognized and clinically significant complication of cervical spine surgery, particularly following procedures for degenerative cervical myelopathy (DCM).[1,2] Postoperative C5NP is characterized by new-onset motor weakness mainly affecting muscles supplied by the C5 nerve root, with or without concurrent sensory changes in the C5 dermatome.

Symptoms typically manifest within a week but they may also have delayed appearance and, in some cases, presentation up to 2 months postoperatively have been described in the literature.[3,4] The severity of symptoms also varies depending on the number of muscle groups involved and their weakness. Usually, functional impairment is due to deltoid and biceps brachii involvement and may lead to mild or severe weakness in shoulder abduction and elbow flexion. This often-unexpected complication can prolong rehabilitation time, impacting activities of daily living (ADL) and overall quality of life (QoL). Having said that, even severe forms of C5NP have a generally good prognosis with spontaneous resolution in most cases.[5]

The incidence of C5NP varies widely in the literature, highlighting disparities in patient populations, surgical techniques, and diagnostic criteria. Reported rates range from 0.58% to approximately 30%,[4,6,7] with a higher incidence following posterior procedures compared to anterior access surgery. More specifically, a recent meta-analysis revealed pooled rates of 8% following noninstrumented laminectomy and 7.03% after posterior cervical decompression and fusion versus a 2.61% rate following anterior cervical discectomy and fusion (ACDF).[8] Those figures differ slightly from those reported in an earlier meta-analysis

[a] School of Medicine, University of Cagliari, Italy; [b] Department of Orthopeadic Surgery, the University of Tokyo, Tokyo, Japan; [c] Department of Neurosurgery, Oxford University Hospitals NHS Foundation Trust, Oxford, UK; [d] Aerospace Medical Institute of Milan "A. Mosso", Italian Air Force, Milan, Italy; [e] Department of Neurosurgery, University of Toronto, Toronto, Canada; [f] Nuffield Department of Clinical Neurosciences, University of Oxford, Oxford, UK; [g] BAU International University Batumi, Batumi, Georgia
* Corresponding author. Neurosciences Offices, West Wing, John Radcliffe Hospital Headley Way, OX3 9DU, Oxford, UK.
E-mail address: Mario.Ganau@alumni.harvard.edu

Neurosurg Clin N Am 37 (2026) 609–621
https://doi.org/10.1016/j.nec.2026.05.015

Abbreviations

ACDF	anterior cervical discectomy and fusion
ADL	activities of daily living
C5NP	C5 nerve palsy
DCM	degenerative cervical myelopathy
EMG	electromyography
ERAS	Early Recovery after Surgery
IONM	intraoperative neuro-monitoring
MEP	motor evoked potential
NCS	nerve conduction studies
OPLL	ossification of the posterior longitudinal ligament
QoL	quality of life

which had revealed a pooled incidence of 5% following anterior cervical surgery versus 6.2% following posterior procedures.[9] The heterogeneity in study design and diagnostic criteria explain why the estimated incidence range remains broad; these inconsistencies also reflect a growing interest in this postoperative complication and emphasize the importance of better mechanistic understanding, risk stratification, and prevention strategies.

Historical Background

Historically, the attention toward postoperative C5NP grew proportionally to the diffusion of cervical decompressive procedures, particularly expansive laminoplasty techniques, in countries such as Japan characterized by a high incidence of DCM secondary to ossification of the posterior longitudinal ligament (OPLL). Cervical laminoplasty was first described by Hirabayashi, who popularized the expansive "open-door" technique (ELAP) using sutures for fixation during the 1970s.[10] Many variations of such technique were proposed afterward, those included Z-shaped expansive laminoplasty, double door laminoplasty, and French door laminoplasty just to list the most famous ones. With the diffusion of those posterior approaches to the cervical spine, so did increase the reported cases of C5NP. Initially, various factors contributed to gather surgeons' interest in this condition. Among them, the recognition that C5NP could arise despite the lack of a direct iatrogenic injury to the nerve root, the occurrence of delayed symptoms and the variable presentations, have all contributed to prompt a growing attention toward C5NP. Several hypotheses started to be formulated, and with time influenced tailored changes to operative techniques.[11–13] While many surgeon scientists now tend to consider more plausible a multifactorial etiology, controversy persists regarding the primary driver initiating the cascade of biochemical events leading to the onset of signs and symptoms typical of C5NP. For all those reasons, a good understanding of the anatomy of the subaxial cervical spine and the cascade of secondary inflammation is first step to deepen our understanding of current practices and knowledge gaps.

RELEVANT ANATOMY AND BIOMECHANICS

It is nowadays accepted that various anatomic features of the C5 nerve root may increase its vulnerability to postoperative damage. Compared with other cervical nerve roots, the C5 root traverses a relatively short course through the intervertebral foramen after exiting the spinal cord at the C4/5 level.[14] Additionally, the anterior rootlets are susceptible to caudal compression by the tip of the superior facet joint at the narrowest part of the foramen. Anatomic studies suggest that the length of the posterior rami is shortest at C4–5, which may be affected by stretching and compression with multifidus muscle retraction in posterior procedures.[14] Delayed symptom onset may be explained by distraction and/or compression of the nerve root by adjacent structures such as the facet joint and vertebral body as patients regain some mobility and begin rehabilitation.[13] Taken together, the short course and narrow intervertebral foramen result in limited mobility and increased tension on the C5 nerve root, potentially predisposing this specific nerve root to injury from traction forces and postoperative shifts.

Multiple other factors, though, including alignment, ligamentous structures, and degree of stenosis, influence the mobility of the cervical spinal cord and cannot be disregarded in the assessment of anatomic reasons for C5NP. In DCM patients, cord mobility may be reduced due to chronic anterior, lateral, or posterior compression to relevant neural structures. Decompressive surgery, particularly posterior approaches,[1] may cause posterior shift of the spinal cord with greater tension on the C5 nerve root.[12,13] Furthermore, the diameter of the intervertebral foramen may be affected by degenerative changes, osteophytes, joint hypertrophy, and ligament thickening. Tethering of the C5 nerve root within a narrow foramen increases the risk of stretch injury even after uneventful surgery. Those postoperative changes reflect a modification of the biomechanical forces acting on each functional spinal unit.[14] As such, the risk of C5NP is increased in any cervical deformity surgery with attempts to restore a physiologic lordosis.[15,16] Evidently, anatomic and biomechanical considerations need to be factored in the risk stratification and decision-making regarding operative techniques to prevent C5NP.

CLINICAL AND NEUROPHYSIOLOGICAL DIAGNOSIS

Other than the typical motor weakness affecting shoulder abduction (deltoid) and elbow flexion (biceps) mentioned above, postoperative C5NP may be accompanied by sensory disturbance such as numbness, tingling, and reduced or altered sensation in the lateral shoulder or upper arm. Neuropathic shoulder pain may also be present.[17,18]

Delayed presentation is common in C5NP and the lag between operation and symptom onset aligns with theories concerning dynamic postoperative changes rather than iatrogenic injuries. While excluding other causes of neurologic dysfunction, such as residual neural compression, epidural hematoma, instrumentation misalignment, including screws/cage pull out, is routinely achievable via postoperative computed tomography (CT) and magnetic resonance imaging (MRI) scans, the diagnosis of C5NP remains purely clinical and further neurophysiological investigations should be performed with the intent of objectively confirming it. The gold standard for neurophysiological investigations in the context of C5NP consists in electromyography (EMG) and nerve conduction studies (NCS), which may help identifying isolated or multilevel root involvement and can assist in the monitoring of recovery. Neurophysiological tests are also important to distinguish C5NP from brachial plexus or peripheral nerve injury associated with positioning on the operating table.[19] EMG in C5NP patients typically shows denervation changes in C5-innervated muscles with those alterations being detectable for many weeks (usually 6 weeks and 6 months) after symptom onset.[20,21] Obviously, continued neurologic monitoring and EMG/NCS follow-up is especially important in patients with unresolved palsy: the slight heterogeneity in the natural course of this condition has been fundamental in guiding surgeons-scientists who attempted to identify mechanistic hypothesis.

PATHOPHYSIOLOGY AND MECHANISTIC HYPOTHESES

Despite considerable research, there is no unifying mechanism to explain the pathogenesis of postoperative C5NP. Several hypotheses have been proposed, which likely overlap and interact to varying degrees in individual patients.

Posterior Spinal Cord Shift and Traction Injury

A leading hypothesis suggests that decompression, especially in posterior procedures, can cause the spinal cord to shift posteriorly. This increases tension on the nerve roots, particularly the C5 root with its comparatively short course. Radiological evidence has revealed greater posterior displacement of the cord in patients who develop postoperative C5NP compared with controls.[3,11,12,22–24]

Foraminal Stenosis and Nerve Root Tethering

Preoperative narrowing of the intervertebral foramen may cause mechanical impingement and tethering of the nerve roots, limiting their capacity to adapt to positional shifts.[3,24–29] Consequently, even minor movement of the spinal cord may theoretically lead to stretch-related injury. For this, some authors proposed routine prophylactic foraminotomy as an attempt to lowering the risk of postoperative C5NP, and other suggested that skin laminectomy or oblique corpectomy could be more respective of the anatomy and function of the nerve roots, C5 included.[30,31] Evidence that such approach can be beneficial reinforced the foraminal theory.[32–35]

Ischemia and Reperfusion Injury

Injury to the C5 nerve root may also result from perioperative ischemia and/or postoperative reperfusion, which can cause neural damage due to reactive oxygen species. Impaired blood flow to the C5 root resulting from operative manipulation of radicular arteries in case of intradural procedures, or decompression-related flow changes in the most common ACDF, laminectomy, and laminoplasty may cause ischemic injury of the nerve root.[32,36,37]

Anterior Horn Cells Injury

Transient or permanent injury to the anterior horn cells of the segmental spinal cord, possibly with contribution from ischemia and reperfusion injury, can cause motor deficits.[13] Although direct evidence for this mechanism is lacking, the anterior horn cells injury hypothesis is supported by data from patients with bilateral weakness or associated anterior cord signal changes on MRI.[38,39]

Direct Intraoperative Nerve Root Injury

Though less frequently implicated, direct mechanical trauma, excessive manipulation, or thermal injury during surgery can contribute to postoperative C5NP. Reports of deficits after specific technical steps, case series, and cadaveric anatomic studies support this as a contributing factor in some cases.[11,40] However, direct iatrogenic axonal injury is less likely to show a delayed presentation, indicating that intraoperative manipulation, together with traction-related neuropraxia, are unlikely to be the sole mechanism in the vast majority of cases.

Focal Inflammation and Edema

Finally, the timeline between surgery and symptoms onset reflect well the progression of physiologic inflammation and postoperative edema following surgery in the cervical spine. Nonetheless postoperative local edema and muscle swelling are known sequelae of surgery and should be considered during postoperative assessment.

Multifactorial Etiology

Overall, most of the evidence currently available supports a multifactorial model integrating anatomic susceptibility, biomechanical changes, and physiologic responses. Original theories postulating a predominance of the roles of posterior cord migration and foraminal tethering have now been replaced by a better understanding that a combination of relevant vascular processes, direct iatrogenic injury, inflammation, and reperfusion injury can all play a contributory role. Altogether they may account for the delayed presentation of C5NP.[41–43] Since mechanistic understanding has clinical relevance for prevention and management of the condition, in **Table 1**, we offer a summary of the critical analysis of the various hypothesis currently available.

RISK FACTORS

By now, it has become clear that various risk factors for postoperative C5NP should be considered, in **Table 2** we have categorized them as per patient-related, anatomic, and surgical factors.

Meta-analyses and cohort studies pointed at advanced age, male sex, OPLL, foraminal stenosis, spinal cord signal change (high signal intensity on T2-weighted MRI), and cervical deformities.[47–50]

Some studies used multivariate analysis or machine learning to identify risk factors and develop predictive models for postoperative C5NP. One of those studies developed an ensemble machine learning model using logistic regression, random forest, AdaBoost, gradient boosting machines, and XGBoost to achieve an area under the receiver operating characteristic curve of 0.773 and create a risk calculator for predicting C5NP after instrumented cervical fusion.[44] Nevertheless the clinical utility of those tools remains unclear due to issues regarding generalizability of the results extrapolated from single-center cohort, and without standardized scoring system for risk stratification. This said, a deeper awareness of common risk factors and epidemiologic trends can help surgeons in their surgical planning and are of paramount importance to ensure a watertight consent process meant to counseling patients and developing preventative strategies tailored around different surgical approaches and individual patient characteristics.

PREVENTION STRATEGIES

Based on existing understanding of postoperative C5NP, including possible underlying mechanisms and contributing factors, several preventive strategies have been proposed. Those aim at an early recognition of patient-related risk factors, which could be amenable to preoperative optimization,[46] and a consideration for surgical techniques that hold a potential to reduce nerve root manipulation and therefore postoperative dysfunction.

Surgical Planning and Technique

During surgical planning for decompression of the cervical spinal cord and nerve roots, a thorough evaluation of cervical alignment (including sagittal vertical alignment, C7 slope, and rule of 9, to name a few), foraminal characteristics (orientation and dimensions), and position of the neural structures (hyperintense intramedullary T2WI signal, viper sign, length of nerve roots, and their direction) should be undertaken. High-risk patients may benefit from individualized approach including long cassette x-rays to assess global spine alignment, flexion-extension x-rays, and dynamic MRI scans. For instance, preoperative imaging can be used to assess the medial line of the C5 facet joint, particularly in patients with advanced degenerative changes and foraminal stenosis.

Various surgical nuances have also been reported to minimize the risk of postoperative C5NP. Avoiding prolonged, excessive retraction and lateral stretch of the paraspinal muscles including the multifidus, with intermittent relaxation of retractors, is advisable to reduce postoperative muscle swelling.[13] Nakakima and colleagues suggested that the ligamentum flavum can be used as an intraoperative anatomic marker, and drilling of the bony gutter should be of sufficient width and not overly lateral to prevent C5 root kinking.[51] A retrospective study of prospectively collected data showed that selective blocking laminoplasty with cervical laminectomy and fusion may be associated with reduced rates of postoperative C5NP in DCM patients, compared with conventional cervical laminectomy and fusion.[52] Gradual decompression, careful handling of the spinal cord, use of cottonoids, gentle aspiration all help avoiding excessive manipulation of the neural elements. As anticipated above, being

Table 1
Mechanistic hypotheses and supporting evidence for postoperative C5 nerve palsy

Mechanistic Hypothesis	Key Supporting Evidence	Limitations or Controversies	Clinical Implications
Posterior spinal cord shift	• Imaging studies showing increased posterior displacement • Higher incidence following posterior surgery	• Less likely after anterior surgery • Not all patients with significant posterior cord shift develop symptoms	• Consider surgical planning and techniques to limit excessive cord shift
Foraminal stenosis and nerve root tethering	• Increased risk of C5 palsy in patients with narrow intervertebral foramen at C4–5 • Studies showing benefit of prophylactic foraminotomy	• Inconsistent evidence across studies • Unclear patient selection	• Evaluate foraminal anatomy on preoperative imaging • Consider prophylactic foraminotomy in selected cases
Segmental spinal cord dysfunction, ischemia/reperfusion injury	• Delayed onset • Bilateral symptoms • MRI signal changes	• Limited direct evidence • Mechanism remains mostly speculative	• Potential role for neuroprotection and neurophysiological monitoring
Direct injury	• Some cases with immediate or early onset	• Does not explain delayed onset which occurs in most cases	• Importance of careful surgical technique • Consider intraoperative neuromonitoring
Multifactorial model	• Variable presentations and clinical findings	• Difficult to identify a single dominant mechanism	• Personalized approach with risk stratification and targeted prevention

mindful of avoiding over-correction may also minimize posterior cord shift and biomechanical changes that can ultimately contribute to C5NP.

While a clinical trial is underway attempting to address the usefulness of routine prophylactic foraminotomy (NCT03023696), recent studies have been less convincing than previous reports in showing the efficacy of bilateral foraminotomy in preventing C5NP.[53,54] Addressing such knowledge gap will certainly inform the surgical community on how to conduct an appropriate patients selection.

Table 2
Risk factors for postoperative C5 nerve palsy

Patient-Related Factors	Anatomic and Radiological Factors (Preoperative)	Surgical Factors
• Older age[24,25,29,44,45] • Male sex[3,5,7,24,25,29,46] • Ossification of the posterior longitudinal ligament (OPLL)[3,9,29,47] • Degenerative cervical myelopathy[29,44] • Preoperative nonmotor neurologic symptoms[44]	• Intervertebral foramen narrowing or stenosis (reduced foraminal diameter at C4–5 or high encroachment ratio)[3,24–29,48,49] • Preoperative spinal cord signal change (eg, high signal intensity on T2-weighted MRI at the C4–5 spinal cord segment)[17,25,29] • Cervical alignment or curvature abnormalities (eg, kyphosis, reduced T1 slope)[25,27,48] • Larger cord-lamina angle[30,50] • Atlantoaxial subluxation[45]	• Posterior surgical approaches[7,9,17,23,29] • Laminectomy (compared with laminoplasty and other procedures)[3,5] • Multilevel decompression[24,45] • Posterior spinal cord shift[3,23,24] • Over-correction or excessive change in cervical curvature[15,25,49] • Increased spinal cord retraction distance[25]

Finally, the use of intraoperative ultrasound can also help surgeons in ruling out residural ventral compression on nerve root or spinal cord during posterior approaches and can serve as a real time neuronavigation tool throughout various stages of the procedure including pedicular screw insertion.[55]

Intraoperative Neuromonitoring

Intraoperative neuro-monitoring (IONM), including somatosensory evoked potentials and motor evoked potentials (MEPs), and spontaneous EMG, have been a longstanding pillar of cervical spine surgery. Several studies have shown that multimodal electrophysiological monitoring of deltoid and biceps muscles during surgery, particularly transcranial electrical stimulation MEP changes, may be useful in predicting postoperative C5NP.[56–61] In a retrospective study, the sensitivity and specificity of MEP alerts in the deltoid or biceps were 100% and 98.4%, respectively.[57] In a prospective multicenter observational study, the sensitivity of transcranial MEP alerts for predicting C5 palsy was 57.1%, and the rescue rate after intervention in response to alerts was 57.9%.[60] Other studies have demonstrated that sustained EMG activity of the C5 root can be considered as a reliable intraoperative indicator of nerve root irritation, being associated with C5NP and deltoid muscle weakness in various reports.[62,63] However, the quality of most of those studies is downgraded by their retrospective nature and the lack of standardized protocols, particularly in response to intraoperative alerts, which currently limit our ability to make stronger recommendations on the utility of IONM as an independent preventative method.[17,64–67] Further collaborative research is therefore needed to better understand how electrophysiological measures can be more specific and how it should be combined with other strategies to reduce the risk of postoperative C5NP.

Pharmacologic Prophylaxis

The use of prophylactic perioperative dexamethasone has been considered to prevent C5NP, however the quality of the evidence is very low. In a retrospective single-center study of patients undergoing multilevel posterior cervical laminectomy and fusion for DCM, the incidence of C5NP was lower in those patients who received perioperative dexamethasone compared with an historical control rate.[68] Even though there are no medications specifically licensed for prevention of this postoperative complication, we can expect that in the near future useful information could be available for extraction from ongoing clinical trials on neuroprotective pharmacologic interventions (e.g. Ibudilast) which proved a good degree of safety and effectiveness in preclinical trials and are currently tested in randomized controlled trials for DCM patients (RECEDE DCM, NCT04631471). To conclude this section of the article, we created **Fig. 1** to show the parallelism between proposed mechanism of injury and suggested prevention strategies for C5NP.

TREATMENT

The treatment of postoperative C5NP is typically nonoperative and a large cohort study indicated that it mostly revolves on clinical observation with physiotherapy (90% of cases), oral corticosteroids (18%), and referral for peripheral nerve surgery (in only 17% of cases).[69] Supportive strategies reported in **Table 3** may change over time and are guided by the clinical evolution.

Early mobilization and physiotherapy are crucial to preserve range of movement, reduce stiffness, and prevent muscle contractures, all aiding functional recovery.[70] Analgesia and a short course of corticosteroids may help addressing the issue of C5NP-associated neuropathic pain.[17,69,71,72] In some patients, adjuvant therapy with neuromuscular or functional electrical stimulation may also help improve motor function, though there is no high-level clinical evidence for their use in standard operating protocols.[73,74]

Riluzole, a glutamate antagonist, showed potential for limiting ischemia-reperfusion injury in cervical spine surgery. In preclinical studies, it reduced oxidative DNA damage in the spinal cord and postoperative deterioration following surgical decompression.[75,76] However, such clinical advantage in DCM patients was not fully captured by the initial report from a phase 3 randomized controlled trial (CSM-PROTECT, NCT01257828).[77] In contrast, a secondary analysis found that patients taking riluzole showed significantly greater global improvement (combining the 36-Item Short Form Health Survey Physical Component Score, arm and neck pain numeric rating scale scores, American Spinal Injury Association motor score, and Nurick grade) compared with placebo at 1-year follow-up.[78] While existing studies have been limited to the broad spectrum of DCM and not the narrow cohort of patients with postoperative C5NP, data on Riluzole provides early promise that this drug could enhance functional recovery even in this latter group of cases.[79]

Peripheral nerve surgery with transfer of the ulnar/median nerve to the biceps or brachialis branches of the musculocutaneous nerve, either in the form of single or double fascicular transfer

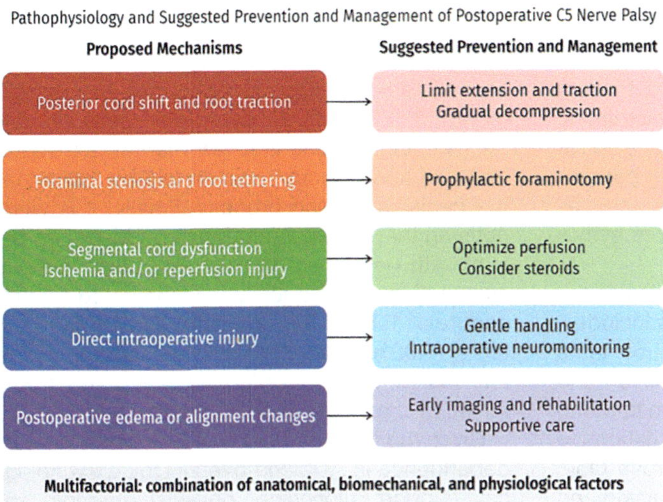

Fig. 1. Proposed pathophysiological mechanisms and suggested prevention and management of postoperative C5 nerve palsy.

has been proposed.[69,] Other techniques include transfer of the radial nerve to the axillary nerve and transfer of the spinal accessory nerve to the suprascapular or axillary nerve.[80] Those options have proven effectiveness in restoring elbow flexion and shoulder abduction, respectively. Nevertheless, they should be considered only as a last resort in patients with persistent neurophysiological evidence of nerve damage refractory to conservative and medical management. This is

Table 3
Phases of management of postoperative C5 nerve palsy

Phase	Management	Purpose and Considerations
Immediate (days)	Detailed neurologic examination	Document MRC grade for muscle power and compare with baseline
	Urgent imaging with MRI (±CT)	Assess for structural abnormalities and exclude compressive causes. Surgical revision may be needed for structural compression
	Consider a short course of steroids	Reduce inflammation and/or edema (no high-level evidence)
Early (weeks)	Observation and reassurance	Most cases recover spontaneously. Counsel patients regarding typically favorable prognosis
	Physiotherapy	Preserve range of motion, facilitate strengthening and stabilization, and prevent stiffness and disuse atrophy
	EMG/NCS	Monitor peripheral nerve function and re-innervation. Guide prognosis (severe denervation predicts slower recovery)
	Consider neuromuscular electrical stimulation	Preserve muscle bulk during re-innervation (adjunctive therapy with limited high-level evidence)
Intermediate (3–6 mo)	Regular follow-up	Monitor symptoms and muscle power
	Structured rehabilitation	Maximize recovery and compensatory strategies
	Consider referral to peripheral nerve specialist	Early evaluation for surgical intervention may be warranted if severe deficits persist, particularly with minimal recovery by 3–6 mo
Late (>6–9 mo)	Peripheral nerve surgery	Consider nerve transfer surgery for persistent severe palsy in selected patients
	Long-term rehabilitation	Optimize strength and functional independence

due to the fact that such operations cannot guarantee functional improvement and come with the risk of additional sensory deficits. Furthermore, with regards to peripheral nerve surgery, there is no established consensus on the optimal timing of intervention, but research suggests that electrophysiological monitoring can help identify patients suitable for nerve transfer surgery as early as 3 months and within 9 to 12 months from symptoms onset.[81]

For all those reasons, rehabilitation remains the cornerstone of C5NP management. This includes, among others, a mix of passive and isometric exercises to aid recovery of muscle function and prevent muscle wasting from inactivity. In tandem, occupational therapy can help with adaptations to ensure independence in ADL and improve QoL. Newer technologies including robotic training and virtual reality have been studied to support rehabilitation by correcting motion patterns, improving efficiency, enhancing motivation, and providing engaging and immersive therapy.[82–84] However, existing evidence is limited to case reports and single-center studies, whereas outcomes-focused research would be useful to refine our propensity to engage with novel technologies alongside well-established physiotherapy training programs.

PROGNOSIS AND OUTCOMES

The recovery trajectory of delayed C5NP can vary in terms of pace (fast vs slow), degree (partial vs complete) and direction (linear vs in waves). A multicenter study found that 57.95% of patients recovered within 6 months.[7] In a retrospective single-center study of patients with C5NP after surgery for DCM, only 50% of those patients who showed persistent severe deficits at 3 months postoperatively regained useful strength by 1 year.[81] In a retrospective single-center study, 89% of patients experienced recovery of deltoid muscle strength to at least grade 4/5 by the final postoperative follow-up at 12 months.[17] In general, the longer C5NP persists, less likely full recovery becomes; a more precise overview of the different trajectories is offered by a very recent study providing a Bayesian modeling of recovery, which revealed an approximately 88% recovery rate by 2 years.[85] While the majority of patients will achieve partial or complete recovery at some point,[1,5,7,17,86] in a small proportion of cases the signs and symptoms will unfortunately persist over time. Such dismal outcome has been associated not only with structural nerve damage but also delayed access to rehabilitation[2,87]

Early severe symptoms tend to be associated with poorer prognosis and may warrant additional radiological and neurophysiological investigations as well as specialist referral for further management.[81,87] Therefore, symptom severity and persistence over the first few months are important prognostic factors and should be factored in the decision-making process. Finally, it is worth noticing that a pooled analysis conducted on patient with permanent deficits revealed a minimal association with the following index surgical procedures: 1.44% for noninstrumented laminectomy, 1.02% posterior cervical decompression and fusion, 0.28%, for laminoplasty, and 1.06% for ACDF, respectively.[8]

Given the impact of persistent symptoms on independence in ADL and overall QoL, psychological support alongside physical therapy and rehabilitation should be considered. Furthermore, optimizing patient education has certainly a role in improving our standards of care.

FUTURE DIRECTIONS

Key areas for future research on postoperative C5NP include: (a) standardizing diagnostic criteria,[88,89] (b) clarifying pathophysiological mechanisms,[90] including understanding whether spinal traumas patients, similarly to DCM cases, should be considered for tailored prophylaxis,[91,92] (c) developing predictive models and risk stratification strategies,[93] (d) assessing the role of new surgical tools, including exoscope-assisted surgery,[79,94] (e) designing high-quality trials on perioperative neuroprotective pharmacologic protocols,[78,88] and (f) integrating big data analysis and machine learning models to enhance neurophysiological monitoring, postoperative rehabilitation and direct educational programs on DCM and complications of its surgical management.[80,84,95]

Future patient-centered approaches should rely on long-term prospective outcomes because most existing evidence is based on retrospective studies. To this regards, developing and validating uniform diagnostic criteria and clinically applicable scoring systems to grade the severity and recovery can help reduce heterogeneity across studies and enable comparable outcome reporting. Large prospective cohorts and pooled data can be used to build validated, multivariable prediction tools incorporating clinical, radiological, and surgical factors, as well as imaging biomarkers, to aid prognosis and identification of patients who would benefit from prophylactic measures. Current knowledge gaps can only be addressed by focusing also on patients' QoL to capture impact and inform shared decision-making.

SUMMARY

Delayed postoperative C5NP is a well-known yet incompletely understood complication of cervical spine surgery. Despite its relatively low incidence, it can result in a significant, although usually transient, functional impairment. Prevention and management should be personalized depending on preexisting risk factors, the type of surgical procedure, and the postoperative course. The complex and multifactorial nature of the condition is reflected by several pathologic theories that have been proposed over time underscoring various noxious mechanisms involving anatomic and surgical factors. While the prognosis is favorable in most cases, a subset of patients might show persistent deficits months or years after the index surgery. A set of radiological and neurophysiological investigations is fundamental to assess patients who develop delayed postoperative C5NP and specialist treatment, including physical and pharmacologic therapy, have proven their efficacy in expediting recovery. Going forward, further advancements can be expected by ongoing research efforts, which have a 3-fold focus:

- Optimizing prevention strategies (namely, surgical planning to achieve adequate decompression of the spinal cord and nerve roots while minimizing excessive manipulation of the neural structures or over-correction of cervical alignment; and ERAS protocols to ensure adequate preoperative preparation and smooth postoperative management).
- Improving our ability to predict the clinical evolution of this condition through nomograms based on data from imaging, electromyography and nerve conduction studies.
- And, ensuring that effective pharmacologic strategies (eg, riluzole) for perioperative management can be tested in multicenter randomized clinical trials including patients with delayed C5NP.

CLINICS CARE POINTS

- Most cases of C5NP have a benign clinical course and its symptoms generally tend to improve over time.
- During diagnostic work up clinicians should try to identify the cause/s of C5NP in order to optimize its management.
- A course of steroids and novel anti-inflammatory drugs (such as riluzole) expedite recovery with negligeable side effects.

DISCLOSURE

No COI or anything else to disclose.

REFERENCES

1. Kato S, Ganau M, Fehlings MG. Surgical decision-making in degenerative cervical myelopathy - anterior versus posterior approach. J Clin Neurosci 2018;58:7–12.
2. Martin AR, Jentzsch T, Wilson JRF, et al. Inter-rater reliability of the modified Japanese orthopedic association score in degenerative cervical myelopathy: a cross-sectional study. Spine (Phila Pa 1976) 2021; 46(16):1063–9.
3. Gu Y, Cao P, Gao R, et al. Incidence and risk factors of C5 palsy following posterior cervical decompression: a systematic review. PLoS One 2014;9(8): e101933.
4. Deshpande N, Stino AM, Smith BW, et al. Defining postoperative C5 palsy and recovery: a systematic review. J Neurosurg Spine 2022;38(4):457–64.
5. Nassr A, Eck JC, Ponnappan RK, et al. The incidence of C5 palsy after multilevel cervical decompression procedures: a review of 750 consecutive cases. Spine (Phila Pa 1976) 2012;37(3):174–8.
6. Epstein NE, Hollingsworth R. C5 nerve root palsies following cervical spine surgery: a review. Surg Neurol Int 2015;6(Suppl 4):S154–63.
7. Oh JK, Hong JT, Kang DH, et al. Epidemiology of C5 palsy after cervical spine surgery: a 21-Center study. Neurospine 2019;16(3):558–62.
8. Stockman IG, Soliman MAR, Quiceno E, et al. Incidence of C5 palsy and recovery rate after cervical spine surgery: a systematic review and meta-analysis. Neurosurgery 2026;98(3):520–42.
9. Wang T, Wang H, Liu S, et al. Incidence of C5 nerve root palsy after cervical surgery: a meta-analysis for last decade. Medicine (Baltim) 2017;96(45):e8560.
10. Hirabayashi S, Kitagawa T, Yamamoto I, et al. Development and achievement of cervical laminoplasty and related studies on cervical myelopathy. Spine Surg Relat Res 2019;4(1):8–17.
11. Sakaura H, Hosono N, Mukai Y, et al. C5 palsy after decompression surgery for cervical myelopathy: review of the literature. Spine (Phila Pa 1976) 2003;28-(21):2447–51.
12. Imagama S, Matsuyama Y, Yukawa Y, et al. C5 palsy after cervical laminoplasty: a multicentre study. J Bone Joint Surg Br 2010;92(3):393–400.
13. Hirabayashi S, Kitagawa T, Yamamoto I, et al. Postoperative C5 palsy: conjectured causes and effective countermeasures. Spine Surg Relat Res 2018; 3(1):12–6.
14. Ganau M, Fehlings MG. Functional anatomy of the spinal cord: chapter 1 in degenerative cervical myelopathy and radiculopathy: treatment approaches and

options. Kaiser MG, Haid RW, Shaffrey CI, et al. Editors 2019: 31-12. doi: 10.1007/978-3-319-97952-6_1.
15. Cherian J, Mayer RR, Haroun KB, et al. Contribution of lordotic correction on C5 palsy following cervical laminectomy and fusion. Neurosurgery 2016;79(6): 816–22.
16. Ogura Y, Dimar JR, Djurasovic M, et al. Etiology and treatment of cervical kyphosis: state of the art review-a narrative review. J Spine Surg 2021;7(3): 422–33.
17. Houten JK, Buksbaum JR, Collins MJ. Patterns of neurological deficits and recovery of postoperative C5 nerve palsy. J Neurosurg Spine 2020;33(6): 742–50.
18. Silver J, Mancini M, Pavano C, et al. C5 nerve root palsy (without prior cervical decompression) case series: 9 patients with critical delay to presentation. J Back Musculoskelet Rehabil 2024;37(3):811–5.
19. Joaquim AF, Makhni MC, Riew KD. Post-operative nerve injuries after cervical spine surgery. Int Orthop 2019;43(4):791–5.
20. Tucker A, Wallbom A, Darling M, et al. Electrodiagnostic findings in postoperative C5 palsy after cervical laminectomy and fusion. Interdisciplinary Neurosurgery 2018;14:39–41.
21. Lubelski D, Pennington Z, Planchard RF, et al. Use of electromyography to predict likelihood of recovery following C5 palsy after posterior cervical spine surgery. Spine J 2021;21(3):387–96.
22. Nakashima H, Imagama S, Yukawa Y, et al. Multivariate analysis of C-5 palsy incidence after cervical posterior fusion with instrumentation. J Neurosurg Spine 2012;17(2):103–10.
23. Krätzig T, Mohme M, Mende KC, et al. Impact of the surgical strategy on the incidence of C5 nerve root palsy in decompressive cervical surgery. PLoS One 2017;12(11):e0188338.
24. Takase H, Murata H, Sato M, et al. Delayed C5 palsy after anterior cervical decompression surgery: preoperative foraminal stenosis and postoperative spinal cord shift increase the risk of palsy. World Neurosurg 2018;120:e1107–19.
25. Zhao R, Yuan D, Li P, et al. Risk factors for C5 nerve root palsy following posterior cervical spinal canal expansion and reconstruction: a systematic review and meta-analysis. BMC Muscoskelet Disord 2026; 27(1):115.
26. Traynelis VC, Fontes RBV, Kasliwal MK, et al. Risk factors for C5 palsy: a systematic review and multivariate analysis. J Neurosurg Spine 2023;40(2): 216–28.
27. Zhu L, Miao Y, Mao Y, et al. Analysis of the risk factors for C5 nerve palsy after cervical posterior open-door laminoplasty for patients with cervical spondylotic myelopathy-from the perspective of cervical sagittal parameters. World Neurosurg 2022; 165:e169–74.
28. Kang KC, Suk KS, Kim HS, et al. Preoperative risk factors of C5 nerve root palsy after laminectomy and fusion in patients with cervical myelopathy: analysis of 70 consecutive patients. Clin Spine Surg 2017;30(9):419–24.
29. Huang M, Chen K, Zhang Y, et al. Risk factors for C5 nerve root palsy following surgery for cervical degenerative disease : a systematic review and meta-analysis. Neurosurg Rev 2026;49(1):120.
30. Lomax JL, Mehta A, Vedantam A, et al. Are skip laminectomy and oblique corpectomy effective options to treat degenerative cervical myelopathy while preserving motion? Results of a scoping review. Global Spine J 2026;16(1_suppl):64S–71S.
31. Chibbaro S, Cornelius JF, Mallereau CH, et al. Lateral approach to the cervical spine to manage degenerative cervical myelopathy and radiculopathy. Acta Neurochir Suppl 2023;135:339–43.
32. Komagata M, Nishiyama M, Endo K, et al. Prophylaxis of C5 palsy after cervical expansive laminoplasty by bilateral partial foraminotomy. Spine J 2004;4(6):650–5.
33. Sasai K, Saito T, Akagi S, et al. Preventing C5 palsy after laminoplasty. Spine (Phila Pa 1976) 2003;28-(17):1972–7.
34. Katsumi K, Yamazaki A, Watanabe K, et al. Can prophylactic bilateral C4/C5 foraminotomy prevent postoperative C5 palsy after open-door laminoplasty?: a prospective study. Spine (Phila Pa 1976) 2012;37(9):748–54.
35. Lee YH, Abdou M, Kwon JW, et al. Posterior preventive foraminotomy before laminectomy combined with pedicle screw fixation may decrease the incidence of C5 palsy in complex cervical spine surgery in patients with severe myeloradiculopathy. J Clin Med 2023;12(6):2227.
36. Chiba K, Toyama Y, Matsumoto M, et al. Segmental motor paralysis after expansive open-door laminoplasty. Spine (Phila Pa 1976) 2002;27(19):2108–15.
37. Malinovic M, Walker J, Lee F. Ischemia-reperfusion injury after posterior cervical laminectomy. Cureus 2021;13(9):e18298.
38. Planchard RF, Maloney PR, Mallory GW, et al. Postoperative delayed cervical palsies: understanding the etiology. Global Spine J 2016;6(6):571–83.
39. Tanaka N, Nakanishi K, Fujiwara Y, et al. Postoperative segmental C5 palsy after cervical laminoplasty may occur without intraoperative nerve injury: a prospective study with transcranial electric motor-evoked potentials. Spine (Phila Pa 1976) 2006;31-(26):3013–7.
40. Alonso F, Voin V, Iwanaga J, et al. Potential mechanism for some postoperative C5 palsies: an anatomical study. Spine (Phila Pa 1976) 2018; 43(3):161–6.
41. Usami Y, Nakaya Y, Hayama S, et al. Impact of multifidus muscle swelling on C5 palsy after cervica

laminoplasty. Spine (Phila Pa 1976) 2020;45(1): E10–7.
42. Khuyagbaatar B, Kim K, Park WM, et al. Biomechanical investigation of post-operative C5 palsy due to ossification of the posterior longitudinal ligament in different types of cervical spinal alignment. J Biomech 2017;57: 54–61.
43. Frazzetta JN, Pecoraro N, Jusue-Torres I, et al. Increased change in cervical lordosis is associated with decreased rate of recovery in patients with C5 palsy. Clin Spine Surg 2025;38(3):E152–9.
44. Shah AA, Devana SK, Lee C, et al. A risk calculator for the prediction of C5 nerve root palsy after instrumented cervical fusion. World Neurosurg 2022;166: e703–10 [Erratum in: World Neurosurg. 2023;173: 282. doi: 10.1016/j.wneu.2023.02.054].
45. Bydon M, Macki M, Kaloostian P, et al. Incidence and prognostic factors of c5 palsy: a clinical study of 1001 cases and review of the literature. Neurosurgery 2014;74(6):595–604 [discussion: 604–5].
46. Zaed I, Bossi B, Ganau M, et al. Current state of benefits of enhanced recovery after surgery (ERAS) in spinal surgeries: a systematic review of the literature. Neurochirurgie 2022;68(1):61–8.
47. Kaneyama S, Sumi M, Kanatani T, et al. Prospective study and multivariate analysis of the incidence of C5 palsy after cervical laminoplasty. Spine (Phila Pa 1976) 2010;35(26):E1553–8.
48. Nakajima H, Honjoh K, Watanabe S, et al. Risk factors and prevention of C5 palsy after anterior cervical decompression and fusion: similarity of the pathomechanism with that after a posterior approach. Clin Spine Surg 2022;35(1):E274–9.
49. Wang H, Zhang X, Lv B, et al. Analysis of correlative risk factors for C5 palsy after anterior cervical decompression and fusion. Int J Clin Exp Med 2015;8(3): 3983–91.
50. Zhou W, Sun B, Wu Z, et al. Cord-lamina angle and foraminal diameter as key predictors of C5 palsy after anterior cervical decompression and fusion surgery. Open Med (Wars) 2025;20(1):20251162.
51. Nakajima H, Kuroda H, Watanabe S, et al. Risk factors and preventive measures for C5 palsy after cervical open-door laminoplasty. J Neurosurg Spine 2019;32(4):592–9.
52. Kim GU, Lee GW. Selective blocking laminoplasty in cervical laminectomy and fusion to prevent postoperative C5 palsy. Spine J 2019;19(4):617–23.
53. Liu G, Reyes MR, Riew KD. Why does C5 palsy occur after prophylactic bilateral C4-5 foraminotomy in open-door cervical laminoplasty? A risk factor analysis. Global Spine J 2017;7(7):696–702.
54. Yamasaki Y, Takeuchi K, Numasawa T, et al. Can prophylactic C4/5 foraminotomy prevent C5 palsy after cervical laminoplasty with and without posterior instrumented fusion with maximal expansion? Eur J Orthop Surg Traumatol 2021;31(6):1037–46.
55. Ganau M, Syrmos N, Martin AR, et al. Intraoperative ultrasound in spine surgery: history, current applications, future developments. Quant Imaging Med Surg 2018;8(3):261–7.
56. Fan D, Schwartz DM, Vaccaro AR, et al. Intraoperative neurophysiologic detection of iatrogenic C5 nerve root injury during laminectomy for cervical compression myelopathy. Spine (Phila Pa 1976) 2002;27(22):2499–502.
57. Oya J, Burke JF, Vogel T, et al. The accuracy of multimodality intraoperative neuromonitoring to predict postoperative neurologic deficits following cervical laminoplasty. World Neurosurg 2017;106:17–25.
58. Bhalodia VM, Schwartz DM, Sestokas AK, et al. Efficacy of intraoperative monitoring of transcranial electrical stimulation-induced motor evoked potentials and spontaneous electromyography activity to identify acute-versus delayed-onset C-5 nerve root palsy during cervical spine surgery: clinical article. J Neurosurg Spine 2013;19(4):395–402.
59. Fujiwara Y, Manabe H, Izumi B, et al. The efficacy of intraoperative neurophysiological monitoring using transcranial electrically stimulated muscle-evoked potentials (TcE-MsEPs) for predicting postoperative segmental upper extremity motor paresis after cervical laminoplasty. Clin Spine Surg 2016;29(4): E188–95.
60. Funaba M, Kanchiku T, Yoshida G, et al. Efficacy of intraoperative neuromonitoring using transcranial motor-evoked potentials for degenerative cervical myelopathy: a prospective multicenter study by the monitoring committee of the Japanese society for spine surgery and related research. Spine (Phila Pa 1976) 2022;47(1):E27–37.
61. Yanase M, Matsuyama Y, Mori K, et al. Intraoperative spinal cord monitoring of C5 palsy after cervical laminoplasty. J Spinal Disord Tech 2010;23(3):170–5.
62. Haghighi SS, Blaskiewicz DJ, Ramirez B, et al. Can intraoperative neurophysiologic monitoring during cervical spine decompression predict post-operative segmental C5 palsy? J Spine Surg 2016;2(3):167–72.
63. Jimenez JC, Sani S, Braverman B, et al. Palsies of the fifth cervical nerve root after cervical decompression: prevention using continuous intraoperative electromyography monitoring. J Neurosurg Spine 2005;3(2):92–7.
64. Clark AJ, Ziewacz JE, Safaee M, et al. Intraoperative neuromonitoring with MEPs and prediction of postoperative neurological deficits in patients undergoing surgery for cervical and cervicothoracic myelopathy. Neurosurg Focus 2013;35(1):E7.
65. Spitz S, Felbaum D, Aghdam N, et al. Delayed postoperative C5 root palsy and the use of neurophysiologic monitoring. Eur Spine J 2015;24(12):2866–71.
66. Wilson JP Jr, Vallejo JB, Kumbhare D, et al. The use of intraoperative neuromonitoring for cervical spine

surgery: indications, challenges, and advances. J Clin Med 2023;12(14):4652.
67. Charalampidis A, Jiang F, Wilson JRF, et al. The use of intraoperative neurophysiological monitoring in spine surgery. Global Spine J 2020;10(1 Suppl): 104S–14S.
68. Dombrowski ME, Morales-Restrepo A, Fourman MS, et al. Prophylactic perioperative dexamethasone decreases the incidence of postoperative C5 palsies after a posterior cervical laminectomy and fusion. Spine J 2019;19(2):253–60.
69. Pennington Z, Lubelski D, Lakomkin N, et al. Timing of referral to peripheral nerve specialists in patients with postoperative C5 palsy. J Clin Neurosci 2021; 92:169–74.
70. Seth NH, Joshi MV Jr, Phansopkar P. C5 nerve root palsy: an uncommon postoperative complication and its management. Cureus 2022;14(9):e28988.
71. Chen G, Wang Y, Wang Z, et al. Analysis of C5 palsy in cervical myelopathy with massive anterior compression following laminoplasty. J Orthop Surg Res 2018;13(1):26.
72. Jeon HS, Kim KN. Delayed bilateral C5 palsy following circumferential decompression and fusion in patient with cervical spondylotic myelopathy. Korean J Spine 2015;12(3):200–3.
73. Hamid S, Hayek R. Role of electrical stimulation for rehabilitation and regeneration after spinal cord injury: an overview. Eur Spine J 2008;17(9):1256–69.
74. Karamian BA, Siegel N, Nourie B, et al. The role of electrical stimulation for rehabilitation and regeneration after spinal cord injury. J Orthop Traumatol 2022;23(1):2.
75. Karadimas SK, Laliberte AM, Tetreault L, et al. Riluzole blocks perioperative ischemia-reperfusion injury and enhances postdecompression outcomes in cervical spondylotic myelopathy. Sci Transl Med 2015;7-(316):316ra194.
76. Moon ES, Karadimas SK, Yu WR, et al. Riluzole attenuates neuropathic pain and enhances functional recovery in a rodent model of cervical spondylotic myelopathy. Neurobiol Dis 2014;62: 394–406.
77. Fehlings MG, Badhiwala JH, Ahn H, et al. Safety and efficacy of riluzole in patients undergoing decompressive surgery for degenerative cervical myelopathy (CSM-Protect): a multicentre, double-blind, placebo-controlled, randomised, phase 3 trial. Lancet Neurol 2021;20(2):98–106.
78. Fehlings MG, Pedro KM, Alvi MA, et al. Riluzole for degenerative cervical myelopathy: a secondary analysis of the CSM-PROTECT trial. JAMA Netw Open 2024;7(6):e2415643.
79. Ganau M, Holly LT, Mizuno J, et al. Future directions and new technologies for the management of degenerative cervical myelopathy. Neurosurg Clin N Am 2018;29(1):185–93.
80. Lubelski D, Hersh AM, Feghali J, et al. Treatment of C5 palsy: an International Survey of peripheral nerve surgeons. Global Spine J 2024;14(8):2225–31.
81. Saadeh YS, Chopra Z, Olsen E, et al. Optimal timing of referral for nerve transfer surgery for postoperative C5 palsy. J Neurosurg Spine 2022;37(4):563–8.
82. Kubota S, Kadone H, Shimizu Y, et al. Robotic shoulder rehabilitation with the hybrid assistive limb in a patient with delayed recovery after postoperative C5 palsy: a case report. Front Neurol 2021;12:676352.
83. Soma Y, Kubota S, Kadone H, et al. Hybrid assistive limb treatment for the shoulder and elbow joints enabled recovery from chronic-phase severe C5 palsy following cervical spine surgery. J Clin Med 2025;14(21):7520.
84. Suk KS, Park J, Choi T, et al. Virtual reality-assisted rehabilitation for postoperative C5 palsy: a pilot exploratory randomized controlled trial. J NeuroEng Rehabil 2025;22(1):178.
85. Krijnen NA, Comerci AJ, Fedor CJ, et al. What is the probability of recovery of C5 palsy after cervical spine surgery over time? A systematic review and meta-analysis. Spine J 2026;26(5):853–62.
86. Thompson SE, Smith ZA, Hsu WK, et al. C5 palsy after cervical spine surgery: a multicenter retrospective review of 59 cases. Global Spine J 2017;7(1 Suppl):64S–70S.
87. Pennington Z, Lubelski D, Westbroek EM, et al. Time to recovery predicted by the severity of postoperative C5 palsy. J Neurosurg Spine 2019;32(2):191–9.
88. Fehlings MG, Evaniew N, Ter Wengel PV, et al. AO spine clinical practice recommendations for diagnosis and management of degenerative cervical myelopathy: evidence based decision making - a review of cutting edge recent literature related to degenerative cervical myelopathy. Global Spine J 2025;15(5):2585–93.
89. Ganau M, Iqbal M, Ligarotti GKI, et al. Letter to the editor. Randomized controlled trials on anterior versus posterior surgical decompression for degenerative cervical myelopathy. J Neurosurg Spine 2021;34(6):957–8.
90. Karamian BA, Schroeder GD, Holas M, et al. Variation in global treatment for subaxial cervical spine isolated unilateral facet fractures. Eur Spine J 2021;30(6):1635–50.
91. Haq IZ, Fehlings MG, Vaccaro AR, et al. Traumatic bilateral cervical facet dislocation:a comprehensive review and evidence-based treatment algorithm. Eur Spine J 2026;35(6):2985–96.
92. Tetreault L, Palubiski LM, Kryshtalskyj M, et al. Significant predictors of outcome following surgery for the treatment of degenerative cervical myelopathy a systematic review of the literature. Neurosurg Clin N Am 2018;29(1):115–27.e35.
93. Ganau L, Ligarotti GKI, Ganau M. Neurological recovery rate and minimal clinically important difference

as metrics for assessing outcomes of decompressive surgery in patients with degenerative cervical myelopathy. Acta Neurochir (Wien) 2022;164(12): 3181–3.
94. Milani D, Zaed I, Ricciardi L, et al. Defining the learning curve of the exoscope in spine surgery. World Neurosurg 2024;182:e1–4.
95. Veremu M, Deakin N, Chauhan RV, et al. Accelerating diagnosis of degenerative cervical myelopathy through improved education: a mixed-methods study protocol from myelopathy.org RECODE-DCM to define stakeholders, knowledge requirements and an optimal intervention strategy. BMJ Open 2026;16(3):e107940.

Genetic and Molecular Biomarkers for Predicting Outcomes in Traumatic and Nontraumatic Spinal Cord Injury

Brendon Wang, BA, Do H. Lim, BA, Shekar N. Kurpad, MD, PhD, Aditya Vedantam, MD*

KEYWORDS

• Spinal cord injury • Degenerative cervical myelopathy • Biomarkers • Neurofilament light chain • GFAP • Prognosis • Genetic markers • Outcome prediction

KEY POINTS

- Neurofilament light chain, glial fibrillary acidic protein, and S100β, are the most consistently validated prognostic biomarkers across both traumatic spinal cord injury and degenerative cervical myelopathy.
- ApoE ε4 reduces neurologic recovery in in tSCI and worsens DCM susceptibility and surgical outcomes, while HIF-1α, SPP1, and BMP4 further modulate DCM prognosis.
- Despite shared marker identities across conditions, absolute biomarker concentrations differ substantially between tSCI and DCM, requiring etiology-specific and timing-specific reference frameworks for accurate clinical interpretation.
- Multimodal panels integrating proteomics, transcriptomics, and cell-free DNA consistently outperform single-marker models, supporting a shift toward biologically composite prognostic frameworks.
- Large-scale, standardized, longitudinal validation studies are needed before genetic and molecular biomarkers can be incorporated into routine clinical management of spinal cord injury and cervical myelopathy.

BACKGROUND

Spinal cord injury is among the most consequential neurologic conditions in clinical medicine, leaving patients with lasting deficits in motor function, sensation, autonomic regulation, and quality of life (QOL).[1] Two prevalent forms, traumatic spinal cord injury (tSCI) and degenerative cervical myelopathy (DCM), arise through fundamentally different mechanisms yet converge on shared pathways of secondary neurodegeneration that ultimately determine functional outcomes.[2] Understanding this shared biology, and where the 2 conditions diverge, is essential context for interpreting the growing body of molecular and genetic prognostic literature.

Traumatic SCI results from acute mechanical forces, most commonly sustained in motor vehicle

Department of Neurosurgery, Medical College of Wisconsin, Milwaukee, WI, USA
* Corresponding author. Department of Neurosurgery, Medical College of Wisconsin, 8701 Watertown Plank Road, Milwaukee, WI 53226.
E-mail address: avedantam@mcw.edu

Neurosurg Clin N Am 37 (2026) 623–647
https://doi.org/10.1016/j.nec.2026.05.011

Abbreviations

AGEs	advanced glycation end-products
AIS	American Spinal Injury Association Impairment Scale
APOE	apolipoprotein E
AUC	area under the curve
CAR	C-reactive protein-to-albumin ratio
cfDNA	cell-free DNA
CSF	cerebrospinal fluid
DCM	degenerative cervical myelopathy
FABP3	fatty acid binding protein 3
GFAP	glial fibrillary acidic protein
GPR	glucose-to-potassium ratio
IL-6	interleukin-6
JOA	japanese orthopedic association score
mJOA	modified Japanese Orthopedic Association
NfL	neurofilament light chain
NLR	neutrophil-to-lymphocyte ratio
pNF-H	phosphorylated neurofilament heavy chain
QOL	quality of life
SCI	spinal cord injury
tSCI	traumatic spinal cord injury
SELENOP	selenoprotein P
SNPs	single nucleotide polymorphisms
UCH-L1	ubiquitin C-terminal hydrolase L1
VEGF	vascular endothelial growth factor

accidents, falls, and sports-related events, that deliver a primary insult to the spinal cord followed by a complex cascade of secondary injury.[3,4] Within hours of the initial impact, excitotoxicity, ischemia, oxidative stress, mitochondrial dysfunction, and neuroinflammation accelerate cell death beyond the zone of direct mechanical damage, and this secondary cascade unfolds over days to weeks.[5,6] The net severity of both the primary and secondary injury determines the final neurologic deficit, making individual outcome prediction challenging using clinical examination and neuroimaging alone.[7,8]

Degenerative cervical myelopathy, by contrast, develops insidiously over months to years as age-related changes to the cervical spine, including disc degeneration, osteophyte formation, ligamentum flavum hypertrophy, and in some patients ossification of the posterior longitudinal ligament, progressively compress the spinal cord.[9,10] The resulting chronic mechanical injury superimposed on repetitive dynamic microtrauma produces ischemia, demyelination, axonal loss, and glial scar formation, ultimately culminating in the gait disturbance, hand dysfunction, and upper motor neuron signs that characterize the clinical syndrome. Unlike the dramatic and unmistakable presentation of acute traumatic injury, DCM is frequently underrecognized and underdiagnosed, and many patients demonstrate considerable cord damage before surgical decompression.[11]

Despite these mechanistic differences, tSCI and DCM share convergent secondary injury pathways involving neuroinflammation, blood–spinal cord barrier disruption, axonal degeneration, and astroglial activation, the same biological processes reflected by the most consistently prognostic molecular markers identified in this review.[3,10] Both conditions also share the fundamental clinical challenge that standard prognostic tools have limited ability to predict individual recovery trajectories. For tSCI, the American Spinal Injury Association Impairment Scale (AIS) and MRI provide a reasonable framework for classifying injury severity but perform poorly as predictors of neurologic conversion, particularly in the acute phase when clinical examination may be confounded by sedation, pain, or polytrauma.[7,8] For DCM, the modified Japanese Orthopedic Association (mJOA) score quantifies functional impairment but does not reliably identify which patients will achieve meaningful postoperative improvement.[12]

It is in this prognostic gap that molecular and genetic biomarkers have generated substantial interest. Proteins released from damaged axons and glia into CSF and blood offer a biologically direct window into injury severity and recovery biology.[13] Inflammatory ratios derivable from routine blood tests can capture systemic physiologic stress.[14] Germline genetic variants can modify injury susceptibility and recovery potential.[15] Lastly, high-dimensional omics technologies, including proteomics, transcriptomics, and epigenomics, have begun to yield composite biomarker signatures whose predictive performance exceeds anything achievable by a single marker alone.[16–19] This article includes a review of studies evaluating these approaches across both tSCI and DCM, with the goal of improving our understanding of the current landscape and the clinical potential of molecular prognostication in spinal cord disease.

DEFINITIONS

In the context of this review, a biomarker is defined as any measurable biological characteristic, including proteins, metabolites, genes, genetic variants, or epigenetic signals, which carries prognostic information about neurologic outcomes in tSCI or DCM.[20] Biomarkers are classified here into 5 categories. Neuroaxonal and glial injury proteins are structural proteins released into biofluids following central nervous system damage, including neurofilament light chain (NfL), glial fibrillary acidic protein (GFAP), S100β, and ubiquitin

C-terminal hydrolase L1 (UCH-L1). Inflammatory and immune response biomarkers encompass systemic inflammatory ratios such as the neutrophil-to-lymphocyte ratio (NLR) and specific cytokines. Metabolic and nutritional signatures include trace elements such as selenium and zinc, as well as nutritional proteins such as albumin. Genetic biomarkers refer to germline variants, including single nucleotide polymorphisms (SNPs) and apolipoprotein E (APOE) genotype, as well as circulating noncoding RNA molecules such as microRNAs. Finally, omics-based and multianalyte panels represent high-dimensional approaches integrating proteomic, transcriptomic, or epigenomic data into composite diagnostic or prognostic signatures.

CURRENT EVIDENCE

A systematic search of PubMed and Embase through October 22, 2025, identified 2782 unique records (**Fig. 1**). After title and abstract screening, 170 articles proceeded to full-text review, and 52 studies ultimately met the prespecified inclusion criteria, each evaluating at least one genetic or molecular biomarker in human participants with tSCI or DCM and reporting associations with neurologic prognosis or clinical outcomes.

Neuroaxonal and Glial Injury Proteins

The most extensively investigated biomarkers across both tSCI and DCM are proteins that are constitutively expressed within neurons and glia and released into biofluids when those cells sustain damage.[13] Their clinical application, however, differs substantially between the 2 conditions, reflecting the distinct temporal dynamics of acute trauma versus chronic neurodegeneration.

In tSCI, these markers are used primarily to characterize the intensity of the acute structural disruption and predict whether meaningful neurologic conversion will occur. One demonstration of their clinical utility comes from Dalkilic and colleagues, who showed that a CSF biomarker panel combining Tau, GFAP, and S100β, measured at approximately 24 hours post injury, outperformed MRI in predicting AIS conversion and achieved a logistic accuracy of 91%.[18] The prognostic value of individual serum markers in tSCI is also meaningfully time-dependent, a nuance that matters for clinical implementation. Raheja and colleagues found that serum GFAP levels at days 2 and 7 post injury were associated with complete injury classification and nonfunctional status, while S100β at day 7 specifically predicted nonfunctional outcomes at 6 months.[21] When the sampling compartment is shifted from serum to CSF, the discriminatory power of S100β improves substantially. Haddadi and colleagues demonstrated that CSF S100β distinguished complete from incomplete injury with an area under the curve (AUC) of 0.823, compared with only 0.586 in serum, a finding that reflects the more direct biological proximity of CSF to the injury microenvironment.[22] Waliullah and colleagues reinforced S100β′s role as a severity correlate by showing that levels were significantly higher in patients with paraplegia compared to paraparesis.[23]

NfL behaves differently from the acute-phase proteins. Rather than peaking immediately and declining, NfL levels in tSCI continue to rise over the first 30 days post injury, reflecting not the initial mechanical impact but the ongoing secondary axonal degeneration that unfolds in the weeks that follow.[24] NfL is not a marker of the injury itself so much as a marker of how aggressively the secondary injury cascade is consuming surviving axons, and its delayed peak means that later sampling windows are needed to capture its full prognostic signal.[25] UCH-L1 occupies a different niche as a trauma-specific marker. Stukas and colleagues observed strong CSF elevations immediately post injury,[7] and Abuhamdah and colleagues reported that lower serum UCH-L1 within 24 hours was statistically associated with improved AIS grades at follow-up, suggesting that patients who sustain less neuronal loss at the outset retain more recovery potential.[26]

In degenerative cervical myelopathy, the same protein family is examined differently. Rather than capturing an acute catastrophic event, biomarker measurements in DCM aim to quantify the accumulated burden of chronic cord injury and predict whether a patient's cord retains the biological capacity to recover following surgical decompression. Takahashi and colleagues found that phosphorylated neurofilament heavy chain (pNF-H) in CSF was highest specifically in patients experiencing acute-on-chronic clinical worsening and correlated with the rate of postoperative japanese orthopedic association score (JOA) score improvement, suggesting that the degree of active axonal injury at the time of surgery influences the speed and extent of neurologic recovery.[27] Vedantam and colleagues, using high-sensitivity immunoassay platforms, showed that preoperative serum NfL and GFAP were both elevated in DCM patients relative to healthy controls, with preoperative NfL specifically correlating with postoperative gains in pinch strength and upper limb function.[28] Tsitsopoulos and colleagues extended this to CSF, finding that elevated NfL and fatty acid binding protein 3 (FABP3) were associated with meaningful improvements in QOL following

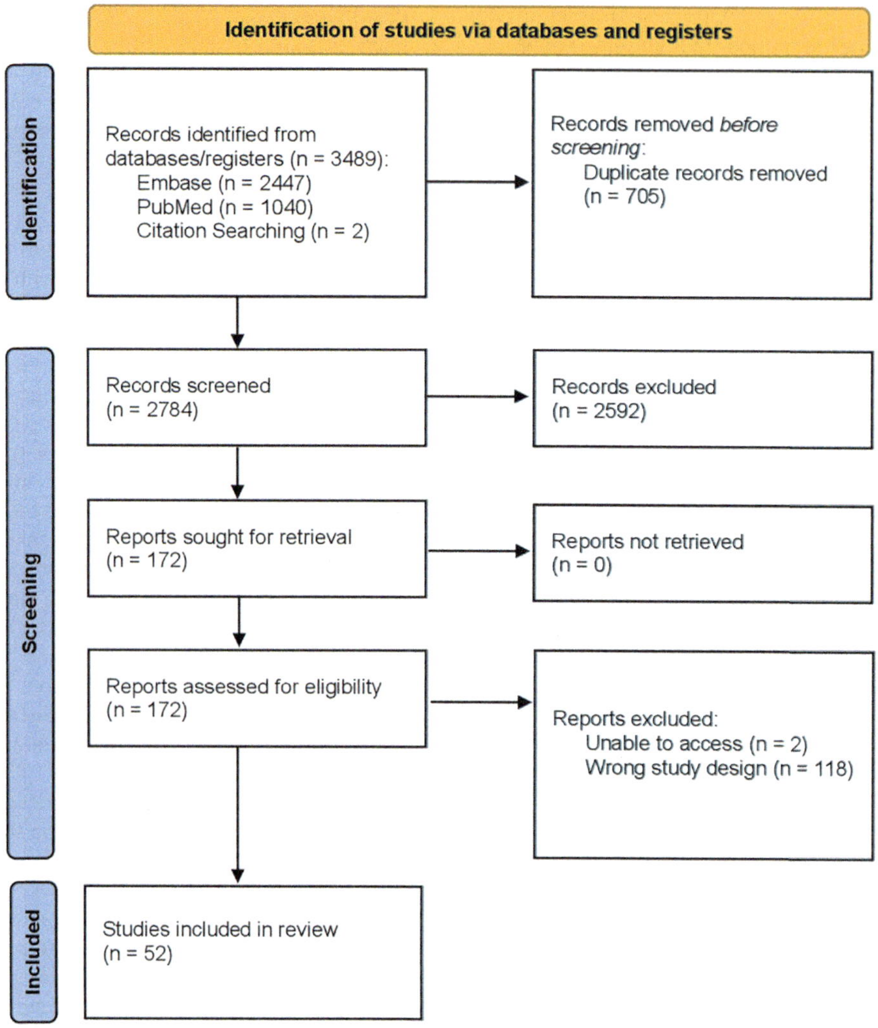

Fig. 1. Preferred Reporting Items for Systematic reviews and Meta-Analyses (PRISMA) flow diagram of study selection. Flow diagram illustrating the identification, screening, eligibility assessment, and inclusion of studies evaluating genetic and biomarker correlates of traumatic and nontraumatic spinal cord injury. (*Created using* PRISMA flow diagram template from https://www.prisma-statement.org/.)

decompressive surgery.[29] A full summary of neuroaxonal and glial injury protein studies is provided in **Table 1**.

Inflammatory and Immune Response Biomarkers

The inflammatory landscape of tSCI and DCM differs sharply. In acute traumatic injury, the systemic inflammatory response is immediate and dramatic, and several studies have demonstrated that routine hematological indices available from standard admission bloodwork carry meaningful prognostic information. Naseri Alavi and colleagues, analyzing a cohort of 600 patients, found that a higher NLR at 24 and 48 hours post injury was independently associated with poorer neurologic outcomes, suggesting that the magnitude of the acute systemic inflammatory response predicts not just physiologic stress but neurologic fate.[30] Tao and colleagues identified the C-reactive protein-to-albumin ratio (CAR) as an independent predictor of poor prognosis, with an AUC of 0.749 correlating with admission AIS grade and 1-year outcomes.[31] Zhou and colleagues examined the glucose-to-potassium ratio (GPR), validating it as a correlate of injury severity and 6-month prognosis with an AUC of 0.842.[32]

Beyond these hematological ratios, specific cytokines add nuance to the inflammatory picture in tSCI. Chen and colleagues found that higher serum interleukin (IL-37) levels correlated with

Table 1
Neuroaxonal and glial injury proteins study characteristics

Study, Year	Population	Design (Level of Evidence)	N (Spinal Cord Injury/ Control)	Biomarker(s)	Timing	Source/Assay	Outcome(s) Tied to Recovery (Key Findings)
Dalkilic et al,[18] 2018	tSCI (cervical)	Prospective cohort (II)	36/0	Tau, GFAP, S100β + IL-6/ IL-8/MCP-1	24 h	CSF/Bio-Plex + ELISA	CSF biomarkers outperformed MRI for predicting AIS conversion and motor score improvement.
Raheja et al,[21] 2018	tSCI	Prospective cohort (II)	26/0	GFAP, S100β, NSE, pNF-H	24 h, 2 d, 7 d	Serum/ELISA	GFAP (2 days/7 d) associated with complete SCI + nonfunctional status; S100β (7 d) predicted nonfunctional/complete injury at 6 mo.
Haddadi et al,[22] 2024	tSCI	Observational cohort (III)	31/0	S100β	24–48 h	Serum + CSF/ECLIA	CSF S100B correlated with complete SCI and outperformed serum in discriminating complete vs incomplete injury.
Waliulla et al,[23] 2025	tSCI (thoracolumbar)	Prospective case-control (III)	26/26	S100β	<24 h, 2 wk, 6 wk	Serum/ELISA	S100β higher in SCI vs controls and is higher in paraplegia vs paraparesis.
Stukas et al,[7] 2021	tSCI	Prospective observational (II)	32/10	UCH-L1	0–96 h	CSF + serum/Simoa	CSF UCH-L1 levels were markedly elevated 10–100 fold in SCI patients compared with controls ($P<.05$).
Abuhamdah et al,[26] 2022	tSCI	Prospective case-control (III)	33/30	UCH-L1, Neuroglobin	<24 h	Serum/ELISA	Lower UCH-L1 associated with improved AIS ($P = .041$); Neuroglobin not significant.

(*continued on next page*)

Table 1 (continued)

Study, Year	Population	Design (Level of Evidence)	N (Spinal Cord Injury/Control)	Biomarker(s)	Timing	Source/Assay	Outcome(s) Tied to Recovery (Key Findings)
Kuhle et al,[65] 2014	tSCI	Prospective cohort (II)	27/67	NfL	Longitudinal (Baseline to 120 h)	Serum/ECL	Baseline/24 h NfL correlated with motor outcome ($r = -0.72$ at 24 h) and differed by complete vs incomplete.
Leister et al,[16] 2023	tSCI	Prospective cohort (III)	41/0	GFAP, NfL	1–4 d, 30 d, 120 d	Serum/R-Plex, ELISA	Steeper GFAP decline over 30 d predicted better recovery; NfL rose until day 30 as ongoing neurodegeneration marker.
Fraussen et al,[61] 2025	tSCI	Prospective cohort (II)	37/22	NfL, GFAP, CNTN-1	0–4 d, 1–2 wk, 3–6 wk, 12 wk, 18 wk	Plasma/Simoa + Luminex	Early NfL + GFAP predicted AIS-A (AUC 0.96); CNTN-1 lower in SCI vs controls.
Paragond et al,[66] 2024	tSCI	Cohort (II)	35/0	NF, NSE, MMP-2, S100B	Presentation, post-operation, 6 wk	Serum/ELISA/ECLIA	Significant differences in NF at presentation ($P = .03$), NSE at 6 wk ($P = .016$), and S-100B at presentation ($P = .016$) and postoperation ($P = .007$) between improved and nonimproved groups.
Fernandez et al,[67] 2020	tSCI	Pilot case series (IV)	27/67	GFAP, S100B, NSE, NF-L + cytokines	<24 h	CSF/ELISA	CSF from patients with no neurologic recovery (AIS A) exhibited distinct biological effects, including reduced oligodendrocyte differentiation, compared with CSF from patients who demonstrated recovery.

Takahashi et al,[27] 2018	DCM	Observational with 1 y follow-up (III)	40/29	pNF-H, Tau, MBP, S100b, NSE	Preoperation	CSF/ELISA + ECLIA	pNF-H was higher in acute myelopathy than in chronic myelopathy or lumbar canal stenosis (P<.01) and correlated with JOA recovery (r = 0.381, P = .018). Tau was higher in acute vs chronic myelopathy (P<.05), MBP was largely undetectable, S100b was similar across groups, and NSE was lower in acute and chronic myelopathy than in lumbar canal stenosis.
Tsitsopoulos et al,[29] 2021	DCM	Prospective cohort with controls (II)	20/63	NF-L, GFAP, tau, FABP3, YKL-40, sAPPα/β, Aβ38/40/42	Preoperative	CSF/ELISA + MSD	NF-L/GFAP higher vs controls; NF-L & FABP3 associated with QoL improvement (EQ-VAS>20).
Vedantam et al,[28] 2024	DCM	Prospective cohort with controls (II)	20/10	NF-L, GFAP, BDNF, tau, Aβ40/42 + cytokines	Preoperation; 3-mo postoperation	Serum/ Quanterix Simoa	NfL and IL-6 were higher in DCM than controls (P = .01, P = .003), with an NfL–IL-6–BDNF panel showing good discrimination (AUC = 0.83, P<.001). At 3 mo postoperatively, BDNF, Aβ42, and TNF-α increased, and presurgical biomarkers (eg, NfL) were associated with functional improvement.
Takahashi et al,[68] 2014	DCM	Pilot cross-sectional (III)	14/37	pNF-H	Pre-operative	CSF/ELISA	pNF-H highest in acute-worsening but did not correlate with JOA recovery rate.

Abbreviations: Aβ38/40/42, amyloid-beta peptides; CNTN-1, contactin-1; ECL/ECLIA, electrochemiluminescence (immunoassay); ELISA, enzyme-linked immunosorbent assay; EQ-VAS, EuroQol Visual Analog Scale; MBP, myelin basic protein; MCP-1, monocyte chemoattractant protein-1; MSD, meso scale discovery; NSE, neuron-specific enolase; S100β, S100 calcium-binding protein beta; sAPPα/β, soluble amyloid precursor protein alpha/beta; Simoa, single molecule array; Tau, microtubule-associated protein tau; TNF-α, tumor necrosis factor alpha; YKL-40, chitinase-3-like protein 1.

worse AIS grades and motor scores at admission, linking this anti-inflammatory cytokine's dysregulation to injury severity.[33] At the cellular level, Heller and colleagues observed that favorable intermediate monocyte dynamics within the first 24 hours, specifically a pattern of early monocyte mobilization reflecting an adaptive rather than dysregulated immune response, were associated with neurologic improvement, pointing toward immune cell phenotyping as a potential prognostic tool.[34]

In DCM, the inflammatory milieu is chronic and localized rather than acute and systemic, and the markers that carry prognostic weight reflect a sustained neuroinflammatory environment rather than an acute stress response. Vedantam and colleagues found that IL-6 and a broad panel of cytokines were elevated in DCM patients relative to controls and were associated with postoperative improvements in pain, disability, and upper limb function, suggesting that the extent of preoperative neuroinflammation influences the trajectory of surgical recovery.[28] Tsitsopoulos and colleagues found that CSF levels of YKL-40, a glycoprotein secreted by activated microglia and astrocytes that serves as a marker of chronic glial inflammation, were linked to both the duration of preoperative impairment and the degree of quality-of-life improvement following decompression.[29] Inflammatory biomarkers in tSCI have also been linked to cognitive outcomes. Meng and colleagues found that lower serum Netrin-1 was associated with cognitive impairment at follow-up,[35] and Liu and colleagues demonstrated that lower circulating Adiponectin independently predicted cognitive decline at 3 months post injury, extending the prognostic reach of these markers beyond purely motor outcomes.[36] A full summary of inflammatory and immune response biomarker studies is provided in **Table 2**.

Metabolic and Nutritional Signatures

A less intuitive but increasingly well-supported category of prognostic biomarkers encompasses metabolic and nutritional markers that reflect the systemic physiologic environment in which spinal cord recovery must occur. In tSCI, the research has focused predominantly on trace elements and nutritional proteins, revealing that the metabolic context of injury significantly influences neurologic fate. Heller and colleagues demonstrated that serum selenium dynamics and selenoprotein P (SELENOP) levels within the first 24 hours predicted AIS conversion with an AUC of 0.90, and that free zinc levels at 24 hours predicted neurologic impairment with an AUC of 0.84.[34] These trace elements are critical components of antioxidant defense systems, and their rapid redistribution following injury likely reflects both the magnitude of oxidative stress and the host's capacity to mount a protective response.[37]

Serum albumin has emerged as a particularly robust and clinically accessible metabolic prognostic marker in tSCI. Vo and colleagues established a threshold of 2.8 g/dL at 30 days post injury for predicting marked neurologic recovery at 1 year,[38] and Tong and colleagues found that higher albumin levels at 1 to 2 weeks post injury approximately doubled the odds of achieving marked recovery.[39] Albumin reflects not only nutritional status but also hepatic synthetic function, the systemic inflammatory burden, and overall physiologic reserve, all of which plausibly influence the biological environment available to support axonal repair and neuroplasticity.[40] Li and colleagues additionally examined calcium, finding that serum calcium trajectories during ICU admission independently predicted mortality with better discrimination than standard ICU severity scores, suggesting that electrolyte homeostasis carries information about systemic injury severity beyond what conventional scoring systems capture.[41]

In DCM, metabolic investigation has taken a different form, reflecting the chronic rather than acute nature of the condition. Doi and colleagues used a noninvasive skin sensor to measure advanced glycation end-products (AGEs), markers of cumulative oxidative and metabolic stress that accumulate in tissues over time, and found that higher skin autofluorescence in DCM patients was associated with worse leg and foot pain, suggesting that chronic systemic metabolic burden contributes to the symptom profile of myelopathy and may identify patients whose cord is operating in a more metabolically compromised environment.[42] A full summary of metabolic and nutritional signature studies is provided in **Table 3**.

Genetic Biomarkers

The genetic architecture of spinal cord injury susceptibility and recovery is an area of growing investigation, with the APOE gene occupying a central position as the most consistently characterized shared genetic modifier across both tSCI and DCM.[43,44] The APOE ε4 allele, long established as a risk factor for Alzheimer's disease and other neurodegenerative conditions, appears to exert a similarly detrimental effect on neurologic recovery in spinal cord pathology.[45] In tSCI, Sun and colleagues and Jha and colleagues independently reported that APOE ε4 carriage was associated with reduced motor recovery and longer rehabilitation lengths of stay, though an intriguing

Table 2
Inflammation and immune response biomarker study characteristics

Study, Year	Population	Design (Level of Evidence)	N (Spinal Cord Injury/Control)	Biomarker(s)	Timing	Source	Outcomes/Prognostic Signal
Naseri Alavi et al,[30] 2023	tSCI	Retrospective cross-sectional (III)	600/0	NLR	Admission, 24 h, 48 h, discharge	Blood	Increased NLR at 24 h and 48 h associated with worse neurologic outcome
Tao et al,[31] 2025	tSCI	Retrospective cohort (III)	402/0	CAR (CRP/ albumin)	<24 h	Serum	CAR correlated with admission AIS and 1 y AIS; independent predictor of poor prognosis (AUC = 0.749)
Zhou et al,[32] 2023	tSCI	Retrospective cohort (III)	520/0	GPR (glucose/ potassium)	Admission (<12 h)	Serum	Admission GPR correlated with AIS severity and 6-mo AIS and differed between good and poor prognosis groups. In multivariable analysis, serum GPR was independently associated with poor outcome, with good discriminatory performance.
Chen et al,[33] 2020	tSCI	Prospective observational (II)	148/0	IL-37	<24 h	Serum	IL-37 was elevated in SCI patients vs controls, increased with worsening ASIA grade (A > B > C > D), and was negatively correlated with ASIA motor score.
Meng et al,[35] 2022	tSCI	Prospective cohort with controls (II)	96/60	Netrin-1	<24 h	Serum	Lower Netrin-1 in patients with SCI and was correlated with cognitive impairment at 3 mo.

(*continued on next page*)

Table 2
(*continued*)

Study, Year	Population	Design (Level of Evidence)	N (Spinal Cord Injury/Control)	Biomarker(s)	Timing	Source	Outcomes/Prognostic Signal
Liu et al,[36] 2022	tSCI	Prospective case-control (II)	92/64	Adiponectin	Immediately after admission	Serum	Lower adiponectin independently predicted cognitive decline (MoCA<26) at 3 mo.
Heller et al,[69] 2021	tSCI	Prospective observational (II)	18/4	Monocyte subsets + IL-10/CXCR4 etc.	Longitudinal (admission to 3 mo)	Blood/plasma	Higher early intermediate monocyte dynamics within 24h linked to neuro improvement (P = .010).
Vedantam et al,[28] 2024	DCM	Prospective cohort with controls (II)	30/0	IL-6 + cytokine panel	Pre-operative, 3 mo post-op	Serum	IL-6 elevated in DCM vs controls; inflammatory markers associated with improvement in pain/disability and upper limb function
Tsitsopoulos et al,[29] 2021	DCM	Prospective cohort with controls (II)	83/0	YKL-40	Pre-operative	CSF	DCM patients had higher CSF NF-L and GFAP and lower FABP3, sAPPα/β, and Aβ38/40/42 vs controls (all P<.05). NF-L correlated with preoperative impairment, MRI changes, and shorter symptom duration, while higher NF-L and FABP3 predicted greater postoperative quality-of-life improvements

Abbreviations: CXCR4, C-X-C chemokine receptor type 4; MoCA, montreal cognitive assessment; YKL-40, chitinase-3-like protein 1.

Table 3
Metabolic and nutritional signature study characteristics

Study, Year	Population	Design (Level of Evidence)	N (Spinal Cord Injury/Control)	Biomarker(s)	Timing	Source/Assay	Outcomes/Prognostic Signal
Heller et al,[34] 2019	tSCI	Prospective cohort with controls (II)	19/10	Selenium, SELENOP, zinc	Longitudinal (0 h to 3 mo)	Serum/TXRF + ELISA	Higher admission Se/SELENOP + early 24-h dynamics predicted AIS conversion.
Seelig et al,[70] 2019	tSCI	Prospective observational (II)	21/31	Se/Cu + SELENOP/CP	0–24 h	Serum/TXRF + ELISA	Early Se/Cu + 24h Se/CP model predicted remission.
Heller et al,[71] 2025	tSCI	Prospective cohort with controls (III)	39/9	Total Zn, free Zn, Zn/fZn	0 h, 4 h, 9 h, 12 h, 24 h, 3 d	Serum/TXRF	Lower Zn/fZn correlated with worse impairment and worse AIS improvement.
Vo et al,[38] 2021	tSCI	Secondary analysis of observational cohort (II)	449/0	Albumin	30 d post injury	Serum	Albumin predicted marked recovery at 1 y but lost significance after adjusting for baseline severity.
Tong et al,[39] 2018	tSCI	Secondary analysis of an RCT (II)	591/0	Albumin	24–72 h, 1–4 wk	Serum	Higher albumin at 1–2 wk predicted marked recovery (OR: 1.9–2.0).
Brown et al,[72] 2020	tSCI	Retrospective cohort (II)	82/0	Live function and acute inflammation markers (albumin, CRP, calcium, and electrolytes)	7±4 d	Blood	Liver function and acute inflammation markers significantly improved prediction of neurologic outcomes at 3 mo and 1 y, modestly increasing 3-mo pain prediction (ΔR^2 = 0.043).

(*continued on next page*)

Table 3
(continued)

Study, Year	Population	Design (Level of Evidence)	N (Spinal Cord Injury/Control)	Biomarker(s)	Timing	Source/Assay	Outcomes/Prognostic Signal
Harrington et al,[73] 2021	Mixed SCI (75% traumatic)	Retrospective cohort (II)	417/0	Hematological (Hb, WBC, Platelets) and biochemical (ALT, GGT, Bilirubin, Albumin, and CRP)	31±30 d	Blood	ALT/GGT added value for SCIM prediction; hematologic markers improved AIS motor/sensory prediction.
Li et al,[41] 2025	tSCI	Retrospective cohort (III)	699/0	Serum calcium trajectories	Every 24 h while in ICU	Serum	Trajectory class independently predicted ICU mortality; improved discrimination vs ICU scores.
Doi et al,[42] 2025	DCM	Prospective cross-sectional (II)	93/0	AGEs (skin autofluorescence)	Pre-operative	Skin sensor	Higher AGE associated with worse leg and foot pain.

Abbreviations: Albumin, serum albumin; ALT, alanine aminotransferase; CP, ceruloplasmin; CRP, C-reactive protein; GGT, gamma-glutamyl transferase; Hb, hemoglobin; ICU, intensive care unit; RCT, randomized controlled trial; SCIM, spinal cord independence measure; TXRF, total reflection X-ray fluorescence; WBC, white blood cell count; Zn/fZn, ratio of total to free zinc.

observation emerged in some cohorts whereby ε4 was associated with better pinprick recovery in certain sensory modalities, a finding that remains mechanistically unexplained and warrants further investigation.[46,47]

In DCM, APOE ε4 plays a dual role as both a susceptibility factor and a surgical outcome modifier. Setzer and colleagues found that ε4 carriage increased the likelihood of developing cervical spondylotic myelopathy and independently predicted the absence of neurologic improvement following anterior cervical decompression and fusion.[48] This was subsequently corroborated by Chintapalli and colleagues in a large genetic case-control study using the UK Biobank cohort, providing population-level evidence for an APOE4-DCM susceptibility association.[49] The mechanism by which APOE ε4 impairs recovery is thought to involve its reduced efficiency in lipid transport and neuronal membrane repair, its promotion of neuroinflammation, and its association with greater amyloid deposition and tau pathology, all factors that reduce the biological machinery available for neuroregeneration.[50]

Beyond APOE, the DCM genetic literature has expanded into disease-specific susceptibility variants that have no parallel in the tSCI literature, reflecting the pathophysiological role of ischemic and ossification pathways in chronic myelopathy. Wang and colleagues identified the , hypoxia-inducible factor 1-alpha (HIF1A) 1790 GG genotype as a modifier of postoperative outcomes, with this hypoxia-inducible factor variant linked to worse surgical results and higher expression of inflammatory and vascular endothelial growth factor (VEGF) pathway proteins, findings that implicate ischemia-related gene expression in the biology of DCM progression.[51] Wu and colleagues found that the SPP1 (osteopontin) rs1126616 CC genotype was associated with poorer JOA recovery following decompression,[52] while Wang and colleagues paradoxically found that specific BMP4 variants were associated with greater DCM susceptibility yet better postoperative improvement, suggesting that the genetic determinants of disease initiation and recovery potential may be partially dissociable.[53] Abodelyamah and colleagues added the BDNF (brain-derived neurotrophic factor) Val66Met polymorphism to the list of DCM outcome modifiers, reflecting the role of neurotrophic signaling in postoperative neuroplasticity.[54]

Alongside germline variants, circulating noncoding RNA molecules have emerged as a dynamic and context-sensitive layer of genetic biomarker information. Laliberte and colleagues demonstrated that elevated preoperative plasma miR-21-5p in DCM patients was independently associated with greater neurologic impairment and predicted poorer postoperative functional recovery, findings supported by parallel animal model data implicating miR-21 in the regulation of neuroinflammatory and sensorimotor pathways in myelopathy.[55] Divi and colleagues extended this to a broader microRNA profile, showing that upregulation of miR-223-3p and downregulation of miR-451a in serum could differentiate DCM patients from healthy controls and correlated with disease severity, providing a blood-based epigenetic signature of the inflammatory disease phenotype.[56] A full summary of genetic biomarker studies is provided in **Table 4**.

Omics and Multianalyte Diagnostic Panels

The most technically sophisticated category of biomarker research involves high-dimensional *omics* approaches that integrate multiple molecular signals into composite diagnostic or prognostic tools.[57] These methods have consistently outperformed single-marker models in both tSCI and DCM, and they represent the direction in which the field is most rapidly evolving.

In traumatic SCI, Azad and colleagues developed a multianalyte blood test that combined spinal cord-derived cell-free DNA (cfDNA) methylation patterns, a tissue-of-origin signal reflecting how much spinal cord parenchymal DNA is being released into the circulation, with plasma proteins including FABP3 and NF-H.[58] This composite *Spinal Cord Injury Index* achieved a diagnostic AUC of 0.91 and predicted 6-month AIS conversion with an AUC of 0.77, demonstrating that integrating epigenomic and proteomic signals yields predictive performance that neither source alone could achieve.[58] Tigchelaar and colleagues took a transcriptomic approach, using small RNA sequencing to identify specific microRNA subsets in CSF and serum, most notably miR-124-3p, which distinguished AIS A from B/C patients and independently predicted motor recovery, establishing a molecular basis for injury severity grading that goes beyond the clinical examination.[8] Garcia-Ovejero and colleagues applied untargeted serum proteomics to identify SERPINE1 and ARHGAP35 as recovery-associated proteins and DEFA1 as a marker of non-recovery, pointing toward novel molecular targets whose biological roles in spinal cord repair biology remain to be fully characterized.[59]

In DCM, Zheng and colleagues applied RNA sequencing to peripheral blood samples and developed a 5-gene diagnostic model that distinguished DCM patients from healthy controls with

Table 4
Genetic biomarker study characteristics

Study, Year	Population	Design (Level of Evidence)	N (Spinal Cord Injury/Control)	Platform	Biomarker(s)	Timing/Source	Outcomes/Prognostic Signal
Azad et al,[58] 2025	tSCI	Prospective cohort with controls (II)	50/20	cfDNA methylation (ddPCR) + proteomics (NULISA)	Spinal cord–derived cfDNA (hypomethylated CpG loci) + FABP3/REST/IL-6/NF-H	0–7 d/plasma	Plasma spinal cord–derived cfDNA, combined with 4 proteins as the SCII, accurately diagnosed acute SCI, reflected injury severity, and predicted 6-mo neurologic improvement, outperforming individual biomarkers.
Tigchelaar et al,[8] 2019	tSCI	Prospective multicenter (II)	39/5	Small RNA-seq	CSF and serum microRNA (eg, miR-9, miR-124, miR-219)	1–5 d/CSF/serum	Subset distinguished AIS A vs B/C and predicted motor recovery at 6 mo.
Bernado Harrington et al,[74] 2025	tSCI	Prospective proteomics (II)	32/0	LC-MS/MS (iTRAQ + label-free)	Candidate proteins (α2M, RBP4, SAA1, PRX-2, ApoA1)	<2 wk and 3 mo/plasma	iTRAQ and label-free proteomics identified 79–87 proteins differing across AIS groups, with RBP4 and PRX-2 as potential binary biomarkers and complement cascade proteins strongly associated with recovery.

Garcia-Overjero et al,[59] 2024	tSCI	Prospective observational cohort with exploratory proteomics (II)	30/50	TMT-MS2 + ELISA	SERPINE1, RAGE, Calumenin, ARHGAP35, DEFA1, CD300a	31 d/serum	High SERPINE1 and ARHGAP35 were associated with recovery, while CD300a/DEFA1 were linked to no recovery.
Li et al,[75] 2024	tSCI	Case-control observational study (II)	16/16	RNA-seq, machine learning + qPCR validation	ANO10, BST1, ZFP36L2	<1 mo/blood	In SCI, ANO10 and BST1 were upregulated and ZFP36L2 downregulated (*P*<.01), with diagnostic AUCs of 0.793, 0.810, and 0.870, respectively.
Picotto et al,[76] 2020	Chronic tSCI	Case-control (III)	6/5	Microarray + qPCR	TMEM176A/B	≥2y/blood	TMEM176A and TMEM176B are dramatically overexpressed in circulating monocytes from chronic SCI patients, suggesting these genes contribute to suppression of dendritic cell maturation and immune dysfunction after SCI.

(*continued on next page*)

Table 4
(*continued*)

Study, Year	Population	Design (Level of Evidence)	N (Spinal Cord Injury/ Control)	Platform	Biomarker(s)	Timing/Source	Outcomes/ Prognostic Signal
Zheng et al,[60] 2025	DCM	Retrospective case-control (III)	30/16	RNA-seq + LASSO/logistic	5-gene diagnostic model (TBCD, TPM2, PNKD, EIF4G2, AP5Z1), Immune cell-type signatures (memory B cells; memory-activated $CD4^+$ T cells)	Pretreatment/ blood	A 5-gene panel (TBCD, TPM2, PNKD, EIF4G2, and AP5Z1) identified DCM with 93.5% accuracy. Immune-cell signatures distinguished single- vs multi-level lesions with 80% accuracy (AUC 0.895).
Laliberte et al,[55] 2021	DCM	Prospective observational cohort (II)	69/0	qRT-PCR	miR21-5p	After neurologic assessment and before surgical intervention/ blood	Higher baseline plasma MIR21-5p correlated with greater baseline neurologic severity (lower mJOA) and predicted worse functional outcome at 1 y after surgical decompression.
Divi et al,[56] 2024	DCM	Prospective case-control (II)	36/35	RT-qPCR + MSD V-PLEX proinflammatory panel	miR-223-3p (upregulated), miR-451a (downregulated); inflammatory cytokines (TNF-α, IL-1β, IL-8, IL-12p70, IL-13, IL-4)	Preoperatively at IV placement/ peripheral venous serum	Circulating miR-223-3p and miR-451a distinguish DCM vs controls and correlate with baseline neurologic severity (mJOA).

Abbreviations: ARHGAP35, Rho GTPase-activating protein 35; ANO10, anoctamin 10; BST1, bone marrow stromal cell antigen 1; CD300a, CD300 antigen-like family member a; ddPCR, droplet digital PCR; DEFA1, defensin alpha 1; iTRAQ, isobaric tags for relative and absolute quantitation; LASSO, least absolute shrinkage and selection operator; LC-MS/MS, liquid chromatography–tandem mass; RAGE, receptor for advanced glycation end-products; SERPINE1, serpin family E member 1TTMEM176A/B, transmembrane protein 176A/BMT-MS2, an AUC of 0.939.[60] Importantly, while the model performed well diagnostically, its capacity to stratify disease severity by mJOA strata was more modest, highlighting that diagnostic and prognostic applications of transcriptomic signatures may require different model architectures and training objectives.[60] A full summary of omics and multianalyte panel studies is provided in **Table 5**.

DISCUSSION

The body of evidence synthesized in this review reveals a field that has moved well beyond exploratory biomarker discovery and is beginning to generate clinically interpretable prognostic signals across the full spectrum of spinal cord pathology.[7,29,61] At the same time, it illustrates the biological and methodological complexity that must be navigated before molecular markers can be routinely integrated into clinical care.

Perhaps the most conceptually important finding is the simultaneous convergence and divergence of biomarker biology across tSCI and DCM. NfL, GFAP, and APOE ε4 emerge as shared prognostic markers across both conditions, reflecting the convergent secondary injury mechanisms that operate in both traumatic and degenerative spinal cord disease.[24,28,29,46–48] Yet the absolute concentrations of these shared markers differ dramatically between conditions. Both Vedantam and colleagues and Stukas and colleagues used comparable high-sensitivity proteomic platforms, demonstrating that circulating NfL and GFAP concentrations in acute tSCI were several-fold higher than those observed in DCM, even among patients with severe myelopathy.[7,28] This quantitative divergence likely reflects the abrupt tissue destruction and widespread axonal transection characteristic of trauma, as opposed to the slower, cumulative neurodegeneration seen in chronic compression. Importantly, DCM is associated with ongoing neuroplasticity and compensatory remodeling, processes that may modulate neuronal protein release and partially attenuate peak biomarker concentrations despite persistent cord injury.[62] These distinctions emphasize that shared biomarkers cannot be interpreted using uniform thresholds across etiologies and instead require context-specific reference ranges and timing considerations.[3]

The question of sampling timing is equally central to biomarker interpretation and equally underappreciated in the clinical literature. In tSCI, GFAP and S100β are most informative in the first 24 to 72 hours post injury, when they reflect the magnitude of the acute primary and early secondary insult.[21,22] NfL, by contrast, continues to rise for weeks as secondary axonal degeneration propagates, meaning that early NfL measurements may underestimate the ultimate neurologic deficit and that later measurements, taken at day 14 or day 30, carry superior prognostic information.[24] UCH-L1 is an acute-phase marker whose prognostic window appears to be within the first 24 hours, making it most useful for early triage.[26] In DCM, the optimal timing question is framed around the surgical encounter. Preoperative biomarker levels predict surgical responsiveness, and the degree to which chronic neuroinflammation and axonal loss have accumulated before decompression appears to influence how much recovery the cord retains the biological capacity to achieve.[28,29] Clinicians who wish to use these markers in practice will need to attend carefully to these timing considerations, which are not intuitive from the clinical presentation alone.[16]

The inflammatory biomarker literature in tSCI is particularly noteworthy for its clinical accessibility. The finding that readily available hematological ratios, including the NLR, CAR, and GPR, carry independent prognostic information about neurologic recovery shifts the focus from identifying specialized tests to more effectively leveraging routinely measured biomarkers.[30–32] These markers require no additional blood draws, no specialized assay platforms, and no additional cost beyond what is already collected in standard acute care.[63] The challenge is to move from observational association to prospective validation with defined clinical thresholds, so that these ratios can be incorporated into structured prognostic algorithms rather than used informally.

The genetic biomarker literature raises a different set of clinical considerations. APOE genotyping is a one-time, germline test whose result does not change over time and whose prognostic implications extend across multiple neurologic conditions.[64] If APOE ε4 carriage independently predicts reduced motor recovery in tSCI and poorer surgical outcomes in DCM, there is a reasonable argument for incorporating this information into preoperative counseling and outcome expectation-setting, even before prospective intervention trials have demonstrated that genotype-modified management changes outcomes.[44] The DCM-specific variant literature, encompassing HIF1A, SPP1, BMP4, and BDNF Val66Met, represents a more heterogeneous body of evidence that is not yet ready for clinical translation but points toward biological pathways (ischemic response, ossification biology, neurotrophic signaling) that may eventually yield actionable prognostic or therapeutic targets.[51–54]

Table 5
Omics and diagnostic panel study characteristics

Study, Year	Population	Design (Level of Evidence)	N (Spinal Cord Injury/Control)	Gene(s)	Variant	Outcome(s)/Prognostic Signal
Sun et al,[46] 2011	tSCI	Genetic association cohort (II)	100/0	APOE	ε4 present vs absent	ε4 associated with less motor recovery, longer rehab LOS, and better pinprick recovery.
Jha et al,[47] 2008	tSCI	Retrospective cohort (II)	89/0	APOE	ε2/ε3/ε4	ε4 associated with less motor recovery, longer rehab LOS, and better pinprick.
Chintapalli et al,[49] 2025	DCM	Population-genetidcs case-control (III)	929/411,933	APOE	rs429358/rs7412 (ε alleles)	APOE ε4ε4 and ε2ε4 genotypes were linked to higher DCM risk (OR 1.48 and 1.43, P = .03 and .047), though ε4 dosage–severity associations were not significant after multiple testing.
Setzer et al,[48] 2008	DCM	Prospective genetic cohort (II)	106/0	APOE	ε4 presence	ε4 presence increased likelihood of developing DCM in stenosis cohort
Setzer et al,[77] 2009	DCM	Prospective cohort (II)	60/0	APOE	ε4 presence	ε4 predicted no neurologic improvement after surgery
Wang et al,[53] 2013	DCM	Case-control + surgical follow-up (II)	499/602	BMP4	SNVs (6007C>T; −5826G>A)	6007C>T associated with susceptibility + better postoperative improvement
Wang et al,[51] 2014	DCM	Case-control + surgical follow-up (III)	230/284	HIF1A	SNVs 1772C>T, 1790G>A	1790GG and G allele increased DCM risk, are linked to earlier onset and greater severity, show elevated disc HIF-1α/VEGF/IL-1/IL-6/NF-κB, and predict poorer ACF outcomes.
Wu et al,[52] 2014	DCM	Case-control + surgical outcomes (III)	187/198	SPP1 (OPN)	SNVs (rs1126616 etc.)	The rs1126616 CC genotype and C allele increase DCM risk (OR 2.04) and predict poorer postoperative neurologic recovery (P = .009).
Abode-Iyamah et al,[54] 2016	DCM	Prospective cohort (II)	48/0	BDNF	Val66Met (rs6265)	No association with baseline or 6-mo postoperative mJOA differences.

Abbreviations: ACF, anterior cervical fusion; APOE isoforms; BMP4, bone morphogenetic protein 4; HIF1A, hypoxia-inducible factor 1-alpha; LOS, length of stay; NF-κB, nuclear factor kappa-light-chain-enhancer of activated B cells; rs1126616, single-nucleotide polymorphism in SPP1; rs429358/rs7412, single-nucleotide polymorphisms defining APOE ε alleles; SNV, single-nucleotide variant; SPP1 (OPN), secreted phosphoprotein 1/osteopontin; Val66Met (rs6265), functional BDNF coding variant.

Table 6
Key biomarkers stratified by spine etiology

Category	Biomarker	Condition	Key Prognostic Signal
Neuroaxonal & Glial Proteins	Tau + GFAP + S100β (panel)	tSCI	CSF panel at 24h outperforms MRI for predicting AIS conversion (91% accuracy)
	GFAP	tSCI	Levels at days 2–7 predict complete injury and non-functional status; declining trajectory over 30 d predicts recovery
	S100β	tSCI	CSF outperforms serum for distinguishing complete vs incomplete injury (AUC 0.82 vs 0.59)
	NfL	tSCI	Rises for 30 d post-injury; later measurements (day 14–30) carry superior prognostic value for AIS conversion
	UCH-L1	tSCI	Lower serum levels within 24h associated with improved AIS at follow-up
	NfL	DCM	Elevated preoperatively vs controls; correlates with upper limb and pinch strength improvement after decompression
	pNF-H	DCM	Highest in acute-on-chronic worsening; correlates with rate of JOA recovery ($r = 0.381$)
Inflammatory & Immune	NLR	tSCI	Higher values at 24–48h independently predict worse neurologic outcomes
	CAR (CRP/albumin)	tSCI	Independent predictor of 1-y AIS outcome (AUC 0.749)
	GPR (glucose/ potassium)	tSCI	Correlates with injury severity and 6-mo prognosis (AUC 0.842)
	IL-6 + cytokine panel	DCM	Elevated vs controls; associated with postoperative improvement in pain and upper limb function
	YKL-40	DCM	Linked to symptom duration and degree of quality-of-life improvement after decompression
Metabolic & Nutritional	Albumin	tSCI	Level $\geq$ 2.8 g/dL at 30 d predicts marked 1-y recovery; higher levels at 1–2 wk doubles odds of recovery
	Selenium/SELENOP	tSCI	Early dynamics at 24h predict AIS conversion (AUC 0.90)
	Free zinc	tSCI	Lower free zinc at 24h predicts neurologic impairment (AUC 0.84)
	AGEs (skin sensor)	DCM	Higher skin autofluorescence associated with worse leg and foot pain
Genetic	APOE ε4 allele	Both	Reduces motor recovery in tSCI; increases DCM susceptibility and predicts absence of improvement after surgery
	miR-21-5p	DCM	Higher preoperative levels predict worse 1-y functional recovery after decompression
	miR-124-3p	tSCI	Distinguishes AIS A from B/C; independently predicts motor recovery at 6 mo
Omics & Panels	SCII (cfDNA + protein panel)	tSCI	Diagnostic AUC 0.91; predicts 6-mo AIS conversion (AUC 0.77)
	NfL + GFAP + CNTN-1	tSCI	Combined panel achieves AUC 0.96 for AIS-A classification within 4 d of injury
	5-gene RNA panel	DCM	Peripheral blood RNA distinguishes DCM from controls (AUC 0.939)

Abbreviations: CBC, complete blood count; CMP, comprehensive metabolic panel; Simoa, single molecule array.

Table 7
Key biomarkers stratified by timing

Timing Window	Biomarker	Condition	Sample Source	Key Prognostic Value
< 24 h post-injury	UCH-L1	tSCI	CSF/Serum	Lower levels within 24h associated with improved AIS grade at follow-up
	S100β	tSCI	CSF/Serum	CSF distinguishes complete vs incomplete injury (AUC 0.82); higher in paraplegia than paraparesis
	Selenium/ SELENOP	tSCI	Serum	Early dynamics predict AIS conversion (AUC 0.90)
	Free zinc	tSCI	Serum	Lower levels predict neurologic impairment (AUC 0.84)
	NLR	tSCI	Blood (CBC)	Higher values at 24–48h independently predict worse neurologic outcomes; derived from routine admission labs
	CAR (CRP/albumin)	tSCI	Serum	Independent predictor of 1-y AIS outcome (AUC 0.749); calculated from routine labs
	GPR (glucose/ potassium)	tSCI	Serum	Correlates with injury severity and 6-mo prognosis (AUC 0.842); calculated from routine labs
Days 2–7 post injury	GFAP	tSCI	Serum	Levels at days 2 and 7 predict complete injury classification and nonfunctional status at 6 mo
	Tau + GFAP + S100β (panel)	tSCI	CSF	Combined panel at 24h outperforms MRI for predicting AIS conversion (91% accuracy)
Days 14–30 post injury	NfL	tSCI	Serum	Continues rising for 30 d reflecting ongoing axonal degeneration; later timepoints carry superior prognostic value
	GFAP trajectory	tSCI	Serum	Steeper decline more than 30 d predicts better neurologic recovery
1–2 wk post injury	Albumin	tSCI	Serum	Higher levels at 1–2 wk approximately doubles the odds of marked 1-y recovery
30 d post injury	Albumin	tSCI	Serum	Level ≥ 2.8 g/dL predicts marked neurologic recovery at 1 y

(*continued on next page*)

Table 7
(continued)

Timing Window	Biomarker	Condition	Sample Source	Key Prognostic Value
Preoperative (DCM)	NfL	DCM	Serum	Elevated vs controls; correlates with postoperative upper limb and pinch strength improvement
	GFAP	DCM	Serum	Elevated vs controls; component of multi-analyte diagnostic panel (AUC 0.83)
	pNF-H	DCM	CSF	Highest in acute-on-chronic worsening; correlates with rate of JOA recovery (r = 0.381)
	IL-6 + cytokine panel	DCM	Serum	Elevated vs controls; associated with postoperative improvement in pain, disability, and upper limb function
	YKL-40	DCM	CSF	Linked to symptom duration and degree of quality-of-life improvement after decompression
	miR-21-5p	DCM	Plasma	Higher preoperative levels predict worse 1-y functional recovery after decompression
	AGEs (skin sensor)	DCM	Skin (noninvasive)	Higher burden associated with worse leg and foot pain
Germline (one-time)	APOE ε4 allele	Both	Blood	Reduces motor recovery in tSCI; increases DCM susceptibility and predicts absence of neurologic improvement after surgery

Several important limitations constrain the conclusions that can be drawn from the current literature. The included studies differ in injury type, biomarker class, assay platform, sampling timing, sample compartment, and outcome measure, making cross-study comparison unreliable. Many studies are single-center observational analyses with sample sizes insufficient to detect modest effects or perform meaningful subgroup analyses, and ethnic and demographic diversities are limited. Reference ranges and diagnostic thresholds established in 1 study population cannot be assumed to transfer to others. Most studies report short-term outcomes, providing limited insight into whether biomarker associations persist over the longer recovery trajectories that matter most to patients and families. Finally, and most critically, no prospective trial has yet demonstrated that biomarker-informed clinical decision-making changes patient outcomes.

SUMMARY

Genetic and molecular biomarkers represent a rapidly maturing frontier in spinal cord injury medicine, one that is moving from exploratory science toward clinically interpretable evidence.

Neurofilament light chain, GFAP, and S100β are the most consistently validated prognostic proteins across both conditions (**Tables 6** and **7**). Their utility is well-established in the tSCI setting for predicting AIS conversion, and growing evidence supports their role in predicting surgical responsiveness in DCM. The APOE ε4 allele is the most robustly characterized shared genetic modifier, reducing motor recovery in tSCI and predicting both disease susceptibility and poorer surgical outcomes in DCM. Routine hematological inflammatory ratios, including NLR, CAR, and GPR, are immediately accessible prognostic tools in the acute tSCI setting that deserve greater clinical attention. Metabolic markers including serum albumin and trace elements such as selenium and zinc reflect the physiologic environment of recovery and carry prognostic information that complements purely injury-severity markers.

Across all categories, multimodal approaches that integrate multiple biomarker signals consistently outperform any single marker. The future of molecular prognostication in spinal cord disease almost certainly lies in composite, biologically informed panels rather than in the discovery of any single definitive biomarker. At the same time, the field faces substantial methodological challenges, including assay standardization, timing-specific reference ranges, diverse and adequately powered validation cohorts, and ultimately prospective demonstration of clinical impact, that must be addressed before these markers can be confidently integrated into routine clinical practice.

CLINICS CARE POINTS

- *Pearl:* Serum neurofilament light chain (NfL) and glial fibrillary acidic protein (GFAP) are elevated in both acute traumatic spinal cord injury (tSCI) and degenerative cervical myelopathy (DCM) relative to healthy controls and correlate with neurologic impairment severity.
- *Pearl:* In acute tSCI, a cerebrospinal fluid biomarker panel combining Tau, glial fibrillary acidic protein, and S100β measured within the first 24 hours has demonstrated prognostic accuracy for AIS conversion exceeding that of MRI alone.
- *Pearl:* The neutrophil-to-lymphocyte ratio, C-reactive protein-to-albumin ratio, serum albumin, and glucose-to-potassium ratio are all derivable from standard admission bloodwork in the acute tSCI setting and carry independent prognostic associations with neurologic recovery.
- *Pearl:* APOE ε4 carrier status is associated with reduced motor recovery in tSCI and predicts a lack of neurologic improvement following cervical decompression in DCM; while genotyping is not yet standard of care, its result can appropriately inform preoperative counseling and recovery expectations for patients and families.
- *Pitfall:* Biomarker interpretation in spinal cord disease is highly context-dependent, and a threshold established for one etiology, sampling compartment, or time point cannot be applied to another.
- *Pitfall:* NfL in traumatic SCI continues to rise for up to 30 days post injury, reflecting ongoing secondary axonal degeneration rather than the initial impact. As a result, early NfL measurements may therefore underestimate ultimate neurologic deficit and should be interpreted with awareness of this trajectory rather than as a static injury severity index.
- *Pitfall:* Most published biomarker data are derived from small single-center observational studies with limited ethnic and demographic diversity. Published thresholds and reference ranges should not be overextrapolated to individual patients until multicenter prospective validation is available.

DISCLOSURE

The authors have nothing to disclose.

REFERENCES

1. Karlsson AK. Overview: autonomic dysfunction in spinal cord injury: clinical presentation of symptoms and signs. Prog Brain Res 2006;152:1–8. Elsevier.
2. Seif M, David G, Huber E, et al. Cervical cord neurodegeneration in traumatic and non-traumatic spinal cord injury. J Neurotrauma 2020;37(6):860–7.
3. David G, Mohammadi S, Martin AR, et al. Traumatic and nontraumatic spinal cord injury: pathological insights from neuroimaging. Nat Rev Neurol 2019;15(12):718–31.
4. McDonald JW, Sadowsky C. Spinal-cord injury. Lancet 2002;359(9304):417–25.
5. Ahuja CS, Nori S, Tetreault L, et al. Traumatic spinal cord injury-repair and regeneration. Neurosurgery 2017;80(3S):S9–22.
6. Hellenbrand DJ, Quinn CM, Piper ZJ, et al. Inflammation after spinal cord injury: a review of the critical timeline of signaling cues and cellular infiltration. J Neuroinflammation 2021;18(1):284.
7. Stukas S, Cooper J, Gill J, et al. Association of CSF and serum neurofilament light and glial fibrillary acidic protein, injury severity, and outcome in spinal cord injury. Neurology 2023;100(12):e1221–33.
8. Tigchelaar S, Gupta R, Shannon CP, et al. MicroRNA biomarkers in cerebrospinal fluid and serum reflect injury severity in human acute traumatic spinal cord injury. J Neurotrauma 2019;36(15):2358–71.

9. Mackiewicz-Milewska M, Cisowska-Adamiak M, Głowacka-Mrotek I, et al. Traumatic vs. non-traumatic spinal cord injury-epidemiology, complications, and neurological status during rehabilitation. J Clin Med 2025;14(15):5209.
10. Fehlings MG, Skaf G. A review of the pathophysiology of cervical spondylotic myelopathy with insights for potential novel mechanisms drawn from traumatic spinal cord injury. Spine 1998;23(24):2730–7.
11. Karadimas SK, Erwin WM, Ely CG, et al. Pathophysiology and natural history of cervical spondylotic myelopathy. Spine 2013;38(22 Suppl 1):S21–36.
12. Friesen AC, Detombe SA, Doyle-Pettypiece P, et al. Characterizing mJOA-defined post-surgical recovery patterns in patients with degenerative cervical myelopathy. World Neurosurg X 2024;21:100267. https://doi.org/10.1016/j.wnsx.2023.100267.
13. Albayar AA, Roche A, Swiatkowski P, et al. Biomarkers in spinal cord injury: prognostic insights and future potentials. Front Neurol 2019;10:27.
14. Jabłońska R, Ślusarz R, Zając M, et al. Neutrophil-to-Lymphocyte Ratio as a prognostic marker for hospital-acquired infections in neurosurgical patients. J Inflamm Res 2025;18:16667–84.
15. Pasternak AL, Ward KM, Luzum JA, et al. Germline genetic variants with implications for disease risk and therapeutic outcomes. Physiol Genomics 2017;49(10):567–81.
16. Leister I, Haider T, Mattiassich G, et al. Biomarkers in traumatic Spinal Cord injury-technical and clinical considerations: a systematic review. Neurorehabil Neural Repair 2020;34(2):95–110.
17. Hulme CH, Brown SJ, Fuller HR, et al. The developing landscape of diagnostic and prognostic biomarkers for spinal cord injury in cerebrospinal fluid and blood. Spinal Cord 2017;55(2):114–25.
18. Dalkilic T, Fallah N, Noonan VK, et al. Predicting injury severity and neurological recovery after acute cervical spinal cord injury: a comparison of cerebrospinal fluid and magnetic resonance imaging biomarkers. J Neurotrauma 2018;35(3):435–45.
19. Pfyffer D, Smith AC, Weber KA, et al. Prognostic value of tissue bridges in cervical spinal cord injury: a longitudinal, multicentre, retrospective cohort study. Lancet Neurol 2024;23(8):816–25.
20. Myrou A, Barmpagiannos K, Ioakimidou A, et al. Molecular biomarkers in neurological diseases: advances in diagnosis and prognosis. Int J Mol Sci 2025;26(5):2231.
21. Raheja A, Sinha S, Mansoori N, et al. Diagnostic and prognostic significance of serum biomarkers in traumatic Spinal Cord injury: a prospective cohort Study. Neurol India 2025;73(6):1180–6.
22. Haddadi K, Abediankenari S, Ehteshami S, et al. The accuracy of the S100B protein biomarker in the prognosis of patients with acute spinal cord injury. Asian J Neurosurg 2024;19(1):58–62.
23. Waliullah S, Kumar N, Kumar B, et al. Serum S100-Beta as a biomarker for neurological recovery in Acute Spinal Cord Injury (ASCI): a prospective case-control Study. Cureus 2025;17(2):e79202.
24. Leister I, Altendorfer B, Maier D, et al. Trajectory of serum levels of glial fibrillary acidic protein within four weeks post-injury is related to neurological recovery during the transition from acute to chronic spinal cord injury. J Neurotrauma 2023;40(9–10):999–1006.
25. Narayanan S, Shanker A, Khera T, et al. Neurofilament light: a narrative review on biomarker utility. Fac Rev 2021;10:46.
26. Abuhamdah S, Saleem TH, Elsadek BE, et al. Circulating ubiquitin Carboxyl Terminal hydrolase L1 and Neuroglobin levels in traumatic spinal cord injuries: relation to severity and outcomes. Int J Graph Multimed 2022;15:5795–805.
27. Takahashi H, Aoki Y, Nakajima A, et al. Axonal damage is remarkable in patients with acutely worsening symptoms of compression myelopathy: biomarkers in cerebrospinal fluid samples. Eur Spine J 2018;27(8):1824–30.
28. Vedantam A, Rahman M, Salam S, et al. Serum protein biomarkers for degenerative cervical myelopathy: a prospective study. J Neurosurg Spine 2025;42(6):718–26.
29. Tsitsopoulos PP, Holmström U, Blennow K, et al. Cerebrospinal fluid biomarkers of glial and axonal injury in cervical spondylotic myelopathy. J Neurosurg Spine 2021;34(4):632–41.
30. Naseri Alavi SA, Kobets AJ, Rezakhah A, et al. Can neutrophil to lymphocyte ratio predict early outcome in patients with spinal cord injury? World Neurosurg 2023;180:e243–9.
31. Tao E, Liu Z, Liu Y, et al. Serum C-Reactive protein-to-albumin ratio as a clinical risk factor for traumatic Spinal Cord injury. World Neurosurg 2025;194:123546. https://doi.org/10.1016/j.wneu.2024.12.005.
32. Zhou W, Liu Y, Wang Z, et al. Serum glucose/potassium ratio as a clinical risk factor for predicting the severity and prognosis of acute traumatic spinal cord injury. BMC Musculoskelet Disord 2023;24(1):870.
33. Chen Y, Wang D, Cao S, et al. Association between Serum IL-37 and Spinal cord injury: a prospective observational Study. Biomed Res Int 2020;2020:6664313. https://doi.org/10.1155/2020/6664313.
34. Heller RA, Seelig J, Bock T, et al. Relation of selenium status to neuro-regeneration after traumatic spinal cord injury. J Trace Elem Med Biol 2019;51:141–9.
35. Meng Y, Sun S, Cao S, et al. Netrin-1: a serum marker predicting cognitive impairment after Spinal cord injury. Dis Markers 2022;2022:1033197. https://doi.org/10.1155/2022/1033197.
36. Liu FJ, Xu HH, Yin Y, et al. Decreased adiponectin levels are a risk factor for cognitive decline in spinal

cord injury. In: Shi WQ, editor. Dis Markers 2022; 2022:1–6.

37. Kristine Koekkoek WAC, van Zanten ARH. Antioxidant vitamins and trace elements in critical illness. Nut in Clin Prac 2016;31(4):457–74.
38. Vo AK, Geisler F, Grassner L, et al. Serum albumin as a predictor of neurological recovery after spinal cord injury: a replication study. Spinal Cord 2021; 59(3):282–90.
39. Tong B, Jutzeler CR, Cragg JJ, et al. Serum albumin predicts long-term neurological outcomes after acute Spinal Cord injury. Neurorehabil Neural Repair 2018;32(1):7–17.
40. Li Y, Chen L, Yang X, et al. Dynamic association of serum albumin changes with inflammation, nutritional status and clinical outcomes: a secondary analysis of a large prospective observational cohort study. Eur J Med Res 2025;30(1):679.
41. Li X, Liu F, Liu Z, et al. Association between prognosis and calcium trajectories in patients with spinal cord injury based on MIMIC-IV data. Sci Rep 2025; 15(1):35941. https://doi.org/10.1038/s41598-025-22280-z.
42. Doi T, Inoue T, Sugaya J, et al. Noninvasive skin autofluorescence of advanced glycation end products in patients with degenerative cervical myelopathy. World Neurosurg 2025;194:123556. https://doi.org/10.1016/j.wneu.2024.12.015.
43. Cheng X, Zheng Y, Bu P, et al. Apolipoprotein E as a novel therapeutic neuroprotection target after traumatic spinal cord injury. Exp Neurol 2018;299(Pt A):97–108.
44. Desimone A, Hong J, Brockie ST, et al. The influence of ApoE4 on the clinical outcomes and pathophysiology of degenerative cervical myelopathy. JCI Insight 2021;6(15):e149227. https://doi.org/10.1172/jci.insight.149227.
45. Shvetcov A, Johnson ECB, Winchester LM, et al. APOE ε4 carriers share immune-related proteomic changes across neurodegenerative diseases. Nat Med 2025;31(8):2590–601.
46. Sun C, Ji G, Liu Q, et al. Apolipoprotein E epsilon 4 allele and outcomes of traumatic spinal cord injury in a Chinese Han population. Mol Biol Rep 2011;38(7): 4793–6.
47. Jha A, Lammertse DP, Coll JR, et al. Apolipoprotein E s4 allele and outcomes of traumatic Spinal Cord injury. J Spinal Cord Med 2008;31(2):171–6.
48. Setzer M, Hermann E, Seifert V, et al. Apolipoprotein E gene polymorphism and the risk of cervical myelopathy in patients with chronic spinal cord compression. Spine 2008;33(5):497–502.
49. Chintapalli R, Mowforth OD, Davies BM. APOE4 and prevalence of degenerative cervical myelopathy: a genetic case-control study in the UK Biobank cohort. J Clin Neurosci 2025;136:111247. https://doi.org/10.1016/j.jocn.2025.111247.
50. Mahley RW, Huang Y. Apolipoprotein E sets the stage: response to injury triggers neuropathology Neuron 2012;76(5):871–85.
51. Wang ZC, Hou XW, Shao J, et al. HIF-1α polymorphism in the susceptibility of cervical spondylotic myelopathy and its outcome after anterior cervica corpectomy and fusion treatment. PLoS One 2014;9(11):e110862. https://doi.org/10.1371/journal.pone0110862.
52. Wu J, Wu D, Guo K, et al. OPN polymorphism is associated with the susceptibility to cervical spondylotic myelopathy and its outcome after anterior cervical corpectomy and fusion. Cell Physiol Biochem 2014;34(2):565–74.
53. Wang D, Liu W, Cao Y, et al. BMP-4 polymorphisms in the susceptibility of cervical spondylotic myelopathy and its outcome after anterior cervical corpectomy and fusion. Cell Physiol Biochem 2013;32(1) 210–7.
54. Abode-Iyamah KO, Stoner KE, Grossbach AJ, et al Effects of brain derived neurotrophic factor Val66Met polymorphism in patients with cervical spondylotic myelopathy. J Clin Neurosci 2016;24:117–21.
55. Laliberte AM, Karadimas SK, Vidal PM, et al. Mir21 modulates inflammation and sensorimotor deficits in cervical myelopathy: data from humans and animal models. Brain Commun 2021;3(1):fcaa234 https://doi.org/10.1093/braincomms/fcaa234.
56. Divi SN, Markova DZ, D'Antonio ND, et al. Circulating microRNAs May be predictive of degenerative cervical myelopathy. Spine 2024;49(20):1393–400.
57. Liu X, Li F, Czosnyka M, et al. Multi-omics and high-spatial-resolution omics: deciphering complexity in neurological disorders. GigaScience 2025;14 giaf137. https://doi.org/10.1093/gigascience/giaf137
58. Azad TD, Ran KR, Materi JD, et al. A multi-analyte blood test for acute spinal cord injury. J Clin Investig 2025;135(5):e185463. https://doi.org/10.1172/JCI185463.
59. Garcia-Ovejero D, Beyerer E, Mach O, et al. Untargeted blood serum proteomics identifies novel proteins related to neurological recovery after human spinal cord injury. J Transl Med 2024;22(1):666.
60. Zheng Z, Chen J, Xu J, et al. Peripheral blood RNA biomarkers can predict lesion severity in degenerative cervical myelopathy. Neural Regen Res 2025 20(6):1764–75.
61. Fraussen J, In't Veld SGJG, van Laake-Geelen CCM et al. Longitudinal plasma biomarker profiles predict neurological outcome in traumatic Spinal Cord injury. Ann Neurol 2025;97(6):1180–9.
62. Akter F, Yu X, Qin X, et al. The pathophysiology of degenerative cervical myelopathy and the physiology of recovery following decompression. Front Neurosci 2020;14:138.
63. Novellino F, Donato A, Malara N, et al. Complete blood cell count-derived ratios can be useful

biomarkers for neurological diseases. Int J Immunopathol Pharmacol 2021;35:20587384211048264. https://doi.org/10.1177/20587384211048264.
64. Rajič Bumber J, Rački V, Mežnarić S, et al. Clinical significance of APOE4 genotyping: potential for personalized therapy and early diagnosis of alzheimer's disease. J Clin Med 2025;14(17):6047.
65. Kuhle J, Gaiottino J, Leppert D, et al. Serum neurofilament light chain is a biomarker of human spinal cord injury severity and outcome. J Neurol Neurosurg Psychiatr 2015;86(3):273–9.
66. Paragond S, Dhatt SS, Kumar V, et al. Prognosticating acute traumatic spinal cord injury using Neurofilament (NF), Neuron Specific Enolase (NSE), Matrix Metalloproteinases (MMPs), and S-100B as biomarkers. Ir J Med Sci 2024;193(2):769–75.
67. Fernández M, Baldassarro VA, Capirossi R, et al. Possible strategies to optimize a biomarker discovery approach to correlate with neurological outcome in patients with spinal cord injury: a pilot Study. J Neurotrauma 2020;37(3):431–40.
68. Takahashi H, Aoki Y, Nakajima A, et al. Phosphorylated neurofilament subunit NF-H becomes elevated in the cerebrospinal fluid of patients with acutely worsening symptoms of compression myelopathy. J Clin Neurosci 2014;21(12):2175–8.
69. Heller RA, Seelig J, Crowell HL, et al. Predicting neurological recovery after traumatic spinal cord injury by time-resolved analysis of monocyte subsets. Brain 2021;144(10):3159–74.
70. Seelig J, Heller RA, Hackler J, et al. Selenium and copper status - potential signposts for neurological remission after traumatic spinal cord injury. J Trace Elem Med Biol 2020;57:126415. https://doi.org/10.1016/j.jtemb.2019.126415.
71. Heller RA, Maares M, Chillon TS, et al. Total and free zinc dynamics as biomarkers for neurological impairment in traumatic Spinal Cord injury. Nutrients 2025;17(3):496.
72. Brown SJ, Harrington GMB, Hulme CH, et al. A preliminary cohort Study assessing routine blood analyte levels and neurological outcome after Spinal cord injury. J Neurotrauma 2020;37(3):466–80.
73. Harrington GMB, Cool P, Hulme C, et al. Routinely measured hematological markers can help to predict American spinal injury Association impairment Scale scores after spinal cord injury. J Neurotrauma 2021;38(3):301–8.
74. Bernardo Harrington GM, Cool P, Hulme C, et al. A comprehensive proteomic and bioinformatic analysis of human spinal cord injury Plasma identifies proteins associated with the complement Cascade and liver function as potential prognostic indicators of neurological outcome. J Neurotrauma 2025;42(3–4):292–306.
75. Li X, Yang Y, Xu S, et al. Screening biomarkers for spinal cord injury using weighted gene coexpression network analysis and machine learning. Neural Regen Res 2024;19(12):2723–34.
76. Picotto G, Morse LR, Nguyen N, et al. TMEM176A and TMEM176B are candidate regulators of inhibition of dendritic cell maturation and function after chronic spinal cord injury. J Neurotrauma 2020;37(3):528–33.
77. Setzer M, Vrionis FD, Hermann EJ, et al. Effect of apolipoprotein E genotype on the outcome after anterior cervical decompression and fusion in patients with cervical spondylotic myelopathy: clinical article. SPI 2009;11(6):659–66.

Neuromodulation in Spinal Cord Injury: Clinical Review

Nadine Mansour, MD, MPH, PhD[a,*], Anastasia Keller, PhD[b], Ann Parr, MD, PhD[c,1], Rajiv Saigal, MD, PhD, FAANS[b,1]

KEYWORDS

• Neuromodulation • Spinal cord injury • Functional electrical stimulation • Epidural spinal stimulation • Vagus nerve stimulation • Transcutaneous spinal stimulation

KEY POINTS

- The past decade has witnessed an expansion in neuromodulation clinical studies spanning over 117 publications.
- Consistant volitional and autonomic improvements across diverse injuries and study designs confirm neuromodulation as a robust spinal cord injury management.
- Early stage neuromodulation research faces limitations from small sample sizes with particular scarce data regarding Vagus nerve stimulation and functional electrical stimulation.

INTRODUCTION

Spinal cord injury (SCI) is a devastating consequence of trauma increasing morbidity and mortality and decreasing quality of life (QoL). It disrupts connections within the spinal cord resulting in a constellation of symptoms including the loss of volitional and autonomic function. Currently, there are over 300,000 individuals with chronic SCI and approximately 18,000 new cases reported each year in the United States.[1–3] Given that SCI commonly affects individuals at a young age and the improved life expectancy of those affected, the lifetime economic burden for an individual injured at age 50 is estimated to range between $1.5 and $3.4 million. This number doubles as the age of onset decreases, thereby placing a significant burden on the health care system and the national economy.[3,4]

Currently, there is no treatment of SCI beyond rehabilitation and the prevention and management of complications. Early interventions, such as surgical decompression and stabilization, duraplasty, corticosteroid therapy, and strict blood pressure control, can help improve perfusion and prevent further insult to the spinal cord.[5–7] Research into pharmacologic neuroprotective agents such as Riluzole; cell and gene therapies, including stem cell transplantation; tissue engineering with scaffolds, and rehabilitative strategies, has not yet been successful in restoring function.[6,8] Furthermore, these approaches are not without inherent risks, particularly in a patient population that is already at significant risk of morbidity and mortality.

However, neuromodulation approaches have shown promising results in restoring volitional and autonomic function.[9] The techniques range from noninvasive transcutaneous spinal cord stimulation (tSCS) and functional electrical stimulation (FES) to implanted epidural spinal cord stimulation (eSCS) and vagus nerve stimulation (VNS).

This review aims to support the translation of neuromodulation into clinical practice. It summarizes the underlying mechanisms and current evidence on the safety and efficacy of the different neuromodulation modalities (FES, tSCS, eSCS,

[a] Department of Neurosurgery & Department of Biomedical Engineering, University of Minnesota, Minneapolis, MN, USA; [b] Department of Neurological Surgery, University of California, San Francisco, CA, USA; [c] Department of Neurosurgery, University of Minnesota, Minneapolis, MN, USA
[1] Both authors have contributed equally.
* Corresponding author. 420 Delware Street SE, Minneapolis, MN 55455.
E-mail address: nmansour@umn.edu

Neurosurg Clin N Am 37 (2026) 649–664
https://doi.org/10.1016/j.nec.2026.05.016
1042-3680/26/

Abbreviations

AD	autonomic dysreflexia
BCI	brain computer interface
CPGs	central pattern generators
eSCS	epidural spinal cord stimulation
FES	functional electrical stimulation
QOL	quality of life
SCI	spinal cord injury
tSCS	transcutaneous spinal cord stimulation
VNS	vagus nerve stimulation

and VNS) in improving volitional and autonomic function in individuals with SCI.

FUNCTIONAL ELECTRICAL STIMULATION

FES was first developed as a neuromodulatory technique for promoting movement after SCI many decades ago. By placing electrodes peripherally near the target muscle, FES allows for activation of motor axons while bypassing the injured cord. More than 40 years ago, Marsolais and Kobetic demonstrated restoration of walking with FES in paralyzed individuals.[10] Many neuroprosthetic devices based on FES followed in the ensuing decades.[11–14]

However, the biophysics of electrical stimulation lead to an inverse recruitment order, where larger fibers are activated first. This inverse recruitment is associated with fatigue and limited the widespread adoption of FES devices for independent use.[15,16] Nonetheless, FES still has important applications and is still in common use as part of a rehabilitation program. For example, FES cycling may contribute to physiologic benefits in cardiovascular, muscle and bone health.[17] There is renewed interest in combining FES with newer technologies such as brain computer interface (BCI). A 2017 paper showed BCI combined with FES helped control graded motion in a paralyzed arm.[18]

EPIDURAL SPINAL CORD STIMULATION

The eSCS works by delivering low intensity electrical impulses into the epidural space. First developed for pain, eSCS can modulate pain signals via *gate control*. This stimulation activates large sensory nerve fibers (Aβ) located in the dorsal columns.[19,20] These activated nerve fibers transmit signals to the dorsal horn of the spinal cord to inhibit the transmission of pain signals carried by smaller C-fibers to the brain. As a result, pain sensation is either reduced.[19,20] This phenomenon is known as the *gate control theory of pain*, which was proposed by Ronald Melzack and Patrick Wall in 1965.[20] It was later established as the basis for an approved treatment approach in pain management.[21–23]

The capacity of eSCS to restore volitional movement was discovered serendipitously.[24,25] Volitional function is increasingly controlled by proprioceptive information.[26] eSCS operates by activating dorsal root afferents, which serve as the primary entry point for sensory input into the spinal cord.[27] This activation increases the excitability of spinal interneuronal circuits, which act as the central processing layer and include spinal reflex pathways and central pattern generators (CPGs).[27,28]

eSCS engages spinal interneurons which facilitates integration of supraspinal and sensory inputs to modulate diverse motor functions and the formation of new supraspinal connections.[24,29] Electrical stimulation of proprioceptive circuits increases the excitability of spared neurons *reawakening* dormant circuitry that remains intact even in chronic SCI. Furthermore, it lowers the activation thresholds of these neurons, thereby preparing them for subsequent supraspinal and propriospinal activation. This cascade of events facilitates the remodeling of these pathways, resulting in enhanced neuronal communication.[28,30,31] The effectiveness of this process is further augmented when combined with a rehabilitation program.[32–38] Rehabilitation enhances neuroplasticity by remodeling neural circuits, enhancing neurogenesis, reducing neuronal apoptosis, stimulating myelinogenesis, and regulating neuroinflammatory responses.[1–7]

Spinal reflexes, including monosynaptic and polysynaptic pathways, are also recruited by eSCS.[39] eSCS works by stimulating sensory fibers, which propagate signals through spinal interneuronal and motoneuronal pathways, thereby recruiting spinal reflexes.[25,40] Initially, eSCS activates monosynaptic reflexes in extensor muscles due to their direct connections.[41] Afterward, it activates polysynaptic pathways in flexor muscles, contributing to locomotor-like electromyography (EMG) activity.[42] Following activation, postactivation depression occurs, evoking muscle responses, in which the second response is significantly decreased.[25,43]

Furthermore, eSCS has been shown to engage CPGs in the cervical and lumbar spine. CPGs are specialized networks of neurons located within the central nervous system. They help produce rhythmic motor patterns in the arms and legs during movement. They consist of interneurons that excite and inhibit each other, creating a pattern of rhythmic outputs without the need for constant inputs from the brain.[44,45] CPGs within the brainstem also regulate essential functions such as respiration, mastication, micturition, defecation, and ejaculation.[46]

In short, the eSCS induces afferent sensory input via the dorsal column that recruits local spinal circuitry including interneurons and reflexes. Subsequently, they activate rhythm and pattern generating neural networks through CPGs. This network of modulation enables the recruitment of motor neurons, which serve as the final common pathway for the restoration of volitional output.[27]

Similar to volitional function, the overall mechanism of eSCS on autonomic function including cardiovascular, respiratory, bowel, and bladder control is not fully understood and complex. Supraspinal and propriospinal regulation and neuroplasticity are recognized as significant mechanisms by which eSCS contributes to restoring function. Stimulation directed at activating spinal motor networks can also affect somatosensory reflexes and visceral systems.[47–49] eSCS aims to connect the autonomic supraspinal centers and spinal circuits and regulate sympathetic reflexes.[24,48,50]

This dual capacity of eSCS to excite and inhibit sympathetic responses is key to its therapeutic versatility. eSCS has been shown to improve blood pressure instability, often experienced with SCI.[51,52] Activation of the propriospinal and dorsal root afferents in the lumbosacral region by eSCS increases the resting membrane potential of sympathetic networks. This increase in excitability increases total peripheral resistance, thereby resulting in vasoconstriction, which helps increase blood pressure and addresses orthostatic hypotension.[40,53]

Conversely, to manage the life threatening autonomic dysreflexia eSCS uses an inhibitory strategy. It inhibits the firing of dorsal neurons involved in sympathetic outflow. It can also activate inhibitory interneurons to suppress sympathetic activities.[54] Another key mechanism for regulating cardiovascular function involves eSCS activating afferent baroreceptors located in the aortic arch and carotid sinus, causing bradycardia, increased vascular tone, and ultimately blood pressure stabilization.[39,53]

Moreover, eSCS inhibits the sympathetic outflow, which reduces the release of catecholamines from the adrenal glands and nerve endings. Applying stimulation, lowers the release of norepinephrine, causing vasodilatation through α-adrenergic receptors. It also lowers the release of epinephrine, resulting in decreased heart rate and contractility through β-adrenergic receptors. Ultimately, blood pressure is lowered.[55,56] The impact of improvement in hemodynamic regulation and blood pressure instability by eSCS directly enhances cerebral blood flow and cerebral perfusion contribution. This would help ameliorate impairments in cognitive function associated with SCI.[1]

The mechanisms underlying respiratory recovery with eSCS involve the activation of spinal neural networks and sensory inputs.[33] Stimulating propriospinal networks activates and regulates inspiratory and expiratory muscles. This is achieved through the excitation and inhibition of respiratory motor neurons and the integration of both slow and fast motor units.[57] Activation of the phrenic nerve through monosynaptic and polysynaptic spinal reflex circuits facilitates the recruitment of motor neuron pools. Such recruitment, activates the diaphragm, thereby improving breathing.[40] Moreover, the effect of cervicothoracic eSCS is hypothesized to recruit paraspinal respiratory circuits and supraspinal respiratory centers.[58]

The mechanisms of action of eSCS on bowel and genitourinary functions are due to their anatomic proximity within the lumbosacral spine and their shared neural pathways.[59,60] Despite the fact that there are specific neural circuits for each function, stimulation of one function often influences the others. Supraspinal control of these functions including cortical and subcortical control of these areas indicates a centralized control system.[61]

Bowel, bladder, and sexual functions rely on sacral spinal reflexes to improve control.[59] Further, the pelvic nerves, which contain both afferent sensory and parasympathetic fibers, play a critical role in all three functions. They innervate the bladder, distal colon, rectum, and reproductive organs.[60] Through GABAergic mechanism, the pudendal nerve is involved in the innervation of the external urethral sphincter, external anal sphincter, and perineal muscles.[62] Pudendal stimulation has been shown to improve neurogenic bowel dysfunction, continence and sexual function.[62,63] Improvements in bladder–bowel synergy have been observed with eSCS.

eSCS is generally considered a safe and effective intervention for restoring function after SCI, with a safety profile similar to its use for chronic pain management.[64–66] The implantation procedure is typically a simple routine fluoroscopy-guided surgery.[64] While severe adverse events are rare (<1%), they are similar to those of any neurosurgical procedure. They include severe infection or epidural hematoma causing myelopathy and spinal cord damage.[66] Lead migration is the most common complication, occurring more often following cervical implantation at 18% compared to 7% following thoracic implantation. Other complications include lead breakage, pain over the implant site, and fibrosis, which may require electrode removal, but are also rare.[64–66] However, the long-term safety profile of eSCS for SCI is still being established.[67]

The fact that volitional movement and autonomic function are not optimized through the same stimulator settings and configurations highlights the complexity of the spinal cord. The spinal cord contains distinct neural circuits for each function meaning that optimizing one may not optimize the other or could even be detrimental to the other.[68] Autonomic effects should be considered when deciding on eSCS for motor activity especially cardiovascular deficits including life threatening autonomic dysreflexial.[24,68] Multisite stimulation or broader coverage might be necessary to achieve comprehensive restoration of function. The combinations of stimulation parameters and electrode configurations available are myriad, as is the selection of stimulation parameters that are task- and individual-specific. All of these challenges regarding the role of eSCS in restoring function require ongoing research to refine eSCS for function restoration.[24,68]

TRANSCUTANEOUS SPINAL CORD STIMULATION

The tSCS offers a noninvasive alternative for spinal cord circuitry neuromodulation. The first observation of the possibility to stimulate spinal cord from the skin surface was published in 1982.[69] The interest in tSCS resurfaced in 2007 when Minassian and colleagues, used single pulse tSCS of the lumbosacral posterior roots to characterize lower limb muscle responses in healthy adults. The study demonstrated that tSCS is a useful neurophysiological tool to examine state- and task-dependent spinal cord modulation at multiple segmental levels.[70] In 2010, Gerasimenko and colleagues, demonstrated that stimulation of lumbosacral spinal cord from the skin surface can activate locomotor central pattern generating circuitry in individuals with intact central nervous system.[71] In 2014, Hofstoetter and colleagues, reported the first use of tSCS in 3 individuals with chronic incomplete (AIS D) SCIs for treatment of spasticity, showing significant improvements in exaggerated reflex responsiveness and improvement in gait.[72] Shortly after, Gerasimenko and colleagues, translated their earlier findings of tSCS-induced locomotor-like movements in a gravity-neutral environment to 5 individuals with complete motor paralysis revealing presence of voluntary control in the lower limb muscles during stimulation that was maintained without tSCS after as little at 4 training sessions.[73]

Since these foundational studies, tSCS has become a key neurophysiological tool as well as a promising therapy for recovery of function after SCI. Most research studies focus on implementation of tSCS for treatment of motor function in upper extremities, trunk and lower extremities employing a wide range of study designs and functional outcome measures. To administer tSCS, small round stimulating electrodes are placed on the skin surface between the vertebral segments. For lumbosacral stimulation targeting lower motoneuronal pools, the electrodes are typically placed between at T11/T12 and L1/L2 spinous process. For cervical tSCS targeting upper extremities motoneuronal pools the electrode placement varies substantially and usually involves multisite stimulation strategy, coupling electrodes at C3/C4 with C6/C7 or C7-T1,[74–76] with a more recent large clinical trial stimulating at C2 and T1, with electrodes placed above and below the lesion level.[77] The anodes are typically placed over the iliac crests, anterior superior iliac spine, paraumbilicaly over the abdomen,[78] or clavicles when grounding cervicaly placed cathodes.[77]

Across studies of tSCS in SCI in the past 10 years, most effective protocols applied 30 to 50 Hz stimulation with intensities between sensory and motor thresholds.[73,77,79–82] Repeated tSCS paired with rehabilitation produced clinically meaningful gains in voluntary motor control (eg, increased limb strength, improved upper/lower extremities motor scores)[74,77,83] and walking performance (eg, faster 10 minute walk test [MWT] and improved gait independence),[79,84–86] with the highest-quality evidence from controlled trials demonstrating significant improvements in motor score and gait outcomes compared to sham controls.[85]

Relatively fewer studies examined the efficacy of tSCS to facilitate autonomic system recovery following SCI although significant improvements in bowel and bladder function often coincide with the locomotor improvements in studies focused on lower extremity recovery.[83] Recently, Samejima and colleagues, published a comprehensive investigation of the lumbosacral tSCS effects on urinary, bowel, sexual, cardiovascular and sensorimotor functions in a single-subject design study.[87] An individual with chronic clinically motor-complete cervical SCI underwent 30 sessions of lumbosacral tSCS (administered in sitting, 60 minutes a day, 5 times per week for 6 weeks), which led to improved urinary bladder compliance, anorectal function and simultaneous reduction in autonomic dysreflexia severity during filling cystometry and anorectal manometry assessments. Following tSCS therapy the participant also reported improved erectile function and sexual satisfaction.[87]

Philips and colleagues, have determined that tSCS applied during orthostatic challenge in individuals who experience orthostatic hypotension due to SCI normalizes blood pressure as well as cerebral blood flow with improved cardiac contractility.[50] On the other hand, Solinsky and colleagues, studied autonomic regulation in a battery of assessments designed to test sympathoinhibition and above/below injury level sympathoexcitation, and found that tSCS did not improve autonomic regulation in individuals with SCI.[88] The authors concluded that, while tSCS can facilitate sympathetic response necessary for maintenance of blood pressure during orthostatic or Valsalva maneuver challenges, it may do so by generating a tonic excitation of the sympathetic nervous system, potentially lowering the threshold for the onset of autonomic dysreflexia (AD).[88] The contradicting evidence may, at least in part, be due to methodological differences. In studies on tSCS showing AD resolution, the electrodes were placed at the T7/T8 spinal segment,[50,89] whereas Solinsky and colleagues, stimulated at the T10/11.[88] In addition, it is not yet clear whether chronic tSCS alone or in combination with activity-based rehabilitation can facilitate adaptive and/or reverse maladaptive neuroplasticity underpinning the pathophysiology of AD[90] long-term. Future studies should focus on elucidating the mechanisms.

Similar to epidural, transcutaneous SCS modulates the spinal circuitry by raising its excitability through the activation of low-threshold afferents within the posterior roots.[67,91,92] With increasing stimulation intensities, tSCS may recruit Ib, II and larger diameter cutaneous afferents as well as interneurons, ultimately lowering the threshold for motoneuronal activation and making them more responsive to any remaining descending input resulting in better supraspinal control.[92,93] However, the properties of the electrical current flow vary substantially between the eSCS and tSCS depending on the electrode position.[91,94] While most of the current during eSCS flows through cerebrospinal fluid with minimal resistance, the current generated by tSCS encounters multiple tissues (skin, fat, and bone) with variable conduction properties which substantially alter the flow and reduce the final charge delivered to the neural targets.[94] This fundamental difference makes eSCS advantageous for more selective and precise activation of motoneuronal pools.[91] With advancements in closed loop technology, epidural SCS implants evolve to incorporate real-time physiologic feedback (eg, evoked compound action potentials, EMG activity, or kinematic signals) to dynamically adjust stimulation parameters and maintain engagement of intended spinal circuits while minimizing off-target activation.[95,96] Closed-loop technology can also be implemented with noninvasive SCS, and is already showing great promise to further advance post-SCI gait rehabilitation.[97] Furthermore, the noninvasive nature of tSCS lowers the accessibility barriers allowing for more rapid implementation of neuromodulation technology into rehabilitation avoiding the inherent risks of surgery. The recent studies translating the success of tSCS therapy from adult to pediatric SCI population are the prime example of this, highlighting how the safety profile and ease of tSCS deployment broaden its therapeutic reach to populations for whom implantable neuromodulation may carry disproportionate risk.[98–102]

VAGUS NERVE STIMULATION

VNS is a relatively newer approach to neuromodulation for SCI patients. By driving phasic release of neurotransmitters such as serotonin and acetylcholine, and noradrenaline, VNS may enhance plasticity. First developed for stroke, phasic VNS combined with rehabilitation has been shown to enhance recovery of paretic upper extremities.[103] More recently, the same approach has been used in humans with incomplete SCI. In 2025, Kilgard and colleagues demonstrated closed loop VNS timed during rehabilitation promoted recovery of upper extremity function in humans with chronic and incomplete SCI.[104] As a new approach for neuromodulation after SCI, further exploration of this technology with larger SCI patient populations is needed.

TRENDS IN CLINICAL STUDIES FOR THE NEUROMODULATION MODALITIES

The past decade has witnessed an expansion in neuromodulation clinical studies spanning over 117 publications as shown in **Fig. 1**. These modalities have demonstrated distinct but complementary approaches for functional recovery after SCI.

The eSCS represents the most invasive and studied approach among this cohort. **Fig. 1**A shows 55 published studies with sample sizes ranging from single-case reports to cohorts. This work builds upon our earlier systematic review,[105] which synthesized the foundational history and early clinical evidence. Early highly cited foundational work, demonstrated that eSCS can enable voluntary movement, standing, and stepping in individuals with SCI.[24,28,33,36,37,106,107] These publications have reshaped the concept of residual spinal network capacity. More recent studies

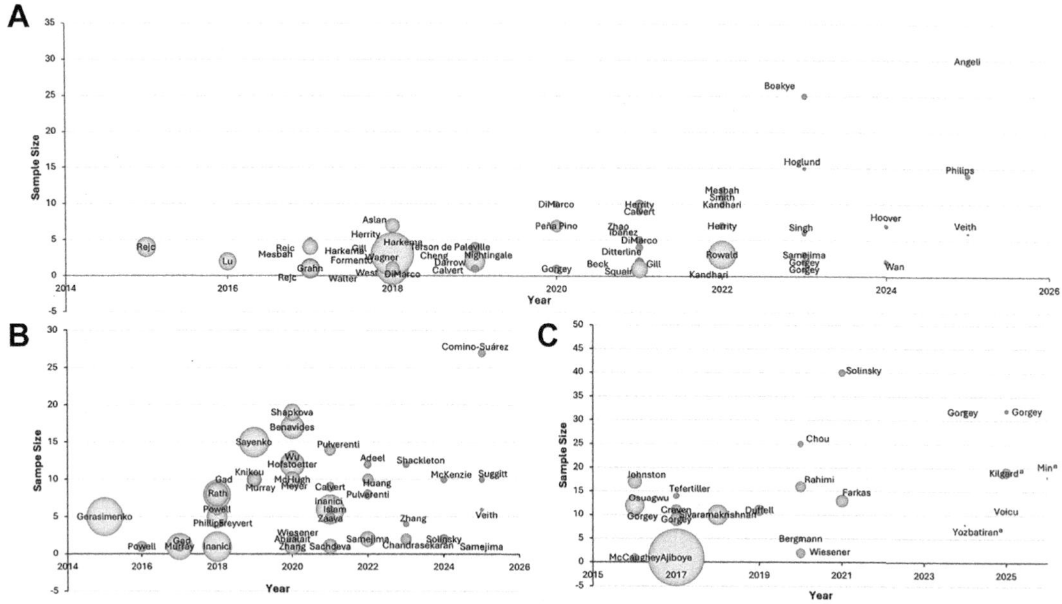

Fig. 1. Trends in clinical literature for the neuromodulation modalities: (*A*) eSCS (*B*) tSCS (*C*) VNS & FES. Note: [a]Indicate VNS studies. Bubble size corresponds to the number of citations.

have shifted toward larger cohorts,[68,108] adopted multimodal approaches,[109,110] refined stimulation parameters and electrode configurations[111–114] (**Table 1**).

In parallel, research on tSCS has expanded rapidly with 42 clinical studies (**Fig. 1**B). Foundational high-impact contributions helped establish the physiologic basis and therapeutic potential of tSCS.[73,74,116,118,119] Subsequent studies expanded sample sizes and refined targets for motor and autonomic function.[117,120,121] Recent studies have shifted toward larger cohorts and standardized outcomes.[77,85,122] Further studies have adapted, multimodal approaches combining tSCS with eSCS or FES.[109,110,123]

Similarly, FES research has progressed from foundational feasibility studies,[124–126] which helped establish the mechanisms of FES for restoring motor function to larger clinical investigations with more refined protocols and specific functional outcomes.[127–129] Recent studies feature larger cohorts and a more standardized methodologies.[130,131] These studies demonstrate the clinical maturation of the field, moving toward optimized, multi-modal approach[123] capable of enhancing metabolic profiles, muscle volume, and overall motor function.[132–134] The body of literature on FES (19 studies) and VNS (3 studies) remains limited (see **Fig. 1**C). The most recent VNS research highlights it as a frontier approach moving toward, *closed-loop* interventions. This recent body of work transitioned VNS from traditional psychiatric and epileptic applications into the realm of physical recovery in SCI.[104,135,136]

Collectively, tSCS,[50,79–81,83,84,87,89,137–156] eSCS,[24,35,53,55,115,149,157–192] FES,[193–198] and VNS studies illustrate a steadily evolving evidence base. Despite heterogeneity in study designs and modest sample sizes, the consistency of motor and autonomic benefits across independent groups and injury severities supports neuromodulation as a robust intervention for SCI management.

COMPARISON BETWEEN THE NEUROMODULATION MODALITIES

Fig. 2A, B show comparison between the different neuromodulation modalities. They show a distinction between invasiveness, primary neuronal targets, applications, and functional outcomes. eSCS represents the most invasive modality that targets spinal circuits. It provides strong motor effects and moderate autonomic and sensory effects. Its effects can be enhanced through intensive, task-specific training and can persist beyond active stimulation.[109,110,199]

In contrast, tSCS is a noninvasive alternative that also targets spinal circuitry. It offers moderate motor and sensory effects but limited autonomic effects. It has a shorter effect duration typically low-to-moderate compared to eSCS.[86,109,110,199,200] While both strategies focus on local circuit excitability, VNS introduces an intermediate level of

Table 1
Summary of pivotal neuromodulation studies

	Key Findings
eSCS Studies	
Harkema et al,[33] 2011	*Proof of concept* showing that the lumbosacral stimulation with locomotor training enabled volitional movement, including standing, and assisted stepping in chronic complete paraplegia.
Gill et al,[106] 2018	Lumbosacral stimulation with locomotor training enabled progression from standing to independent stepping in chronic complete paraplegia.
Darrow et al,[24] 2019	Lumbosacral epidural stimulation restored volitional, cardiovascular, bowel, bladder, and sexual function in individuals with chronic complete SCI without locomotor training.
West et al,[115] 2018	Lumbosacral epidural stimulation in chronic complete cervical SCI resolved orthostatic hypotension, and improved cardiovascular circulation and neurovascular coupling.
Phillips et al, 2024[114]	Updated evidence demonstrating that lower thoracic stimulation is superior to lumbosacral targets for restoring blood pressure and resolving hemodynamic instability identifies the optimal stimulation site for orthostatic hypotension.
tSCS Studies	
Gerasimenko et al,[92] 2015	Demonstrated that noninvasive stimulation could enable voluntary leg movements and standing in complete paraplegia. It introduced a 10 kHz carrier frequency to lessen pain and allow for the high energy needed to reach spinal networks through the skin.
Inanici et al,[74] 2018	Pivotal study on tSCS over the cervical spinal cord. It demonstrated that tSCS combined with hand training significantly improved upper-limb strength and fine motor control (grasp/pinch) in chronic tetraplegia.
Gad et al,[116] 2017	Demonstrated the feasibility of using tSCS to facilitate complex motor tasks and highlighting the potential for tSCS in locomotor rehabilitation. It showed that combining tSCS with robotic assistance enable weight-bearing and stepping in complete paraplegia.
Sayenko et al,[117] 2019	Established that tSCS targets spinal circuits to restore postural control and trunk stability, enabling independent standing in individuals with chronic SCI.
Inanici et al,[118] 2021; Moritz et al,[77] 2024	Building on earlier work, these papers provided definitive clinical evidence for the effectiveness of tSCS in improving upper extremity function. They found that 72% of participants with chronic SCI experienced meaningful, durable improvements in arm and hand function.

invasiveness that targets supraspinal centers. VNS is potent in modulating autonomic function and inducing neuroplasticity. Although, its direct motor and sensory effects are limited compared to those of eSCS & tSCS.[104,135,136]

Finally, FES is another noninvasive alternative. It acts on peripheral nerves and muscles, producing strong, task-dependent motor effects. However, it only offers moderate sensory and minimal autonomic effects. Further, its benefits are often limited to the duration of the activity itself, with no carry over effect.[86,199,200] Together, these modalities offer a spectrum of tools that can be tailored to a patient's specific functional recovery goals.

CONCLUSION AND FUTURE DIRECTION

Current treatment of SCI is multidisciplinary and includes a combination of medical, surgical, and neuro-rehabilitation strategies. Despite these approaches, the functional improvement after SCI typically plateaus. Neuromodulation for SCI has emerged as a promising modality. Specifically, eSCS and tSCS can activate neuronal circuits and leverage neuroplasticity below the level of injury promoting functional recovery. Despite its promising potential, the underlying mechanisms of neuromodulation are not fully understood. Further, clinical outcomes vary between individuals.

A

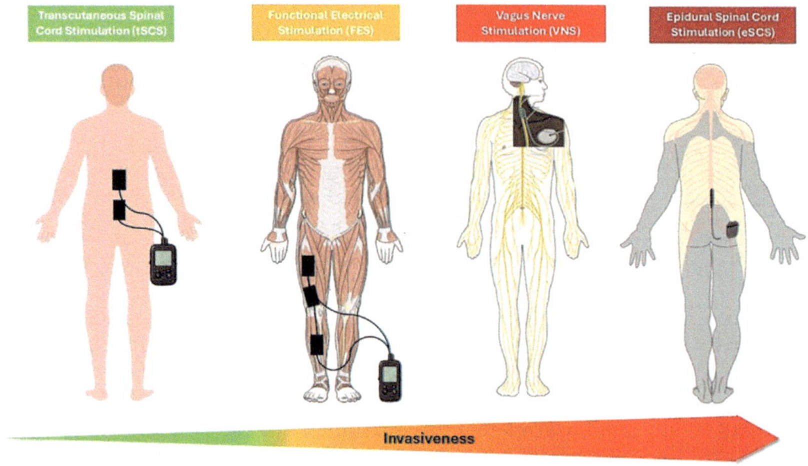

Device Invasiveness	Low (portable external)	Low (portable external)	Moderate (implanted)	High (implanted)
Neuronal target	Transcutaneous spinal cord	Peripheral nerves & muscles	Vagus nerve	Epidural space of spinal cord
Use in SCI	Volitional function, sensorimotor integration, & training enhancement	Primarily rehab enhancement	Rehabilitation & plasticity enhancement	Volitional & autonomic function restoration

B

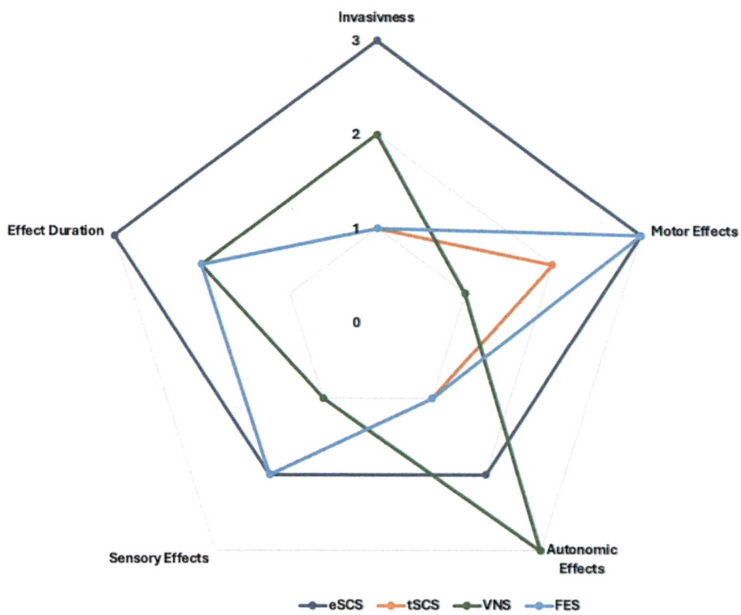

Fig. 2. (*A*) Neuromodulation modalities comparison; (*B*) Neuromodulation modalities and their comparative efficacy for functional restoration.

Research on neuromodulation is still in the early stages, and many studies have small -sample sizes. Research on VNS is an interesting new approach, but has limited data to date. Further research is needed on the mechanisms of action, the optimization of stimulation parameters and strategies, and the long-term effects of the different neuromodulation modalities More studies are needed to move to the next phase of randomized clinical trials to ultimately facilitate the approval of spinal cord stimulation as a treatment option for SCI, maximize functional benefits and improve QoL of the SC population.

CLINICS CARE POINTS

- Expand the pool of SCI population who can benefit from the intervetion by including individuals with higher injury levels and those in the ASIA A & B cohorts.
- Choose the neuromodulation modality that fits the functional target. For example, eSCS targeting lumbusacral circuits can improve cardiovascular function, upper extremity motor control, locomotion, and standing. Meanwhile, eSCS & FES can enhance upper extrmity function including reaching and grasping.
- Individualize stimulation parameters according to each patient's spinal cord anatomy and neurophysiological targets. Continuously fine tuning paramaters to accomodate changes in neural circuits in response to neurospasticity.
- Neuromodulation is a tool to improve independence and quality of life. Utilize neuromodulation to augment rehabilitation training, rather than as a replacement.
- Standarize stimulation protocols and functional biomarkers prior to moving into larger-scale randomized controlled trials. Moreover, assessment of the long term effects of the intervention is required.

DISCLOSURE

The article was supported by the NIH, United States T32 Translational Neuromodulation Training Program (T32-NS121920).

REFERENCES

1. Jain NB, Ayers GD, Peterson EN, et al. Traumatic spinal cord injury in the United States, 1993-2012. JAMA 2015;313:2236–43.
2. Lasfargues JE, Custis D, Morrone F, et al. A model for estimating spinal cord injury prevalence in the United States. Paraplegia 1995;33:62–8.
3. University of Alabama at Birmingham. NSCISC | National Spinal cord injury statistical Center. National Spinal cord injury statistical center. 2025. Available at: https://sites.uab.edu/nscisc/.
4. DeVivo M, Chen Y, Mennemeyer S, et al. Costs of care following spinal cord injury. Top Spinal Cord Inj Rehabil 2011;16:1–9.
5. Carroll AH, Fakhre E, Quinonez A, et al. An update on spinal cord injury and current management. JBJS Rev 2024;12(10). https://doi.org/10.2106/JBJS.RVW.24.00124.
6. Zhong H, Wang H, Huang B, et al. Current frontier technologies in spinal cord injury research: a narrative review. Ovid 2025;2(4):173–86.
7. Greil ME, Hunt ER, Torres Espin A, et al. Retrospective analysis of expansile duraplasty as surgical adjunct after acute traumatic spinal cord injury. Glob Spine J 2025;16:1212–20.
8. Fehlings MG, Moghaddamjou A, Harrop JS, et al. Safety and efficacy of riluzole in acute spinal cord injury study (RISCIS): a multi-center, randomized, placebo-controlled, double-blinded trial. J Neurotrauma 2023;40:1878–88.
9. James ND, McMahon SB, Field-Fote EC, et al. Neuromodulation in the restoration of function after spinal cord injury. Lancet Neurol 2018;17:905–17.
10. Marsolais EB, Kobetic R. Functional walking in paralyzed patients by means of electrical stimulation. Clin Orthop Relat Res 1983;175:30–6.
11. González-Graniel E, Mercado-Gutierrez JA, Martínez-Díaz S, et al. Sensing and control strategies used in FES systems aimed at assistance and rehabilitation of foot drop: a systematic literature review. J Personalized Med 2024;14:874.
12. He R, Dong Y, Li Y, et al. Therapeutic and orthotic effects of an adaptive functional electrical stimulation system on gait biomechanics in participants with stroke. J NeuroEng Rehabil 2025;22:62.
13. Blue Cross Blue Shield of Massachusetts. Functional neuromuscular electrical stimulation. Medical Policy No. 201. 2010. Available at: https://www.bluecrossma.org/medical-policies/ (Accessed 29 April 2026).
14. Popović DB, Popović MB. Advances in the use of electrical stimulation for the recovery of motor function. Prog Brain Res 2011;194:215–25.
15. Saigal R, Renzi C, Mushahwar VK. Intraspinal microstimulation generates functional movements after spinal-cord injury. IEEE Trans Neural Syst Rehabil Eng 2004;12:430–40.
16. Musselman KE, Jervis-Rademeyer H, Nezon E. Functional electrical stimulation as a tool to restore motor control after spinal cord injury: translation to clinical practice. Expert Rev Med Dev 2025;22:845–56.
17. Newham DJ, Donaldson Nde N. FES cycling. Acta Neurochir Suppl 2007;97(Pt 1):395–402.
18. Friedenberg DA, Schwemmer MA, Landgraf AJ, et al. Neuroprosthetic-enabled control of graded arm muscle contraction in a paralyzed human. Sci Rep 2017;7:8386.
19. Sdrulla A, Guan Y, Raja S. Spinal cord stimulation: clinical efficacy and potential mechanisms. Pain Pract 2018;18:1048–67.
20. Melzack R. Gate control theory: on the evolution of pain concepts. Pain Forum 1996;5:128–38.
21. Mortimer JT, Shealy CN, Wheeler C. Experimental nondestructive electrical stimulation of the brain and spinal cord. J Neurosurg 1970;32:553–9.
22. Shealy CN, Mortimer JT, Hagfors NR. Dorsal column electroanalgesia. J Neurosurg 1970;32:560–4.

23. Shealy CN, Mortimer JT, Reswick JB. Electrical inhibition of pain by stimulation of the dorsal columns: preliminary clinical report. Anesth Analg 1967;46:489–91.
24. Darrow D, Balser D, Netoff TI, et al. Epidural spinal cord stimulation facilitates immediate restoration of dormant motor and autonomic supraspinal pathways after chronic neurologically complete spinal cord injury. J Neurotrauma 2019;36:2325–36.
25. Hofstoetter US, Freundl B, Binder H, et al. Common neural structures activated by epidural and transcutaneous lumbar spinal cord stimulation: elicitation of posterior root-muscle reflexes 2018;13(1): e0192013.
26. Takeoka A, Arber S. Functional local proprioceptive feedback circuits initiate and maintain locomotor recovery after spinal cord injury. Cell Rep 2019; 27:71–85.e3.
27. Hachmann JT, Yousak A, Wallner JJ, et al. Epidural spinal cord stimulation as an intervention for motor recovery after motor complete spinal cord injury. J Neurophysiol 2021;126:1843–59.
28. Formento E, Minassian K, Wagner F, et al. Electrical spinal cord stimulation must preserve proprioception to enable locomotion in humans with spinal cord injury. Nat Neurosci 2018;21:1728–41.
29. Li T, Chen J. Spinal cord stimulation for functional restoration in spinal cord injury. A Narrative Review 2025;17(2):1–13.
30. Aman JE, Elangovan N, Yeh I-L, et al. The effectiveness of proprioceptive training for improving motor function: a systematic review. Front Hum Neurosci 2015;8:1075.
31. Jack AS, Hurd C, Martin J, et al. Electrical stimulation as a tool to promote plasticity of the injured spinal cord. J Neurotrauma 2020;37:1933–53.
32. Herman R, He J, D'Luzansky S, et al. Spinal cord stimulation facilitates functional walking in a chronic, incomplete spinal cord injured. Spinal Cord 2002;40:65–8.
33. Harkema S, Gerasimenko Y, Hodes J, et al. Effect of epidural stimulation of the lumbosacral spinal cord on voluntary movement, standing, and assisted stepping after motor complete paraplegia: a case study. Lancet 2011;377:1938–47.
34. Angeli CA, Edgerton VR, Gerasimenko YP, et al. Altering spinal cord excitability enables voluntary movements after chronic complete paralysis in humans. Brain 2014;137:1394–409.
35. Rejc E, Angeli CA, Bryant N, et al. Effects of stand and step training with epidural stimulation on motor function for standing in chronic complete paraplegics. J Neurotrauma 2017;34:1787–802.
36. Rejc E, Angeli CA, Atkinson D, et al. Motor recovery after activity-based training with spinal cord epidural stimulation in a chronic motor complete paraplegic. Sci Rep 2017;7:13476.
37. Grahn PJ, Lavrov IA, Sayenko DG, et al. Enabling task-specific volitional motor functions via spinal cord neuromodulation in a human with paraplegia 2017;92(4):544–54.
38. Angeli CA, Boakye M, Morton RA, et al. Recovery of over-ground walking after chronic motor complete spinal cord injury. N Engl J Med 2018;379: 1244–50.
39. Chalif JI, Chavarro VS, Mensah E, et al. Epidural spinal cord stimulation for spinal cord injury in humans: a systematic review. J Clin Med 2024;13:1090.
40. Zhang T, Jia Y, Wang N, et al. Recent advances in potential mechanisms of epidural spinal cord stimulation for movement disorders. Exp Neurol 2025; 392:115330.
41. Lundberg A. Multisensory control of spinal reflex pathways. Prog Brain Res 1979;50:11–28.
42. Minassian K, Jilge B, Rattay F, et al. Stepping-like movements in humans with complete spinal cord injury induced by epidural stimulation of the lumbar cord: electromyographic study of compound muscle action potentials. Spinal Cord 2004;42:401–16.
43. Vargas Luna JL, Brown J, Krenn MJ, et al. Neurophysiology of epidurally evoked spinal cord reflexes in clinically motor-complete posttraumatic spinal cord injury. Exp Brain Res 2021;239:2605–20.
44. Steuer I, Guertin PA. Central pattern generators in the brainstem and spinal cord: an overview of basic principles, similarities and differences 2019; 30(2):107–64.
45. Marder E, Bucher D. Central pattern generators and the control of rhythmic movements 2001;11 (23):R986–96.
46. Guertin PA, Steuer I. Key central pattern generators of the spinal cord. J Neurosci Res 2009;87(11) 2399–405.
47. Moshonkina TR, Stolbkov YK, Kozlovskaya IB, et al Mechanisms of spinal cord electrical stimulation action on autonomic functions. Hum Physiol 2017 42:694–704.
48. Samejima S, Shackleton C, Miller T, et al. Mapping the iceberg of autonomic recovery: mechanistic underpinnings of neuromodulation following spinal cord injury. Neuroscientist 2024;30:378–89.
49. Kupari J, Ernfors P. Pricking into autonomic reflex pathways by electrical acupuncture. Neuron 2020 108(3):395–7.
50. Phillips AA, Squair JW, Sayenko DG, et al. An autonomic neuroprosthesis: noninvasive electrical spinal cord stimulation restores autonomic cardiovascular function in individuals with spinal cord injury J Neurotrauma 2018;35:446–51.
51. Flett S, Garcia J, Cowley KC. Spinal electrical stimulation to improve sympathetic autonomic functions needed for movement and exercise after spinal cord injury: a scoping clinical review J Neurophysiol 2022;128:649–70.

52. Burns M, Solinsky R. Towards rebalancing blood pressure instability after spinal cord injury with spinal cord electrical stimulation: a mini review and critique of the evolving literature. Auton Neurosci Basic Clin 2022;237:102905.
53. Harkema SJ, Wang S, Angeli CA, et al. Normalization of blood pressure with spinal cord epidural stimulation after severe spinal cord injury. Front Hum Neurosci 2018;12:83.
54. Partida E, Mironets E, Hou S, et al. Cardiovascular dysfunction following spinal cord injury. Neural Regen Res 2016;11:189–94.
55. Aslan SC, Legg Ditterline BE, Park MC, et al. Epidural spinal cord stimulation of Lumbosacral networks modulates arterial blood pressure in individuals with spinal cord injury-induced cardiovascular deficits. Front Physiol 2018;9:565.
56. Burns M, Solinsky R. Toward rebalancing blood pressure instability after spinal cord injury with spinal cord electrical stimulation: a mini review and critique of the evolving literature. Auton Neurosci 2022;237:102905.
57. Brown R, DiMarco AF, Hoit JD, et al. Respiratory dysfunction and management in spinal cord injury. Respir Care 2006;51:853–70.
58. Huang R, Yamamoto MT, Zhou Y, et al. Lumbar epidural electrical stimulation enhances respiration in mice. Physiology 2024;39:1942.
59. Sinha S, Vasudeva P, Bharadwaj S, et al. Role of pelvic organ crosstalk in dysfunction of the bowel and bladder. Curr Bladder Dysfunct Rep 2022;17:91–103.
60. Daneshgari F, Paspulati RM, Simon JH. Bladder, bowel, and sexual dysfunction. In: Imaging acute neurologic disease: a symptom-based approach. Cambridge: Cambridge University Press; 2014. p. 260–9. https://doi.org/10.1017/CBO9781139565653.017.
61. Coolen RL, Groenendijk IM, Blok BFM. Recent advances in neuroimaging of bladder, bowel and sexual function. Curr Opin Urol 2020;30:480–5.
62. McGee MJ, Danziger ZC, Bamford JA, et al. A spinal GABAergic mechanism is necessary for bladder inhibition by pudendal afferent stimulation. Am J Physiol Ren Physiol 2014;307:F921–30.
63. Calabrò RS, Leo A, Bramanti P. Pudendal nerve stimulation: a potential tool for neurogenic bowel dysfunction. Neurourol Urodyn 2014;33:358–9.
64. Pino IP, Nightingale TE, Hoover C, et al. The safety of epidural spinal cord stimulation to restore function after spinal cord injury: post-surgical complications and incidence of cardiovascular events. Spinal Cord 2022;1–8. https://doi.org/10.1038/s41393-022-00822-w.
65. Baranidharan G, Edgar D, Bretherton B, et al. Efficacy and safety of 10 kHz spinal cord stimulation for the treatment of chronic pain: a systematic review and narrative synthesis of real-world retrospective studies. Biomedicines 2021;9:180.
66. Luz A, Rupp R, Ahmadi R, et al. Beyond treatment of chronic pain: a scoping review about epidural electrical spinal cord stimulation to restore sensorimotor and autonomic function after spinal cord injury. Neurol Res Pract 2023;5:14.
67. Ward AR, Robertson VJ. Sensory, motor, and pain thresholds for stimulation with medium frequency alternating current. Arch Phys Med Rehabil 1998;79:273–8.
68. Angeli C, Rejc E, Boakye M, et al. Targeted selection of stimulation parameters for restoration of motor and autonomic function in individuals with spinal cord injury. Neuromodulation Technol Neural Interface 2024;27:645–60.
69. Merton PA, Morton HB, Hill DK, et al. Scope of a technique for electrical stimulation of human brain, spinal cord, and muscle. Lancet 1982;320:597–600.
70. Minassian K, Persy I, Rattay F, et al. Posterior root–muscle reflexes elicited by transcutaneous stimulation of the human lumbosacral cord. Muscle Nerve 2007;35:327–36.
71. Gerasimenko Y, Gorodnichev R, Machueva E, et al. Novel and direct access to the human locomotor spinal circuitry. J Neurosci 2010;30:3700–8.
72. Hofstoetter US, McKay WB, Tansey KE, et al. Modification of spasticity by transcutaneous spinal cord stimulation in individuals with incomplete spinal cord injury. J Spinal Cord Med 2014;37:202–11.
73. Gerasimenko YP, Lu DC, Modaber M, et al. Noninvasive reactivation of motor descending control after paralysis. J Neurotrauma 2015;32:1968–80.
74. Inanici F, Samejima S, Gad P, et al. Transcutaneous electrical spinal stimulation promotes long-term recovery of upper extremity function in chronic tetraplegia. IEEE Trans Neural Syst Rehabil Eng Publ IEEE Eng Med Biol Soc 2018;26:1272–8.
75. Zhang F, Momeni K, Ramanujam A, et al. Cervical spinal cord transcutaneous stimulation improves upper extremity and hand function in people with complete tetraplegia: a case study. IEEE Trans Neural Syst Rehabil Eng Publ IEEE Eng Med Biol Soc 2020;28:3167–74.
76. Gad P, Lee S, Terrafranca N, et al. Non-invasive activation of cervical spinal networks after severe paralysis. J Neurotrauma 2018;35:2145–58.
77. Moritz C, Field-Fote EC, Tefertiller C, et al. Non-invasive spinal cord electrical stimulation for arm and hand function in chronic tetraplegia: a safety and efficacy trial. Nat Med 2024;30:1276–83.
78. Taylor C, McHugh C, Mockler D, et al. Transcutaneous spinal cord stimulation and motor responses in individuals with spinal cord injury: a methodological review. PLoS One 2021;16:e0260166.
79. McHugh LV, Miller AA, Leech KA, et al. Feasibility and utility of transcutaneous spinal cord stimulation

combined with walking-based therapy for people with motor incomplete spinal cord injury. Spinal Cord Ser Cases 2020;6:104.
80. Huang R, Nikooyan AA, Moore LD, et al. Minimal handgrip force is needed for transcutaneous electrical stimulation to improve hand functions of patients with severe spinal cord injury. Sci Rep 2022;12:7733.
81. Freyvert Y, Yong NA, Morikawa E, et al. Engaging cervical spinal circuitry with non-invasive spinal stimulation and buspirone to restore hand function in chronic motor complete patients. Sci Rep 2018; 8:15546.
82. Knikou M. Transpinal and transcortical stimulation alter corticospinal excitability and increase spinal output. PLoS One 2014;9:e102313.
83. Samejima S, Caskey CD, Inanici F, et al. Multisite transcutaneous spinal stimulation for walking and autonomic recovery in motor-incomplete tetraplegia: a single-subject design. Phys Ther 2022;102: pzab228.
84. Abualait TS, Ibrahim AI. Spinal direct current stimulation with locomotor training in chronic spinal cord injury. Saudi Med J 2020;41:88–93.
85. Comino-Suárez N, Moreno JC, Megía-García Á, et al. Transcutaneous spinal cord stimulation combined with robotic-assisted body weight-supported treadmill training enhances motor score and gait recovery in incomplete spinal cord injury: a double-blind randomized controlled clinical trial. J Neuroengineering Rehabil 2025;22:15.
86. Wiesener C, Spieker L, Axelgaard J, et al. Supporting front crawl swimming in paraplegics using electrical stimulation: a feasibility study. J Neuroengineering Rehabil 2020;17:51.
87. Samejima S, Shackleton C, Malik RN, et al. Multisystem benefits of non-invasive spinal cord stimulation following cervical spinal cord injury: a case study. Bioelectron Med 2025;11:20.
88. Solinsky R, Burns K, Tuthill C, et al. Transcutaneous spinal cord stimulation and its impact on cardiovascular autonomic regulation after spinal cord injury. Am J Physiol Heart Circ Physiol 2024;326:H116–22.
89. Sachdeva R, Nightingale TE, Pawar K, et al. Noninvasive neuroprosthesis promotes cardiovascular recovery after spinal cord injury. Neurotherapeutics 2021;18:1244–56.
90. Krassioukov A. Autonomic function following cervical spinal cord injury. Respir Physiol Neurobiol 2009;169:157–64.
91. Hofstoetter US, Freundl B, Binder H, et al. Common neural structures activated by epidural and transcutaneous lumbar spinal cord stimulation: elicitation of posterior root-muscle reflexes. PLoS One 2018;13:e0192013.
92. Gerasimenko Y, Gorodnichev R, Moshonkina T, et al. Transcutaneous electrical spinal-cord stimulation in humans. Ann Phys Rehabil Med 2015;58:225–31.
93. Lavrov I, Gerasimenko YP, Ichiyama RM, et al. Plasticity of spinal cord reflexes after a complete transection in adult rats: relationship to stepping ability. J Neurophysiol 2006;96:1699–710.
94. Ladenbauer J, Minassian K, Hofstoetter US, et al. Stimulation of the human lumbar spinal cord with implanted and surface electrodes: a computer simulation study. IEEE Trans Neural Syst Rehabil Eng 2010;18:637–45.
95. Malone IG, Kelly MN, Nosacka RL, et al. Closed-loop, cervical, epidural stimulation elicits respiratory neuroplasticity after spinal cord injury in freely behaving rats. eNeuro 2022;9. ENEURO.0426-21. 2021.
96. Vallejo R, Chakravarthy K, Will A, et al. A new direction for closed-loop spinal cord stimulation: combining contemporary therapy paradigms with evoked compound action potential sensing. J Pain Res 2021;14:3909–18.
97. Tazoe T, Sasada S, Murayama T, et al. Non-invasive closed-loop spinal stimulation restores leg stepping control in humans with paraplegia. Brain 2026;149: 274–89.
98. Keller A, Singh G, Sommerfeld JH, et al. Noninvasive spinal stimulation safely enables upright posture in children with spinal cord injury. Nat Commun 2021;12:1–11.
99. Amirova L, Keller A, Singh G, et al. Cumulative transcutaneous spinal stimulation with locomotor training safely improves trunk control in children with spinal cord injury: pilot study. Children 2025; 12:817.
100. Singh G, Keller A, Lucas K, et al. Safety and feasibility of cervical and thoracic transcutaneous spinal cord stimulation to improve hand motor function in children with chronic spinal cord injury. Neuromodulation J Int Neuromodulation Soc 2024;27:661–71.
101. Singh G, Lucas K, Keller A, et al. Transcutaneous spinal stimulation from adults to children: a review. Top Spinal Cord Inj Rehabil 2023;29:16–32.
102. Lucas K, Singh G, Alvarado LR, et al. Non-invasive spinal neuromodulation enables stepping in children with complete spinal cord injury. Brain J Neurol 2025;148:3290–9.
103. Engineer ND, Kimberley TJ, Prudente CN, et al. Targeted vagus nerve stimulation for rehabilitation after stroke. Front Neurosci 2019;13:280.
104. Kilgard MP, Epperson JD, Adehunoluwa EA, et al. Closed-loop vagus nerve stimulation aids recovery from spinal cord injury. Nature 2025;643:1030–6.
105. Mansour NM, Peña Pino I, Freeman D, et al. Advances in epidural spinal cord stimulation to restore function after spinal cord injury: history and systematic review. J Neurotrauma 2022;39: 1015–29.

106. Gill ML, Grahn PJ, Calvert JS, et al. Neuromodulation of Lumbosacral spinal networks enables independent stepping after complete paraplegia. Nat Med 2018;24:1677–82.
107. Wagner FB, Mignardot JB, Le Goff-Mignardot CG, et al. Targeted neurotechnology restores walking in humans with spinal cord injury. Nature 2018; 563:65–71.
108. Boakye M, Ball T, Dietz N, et al. Spinal cord epidural stimulation for motor and autonomic function recovery after chronic spinal cord injury: a case series and technical note. Surg Neurol Int 2023;14:87.
109. Calvert JS, Gill ML, Linde MB, et al. Voluntary modulation of evoked responses generated by epidural and transcutaneous spinal stimulation in humans with spinal cord injury. J Clin Med 2021;10:4898.
110. Veith DD, Gill ML, Beck LA, et al. Functional outcomes and participants' perspectives during short-term application of spinal stimulation in individuals with spinal cord injury. J Spinal Cord Med 2025;48:978–89.
111. Hoglund BK, Zurn CA, Madden LR, et al. Mapping spinal cord stimulation-evoked muscle responses in patients with chronic spinal cord injury. Neuromodulation J Int Neuromodulation Soc 2023;26: 1371–80.
112. Mesbah S, Herrity A, Ugiliweneza B, et al. Neuroanatomical mapping of the lumbosacral spinal cord in individuals with chronic spinal cord injury. Brain Commun 2022;5:fcac330.
113. Zhao Z, Ahmadi A, Hoover C, et al. Optimization of spinal cord stimulation using bayesian preference learning and its validation. IEEE Trans Neural Syst Rehabil Eng Publ IEEE Eng Med Biol Soc 2021; 29:1987–97.
114. Phillips AA, Gandhi AP, Hankov N, et al. An implantable system to restore hemodynamic stability after spinal cord injury. Nat Med 2025;31:2946–57.
115. West CR, Phillips AA, Squair JW, et al. Association of epidural stimulation with cardiovascular function in an individual with spinal cord injury. JAMA Neurol 2018;75:630–2.
116. Gad P, Gerasimenko Y, Zdunowski S, et al. Weight bearing over-ground stepping in an exoskeleton with non-invasive spinal cord neuromodulation after motor complete paraplegia. Front Neurosci 2017;11:333.
117. Sayenko DG, Rath M, Ferguson AR, et al. Self-assisted standing enabled by non-invasive spinal stimulation after spinal cord injury. J Neurotrauma 2019;36:1435–50.
118. Inanici F, Brighton LN, Samejima S, et al. Transcutaneous spinal cord stimulation restores hand and arm function after spinal cord injury. IEEE Trans Neural Syst Rehabil Eng 2021;29:310–9.
119. Gad P, Lee S, Terrafranca N, et al. Non-invasive activation of cervical spinal networks after severe paralysis. J Neurotrauma 2018;35(18):2145–58.
120. Hofstoetter US, Freundl B, Danner SM, et al. Transcutaneous spinal cord stimulation induces temporary attenuation of spasticity in individuals with spinal cord injury. J Neurotrauma 2020;37(3): 481–93.
121. Benavides FD, Jo HJ, Lundell H, et al. Cortical and subcortical effects of transcutaneous spinal cord stimulation in humans with tetraplegia. J Neurosci 2020;40:2633–43.
122. McKenzie K, Veit N, Aalla S, et al. Combining neuromodulation strategies in spinal cord injury gait rehabilitation: a proof of concept, randomized, crossover trial. Arch Phys Med Rehabil 2024;105: 1930–7.
123. Wiesener C, Spieker L, Axelgaard J, et al. Supporting front crawl swimming in paraplegics using electrical stimulation: a feasibility study. J NeuroEngineering Rehabil 2020;17:51.
124. Ajiboye AB, Willett FR, Young DR, et al. Restoration of reaching and grasping movements through brain-controlled muscle stimulation in a person with tetraplegia: a proof-of-concept demonstration. Lancet Lond Engl 2017;389:1821–30.
125. McCaughey EJ, McLean AN, Allan DB, et al. Abdominal functional electrical stimulation to enhance mechanical insufflation-exsufflation. J Spinal Cord Med 2016;39:720–5.
126. Osuagwu BCA, Wallace L, Fraser M, et al. Rehabilitation of hand in subacute tetraplegic patients based on brain computer interface and functional electrical stimulation: a randomised pilot study. J Neural Eng 2016;13:065002.
127. Rahimi M, Torkaman G, Ghabaee M, et al. Advanced weight-bearing mat exercises combined with functional electrical stimulation to improve the ability of wheelchair-dependent people with spinal cord injury to transfer and attain independence in activities of daily living: a randomized controlled trial. Spinal Cord 2020;58:78–85.
128. Duffell LD, Paddison S, Alahmary AF, et al. The effects of FES cycling combined with virtual reality racing biofeedback on voluntary function after incomplete SCI: a pilot study. J NeuroEngineering Rehabil 2019;16:149.
129. Sivaramakrishnan A, Solomon JM, Manikandan N. Comparison of transcutaneous electrical nerve stimulation (TENS) and functional electrical stimulation (FES) for spasticity in spinal cord injury - a pilot randomized cross-over trial. J Spinal Cord Med 2018;41:397–406.
130. Solinsky R, Mercier H, Picard G, et al. Cardiometabolic effects of high-intensity hybrid functional electrical stimulation exercise after spinal cord injury. Pharm Manag PM R 2021;13:937–44.

131. Bergmann M, Zahharova A, Ereline J, et al. Single session exercises and concurrent functional electrical stimulation are more effective on muscles' force generation than only exercises in spinal cord injured persons: a feasibility study. J Musculoskelet Neuronal Interact 2020;20:472–9.
132. Gorgey AS, Venigalla S, Deitrich JN, et al. Electrical stimulation paradigms on muscle quality and bone mineral density after spinal cord injury. Osteoporos Int 2025;36:1039–51.
133. Gorgey AS, Khalil RE, Carter W, et al. Skeletal muscle hypertrophy and enhanced mitochondrial bioenergetics following electrical stimulation exercises in spinal cord injury: a randomized clinical trial. Eur J Appl Physiol 2024;125:1075–89.
134. Voicu R, Kuchen DB, Perret C, et al. Influence of gait-synchronized functional electrical stimulation during exoskeleton-assisted ambulation on cardiorespiratory outcomes in individuals with incomplete spinal cord injury. J Rehabil Med 2025;57:jrm43423.
135. Yozbatiran N, Francisco GE, Korupolu R. Safety and feasibility of paired vagus nerve stimulation with rehabilitation for improving upper extremity function in people with cervical spinal cord injury: study protocol for a pilot randomized controlled trial. Front Neurol 2024;15:1465764.
136. Min L, Cheng C, Chen J, et al. Transcutaneous auricular vagus nerve stimulation promotes post-spinal cord injury remyelination via α7nAChR-mediated activation of oligodendrocyte precursor cells. Neurosci Lett 2026;871:138466.
137. Powell ES, Carrico C, Salyers E, et al. The effect of transcutaneous spinal direct current stimulation on corticospinal excitability in chronic incomplete spinal cord injury. NeuroRehabilitation 2018;43:125–34.
138. Powell ES, Carrico C, Raithatha R, et al. Transvertebral direct current stimulation paired with locomotor training in chronic spinal cord injury: a case study. NeuroRehabilitation 2016;38(1):27–35.
139. Murray LM, Knikou M. Remodeling brain activity by repetitive cervicothoracic transspinal stimulation after human spinal cord injury. Front Neurol 2017;8:50.
140. Murray LM, Knikou M. Transspinal stimulation increases motoneuron output of multiple segments in human spinal cord injury. PLoS One 2019;14:e0213696.
141. Adeel M, Lai CH, Lin BS, et al. Effects of paired stimulation with specific waveforms on cortical and spinal plasticity in subjects with a chronic spinal cord injury. J Formos Med Assoc 2022;121:2044–56.
142. Chandrasekaran S, Bhagat NA, Ramdeo R, et al. Targeted transcutaneous spinal cord stimulation promotes persistent recovery of upper limb strength and tactile sensation in spinal cord injury: a pilot study. Front Neurosci 2023;17:1210328.
143. Islam MdA, Pulverenti TS, Knikou M. Neurona actions of transspinal stimulation on locomotor networks and reflex excitability during walking in humans with and without spinal cord injury. Front Hum Neurosci 2021;15:620414.
144. Knikou M, Murray LM. Repeated transspinal stimulation decreases soleus H-reflex excitability and restores spinal inhibition in human spinal cord injury. PLoS One 2019;14:e0223135.
145. Meyer C, Hofstoetter US, Hubli M, et al. Immediate effects of transcutaneous spinal cord stimulatior on motor function in chronic, sensorimotor incomplete spinal cord injury. J Clin Med 2020;9:3541.
146. Pulverenti TS, Zaaya M, Grabowski M, et al. Neurophysiological changes after paired brain and spina cord stimulation coupled with locomotor training ir human spinal cord injury. Front Neurol 2021;12 627975.
147. Pulverenti TS, Zaaya M, Knikou M. Brain and spina cord paired stimulation coupled with locomoto training affects polysynaptic flexion reflex circuits in human spinal cord injury. Exp Brain Res 2022 240:1687–99.
148. Rath M, Vette AH, Ramasubramaniam S, et al. Trunk stability enabled by noninvasive spinal electrica stimulation after spinal cord injury. J Neurotrauma 2018;35:2540–53.
149. Shackleton C, Samejima S, Williams AM, et al. Moto and autonomic concomitant health improvements with neuromodulation and exercise (MACHINE) training: a randomised controlled trial in individuals with spinal cord injury. BMJ Open 2023;13:e070544
150. Shapkova EY, Pismennaya EV, Emelyannikov DV et al. Exoskeleton walk training in paralyzed individuals benefits from transcutaneous lumbar corc tonic electrical stimulation. Front Neurosci 2020 14:416.
151. Solinsky R, Burns K, Tuthill C, et al. Transcutaneous spinal cord stimulation and its impact on cardiovascular autonomic regulation after spinal cord injury Am J Physiol Heart Circ Physiol 2024;326:H116–22
152. Suggitt J, Symonds J, D'Amico JM. Safety and effectiveness of multisite transcutaneous spina cord stimulation combined with activity-based therapy when delivered in a community rehabilitatior setting: a real-world pilot study. Neuromodulatior J Int Neuromodulation Soc 2025;28:1144–56.
153. Wu YK, Levine JM, Wecht JR, et al. Posteroanterio cervical transcutaneous spinal stimulation targets ventral and dorsal nerve roots. Clin Neurophysic 2020;131:451–60.
154. Zaaya M, Pulverenti TS, Knikou M. Transspina stimulation and step training alter function of spina networks in complete spinal cord injury. Spina Cord Ser Cases 2021;7:55.
155. Zhang F, Carnahan J, Ravi M, et al. Combining spinal cord transcutaneous stimulation with activity

based training to improve upper extremity function following cervical spinal cord injury. Annu Int Conf IEEE Eng Med Biol Soc 2023;1–4.

156. Zhang F, Momeni K, Ramanujam A, et al. Cervical spinal cord transcutaneous stimulation improves upper extremity and hand function in people with complete tetraplegia: a case study. IEEE Trans Neural Syst Rehabil Eng 2020;28:3167–74.
157. Beck L, Veith D, Linde M, et al. Impact of long-term epidural electrical stimulation enabled task-specific training on secondary conditions of chronic paraplegia in two humans. J Spinal Cord Med 2021;44: 800–5.
158. Bloom O, Wecht JM, Legg Ditterline BE, et al. Prolonged targeted cardiovascular epidural stimulation improves immunological molecular profile: a case report in chronic severe spinal cord injury. Front Syst Neurosci 2020;14:571011.
159. Calvert JS, Grahn PJ, Strommen JA, et al. Electrophysiological guidance of epidural Electrode array implantation over the human Lumbosacral spinal cord to enable motor function after chronic paralysis. J Neurotrauma 2019;36:1451–60.
160. Cheng R, Sui Y, Sayenko D, et al. Motor control after human SCI through activation of muscle synergies under spinal cord stimulation. IEEE Trans Neural Syst Rehabil Eng 2019;27:1331–40.
161. DiMarco AF, Geertman RT, Tabbaa K, et al. Effects of lower thoracic spinal cord stimulation on bowel management in individuals with spinal cord injury. Arch Phys Med Rehabil 2021;102: 1155–64.
162. DiMarco AF, Geertman RT, Tabbaa K, et al. Restoration of cough via spinal cord stimulation improves pulmonary function in tetraplegics. J Spinal Cord Med 2020;43:579–85.
163. DiMarco AF, Geertman RT, Tabbaa K, et al. Case report: minimally invasive method to activate the expiratory muscles to restore cough. J Spinal Cord Med 2018;41:562–6.
164. Ditterline BEL, Aslan SC, Wang S, et al. Restoration of autonomic cardiovascular regulation in spinal cord injury with epidural stimulation: a case series. Clin Auton Res 2021;31:317–20.
165. Gill ML, Linde MB, Hale RF, et al. Alterations of spinal epidural stimulation-enabled stepping by descending intentional motor commands and proprioceptive inputs in humans with spinal cord injury. Front Syst Neurosci 2021;14:590231.
166. Gorgey AS, Trainer R, Sutor TW, et al. A case study of percutaneous epidural stimulation to enable motor control in two men after spinal cord injury. Nat Commun 2023;14:2064.
167. Gorgey A, Gill S, Holman ME, et al. The feasibility of using exoskeletal assisted walking with epidural stimulation: a case report study. Ann Clin Transl Neurol 2020;7:259–65.
168. Gorgey A, Goldsmith J, Alazzam A, et al. Effects of percutaneously-implanted epidural stimulation on cardiovascular autonomic function and spasticity after complete spinal cord injury: a case report. Front Neurosci 2023;17:2064.
169. Harkema SJ, Legg Ditterline B, Wang S, et al. Epidural spinal cord stimulation training and sustained recovery of cardiovascular function in individuals with chronic cervical spinal cord injury. JAMA Neurol 2018;75:1569–71.
170. Herrity AN, Aslan SC, Ugiliweneza B, et al. Improvements in bladder function following activity-based recovery training with epidural stimulation after chronic spinal cord injury. Front Syst Neurosci 2021;14:614691.
171. Herrity AN, Williams CS, Angeli CA, et al. Lumbosacral spinal cord epidural stimulation improves voiding function after human spinal cord injury. Sci Rep 2018;8:8688.
172. Herrity AN, Aslan SC, Mesbah S, et al. Targeting bladder function with network-specific epidural stimulation after chronic spinal cord injury. Sci Rep 2022;12:11179.
173. Hoover C, Schuerger W, Balser D, et al. Neuromodulation through spinal cord stimulation restores ability to voluntarily cycle after motor complete paraplegia. J Neurotrauma 2024;41(9–10):1163–71.
174. Ibáñez J, Angeli CA, Harkema SJ, et al. Recruitment order of motor neurons promoted by epidural stimulation in individuals with spinal cord injury. J Appl Physiol 2021;131:1100–10.
175. Kandhari S, Sharma D, Tomar AK, et al. Epidural electrical spinal cord stimulation of the thoracic segments (T2-T5) facilitates respiratory function in patients with complete spinal cord injury. Respir Physiol Neurobiol 2022;300:103885.
176. Kandhari S, Sharma D, Samuel S, et al. Epidural spinal stimulation enables global sensorimotor and autonomic function recovery after complete paralysis: 1st Study from India. IEEE Trans Neural Syst Rehabil Eng 2022;30:2052–9.
177. Lu DC, Edgerton VR, Modaber M, et al. Engaging cervical spinal cord networks to re-enable volitional control of hand function in tetraplegic patients. Neurorehabil Neural Repair 2016;30:951–62.
178. Mesbah S, Angeli CA, Keynton RS, et al. A novel approach for automatic visualization and activation detection of evoked potentials induced by epidural spinal cord stimulation in individuals with spinal cord injury. PLoS One 2017;12:e0185582.
179. Mesbah S, Ball T, Angeli C, et al. Predictors of volitional motor recovery with epidural stimulation in individuals with chronic spinal cord injury. Brain 2021;144:420–33.
180. Nightingale TE, Walter M, Williams AMM, et al. Ergogenic effects of an epidural neuroprosthesis in

one individual with spinal cord injury. Neurology 2019;92:338–40.
181. Peña Pino I, Hoover C, Venkatesh S, et al. Long-term spinal cord stimulation after chronic complete spinal cord injury enables volitional movement in the absence of stimulation. Front Syst Neurosci 2020;14:35.
182. Pino IP, Nightingale TE, Hoover C, et al. The safety of epidural spinal cord stimulation to restore function after spinal cord injury: post-surgical complications and incidence of cardiovascular events. Spinal Cord 2022;60:903–10.
183. Rowald A, Komi S, Demesmaeker R, et al. Activity-dependent spinal cord neuromodulation rapidly restores trunk and leg motor functions after complete paralysis. Nat Med 2022;28:260–71.
184. Rybka V, Sediva K, Spackova L, et al. Epidural spinal cord stimulation can facilitate ejaculatory response in spinal cord injury individuals: a report of two cases. Int J Neurosci 2024;134:1357–64.
185. Singh RE, Ahmadi A, Parr AM, et al. Epidural stimulation restores muscle synergies by modulating neural drives in participants with sensorimotor complete spinal cord injuries. J NeuroEngineering Rehabil 2023;20:59.
186. Smith AC, Angeli CA, Ugiliweneza B, et al. Spinal cord imaging markers and recovery of standing with epidural stimulation in individuals with clinically motor complete spinal cord injury. Exp Brain Res 2022;240:279–88.
187. Squair JW, Gautier M, Mahe L, et al. Neuroprosthetic baroreflex controls haemodynamics after spinal cord injury. Nature 2021;590:308–14.
188. Terson de Paleville DGL, Harkema SJ, Angeli CA. Epidural stimulation with locomotor training improves body composition in individuals with cervical or upper thoracic motor complete spinal cord injury: a series of case studies. J Spinal Cord Med 2019;42:32–8.
189. Walter M, Lee AHX, Kavanagh A, et al. Epidural spinal cord stimulation acutely modulates lower urinary tract and bowel function following spinal cord injury: a case report. Front Physiol 2018;9:1816.
190. Rejc E, Angeli C, Harkema S. Effects of Lumbosacral spinal cord epidural stimulation for standing after chronic complete paralysis in humans. PLoS One 2015;10:e0133998.
191. Samejima S, Shackleton C, Malik RN, et al. Spinal cord stimulation prevents autonomic dysreflexia in individuals with spinal cord injury: a case series. J Clin Med 2023;12:2897.
192. Wan KR, Ng ZYV, Wee SK, et al. Recovery of volitional motor control and overground walking in participants with chronic clinically motor complete spinal cord injury: restoration of rehabilitative function with Epidural Spinal Stimulation (RESTORES) Trial-A preliminary Study. J Neurotrauma 2024;41:1146–62.
193. Chou RC, Taylor JA, Solinsky R. Effects of hybrid-functional electrical stimulation (FES) rowing whole-body exercise on neurologic improvement in subacute spinal cord injury: secondary outcomes analysis of a randomized controlled trial. Spinal Cord 2020;58:914–20.
194. Craven BC, Giangregorio LM, Alavinia SM, et al. Evaluating the efficacy of functional electrical stimulation therapy assisted walking after chronic motor incomplete spinal cord injury: effects on bone biomarkers and bone strength. J Spinal Cord Med 2017;40:748–58.
195. Farkas GJ, Gorgey AS, Dolbow DR, et al. Energy expenditure, cardiorespiratory fitness, and body composition following arm cycling or functional electrical stimulation exercises in spinal cord injury: a 16-Week randomized controlled trial. Top Spinal Cord Inj Rehabil 2021;27:121–34.
196. Johnston TE, Marino RJ, Oleson CV, et al. Musculoskeletal effects of 2 functional electrical stimulation cycling paradigms conducted at different cadences for people with spinal cord injury: a pilot study. Arch Phys Med Rehabil 2016;97:1413–22.
197. Tefertiller C, Gerber D. Step ergometer training augmented with functional electrical stimulation in individuals with chronic spinal cord injury: a feasibility study. Artif Organs 2017;41:E196–202.
198. Gorgey AS, Graham ZA, Bauman WA, et al. Abundance in proteins expressed after functional electrical stimulation cycling or arm cycling ergometry training in persons with chronic spinal cord injury. J Spinal Cord Med 2017;40:439–48.
199. Duffell LD, Donaldson NN. A comparison of FES and SCS for neuroplastic recovery after SCI: historical perspectives and future directions. Front Neurol 2020;11:607.
200. Spieker L, Wiesener C, Niedeggen A, et al. Motor and sensor recovery in a paraplegic by transcutaneous spinal cord stimulation in water. Proceedings on Automation in Medical Engineering 2020;1:22.

Future Directions Related to Spinal Cord Compression
Where Will we be in the Next 10 Years?

Shintaro Honda, MD, PhD[a], Jefferson R. Wilson, MD, PhD[b,c], Michael G. Fehlings, MD, PhD, FRCSC, FRSC, FCAHS[a,b,d,*]

KEYWORDS

• Spinal cord compression • Degenerative cervical myelopathy • Spinal cord injury • Neuroprotection • Perfusion • Artificial intelligence

KEY POINTS

- Early surgical decompression is central to acute spinal cord injury care, with growing focus on identifying patients who benefit most from early intervention.
- AI-based MRI quantification, advanced imaging, and molecular biomarkers are poised to improve early diagnosis, risk stratification, and personalized decision-making in degenerative cervical myelopathy.
- Progress in neuroprotection, neuromodulation, and stem cell–based regeneration is shifting toward integrated, patient-specific approaches that combine multiple approaches to support recovery and long-term function.

INTRODUCTION

Spinal cord compression includes a spectrum of acute and chronic disorders, most notably traumatic spinal cord injury (SCI) and degenerative cervical myelopathy (DCM). Recent advances in the field include growing evidence supporting the efficacy of early surgical decompression for SCI,[1–3] an improved understanding of secondary injury cascades following spinal cord damage,[4] and technological progress in cervical operative devices for DCM.[5,6]

Despite these developments, major challenges remain, including the lack of effective therapies for injured spinal cord tissue, the difficulty of accurately quantifying spinal cord compression, and the limited ability to predict postoperative neurologic outcomes. In this review, we outline key areas expected to advance over the next decade and highlight future directions for translational research aimed at improving the care of patients with spinal cord compression (**Table 1**).

Decompression: Timing × Quality in Spinal Cord Injury

Mounting clinical evidence has firmly established early surgical decompression as a cornerstone of

[a] Division of Genetics and Development, Krembil Brain Institute, University Health Network, Toronto, Ontario, Canada; [b] Division of Neurosurgery and Spine Program, Department of Surgery, University of Toronto, Toronto, Ontario, Canada; [c] Division of Neurosurgery, Department of Surgery, St. Michael's Hospital, Toronto, Ontario, Canada; [d] Division of Neurosurgery, Krembil Neuroscience Centre, Toronto Western Hospital, University Health Network, Toronto, Ontario, Canada
* Corresponding author. Division of Neurosurgery and Spinal Program, Department of Surgery, University of Toronto, Krembil Neuroscience Center, Toronto Western Hospital, 399 Bathurst Street, Suite 4W-449, Toronto, Ontario M5T 2S8, Canada.
E-mail address: michael.fehlings@uhn.ca

Neurosurg Clin N Am 37 (2026) 665–671
https://doi.org/10.1016/j.nec.2026.05.014

Abbreviations

DBS	deep brain stimulation
DCM	degenerative cervical myelopathy
EES	epidural electrical stimulation
mJOA	modified Japanese Orthopaedic Association
SCI	spinal cord injury

acute SCI management.[2,7] This concept, often summarized by the phrase "time is spine," is now strongly supported by contemporary clinical practice guidelines.[8] The 2024 AO Spine-Praxis guidelines update recommends that adult patients with acute SCI undergo surgical decompression within 24 hours of injury.[9] In contrast, the role of ultraearly decompression—typically defined as surgery within 12 hours or less after injury—remains an area of active investigation. While some cohort studies suggest potential neurologic benefits with very early intervention,[10,11] the updated guidelines conclude that the current evidence is insufficient to support a recommendation for ultraearly surgery. Limitations include small sample sizes, inconsistent definitions of *ultraearly*, baseline neurologic assessment confounded by spinal

Table 1
Key areas of future development in spinal cord compression disorders

	Current State	Key Limitations	Future Directions
Decompression: Timing × Quality in SCI	Early surgical decompression established as standard of care (*time is spine*).	System-related delays; limited evidence for ultraearly surgery; uncertainty regarding decompression adequacy.	Knowledge translation and system-level implementation; standardized care pathways; regionalized SCI networks; physiologically optimized decompression including evaluation of expansile duroplasty.
Diagnostics and Phenotyping in DCM	MRI and mJOA score guide decision-making.	Limited sensitivity for early disease; poor risk stratification among mild DCM.	AI-based quantitative MRI and automated segmentation; quantitative MRI, electrophysiology, and molecular biomarkers enabling precision phenotyping and earlier intervention.
Neuroprotection and Neuromodulation in SCI	Neuroprotection primarily supportive; neuromodulation emerging.	Heterogeneous trial results; limited patient selection; single-outcome focus.	Precision, phase-specific neuroprotection including real-world evaluation of riluzole; circuit-specific neuromodulation integrated with intensive rehabilitation.
Stem Cell–Based Therapy for SCI Regeneration	Feasibility and safety established in early-phase trials.	Modest and variable efficacy; heterogeneous injury profiles; limited circuit integration.	Biologically informed, multimodal regenerative strategies incorporating regionally specified cells, bioengineering, immune modulation, and combination with neuromodulation.
Clinical Trial Design and Outcome Assessment	Conventional randomized controlled trials with single primary endpoints.	Insufficient sensitivity to heterogeneous recovery; ceiling effects.	Adaptive and platform trial designs; biomarker-based stratification; multidimensional outcome assessment frameworks such as the global statistical test.

shock, and methodological heterogeneity.[9] In addition, the role and timing of early surgery in acute central cord syndrome, the most common form of incomplete SCI, remains a key knowledge gap. An international survey of spine surgeons demonstrated persistent uncertainty regarding surgical timing for this population, particularly in stable injuries with cord compression and less severe neurologic deficits, and prospective trials are needed to establish evidence-based recommendations.[12] Looking ahead, a major challenge will not be generating further evidence for early decompression, but rather ensuring effective knowledge translation and implementation of the *time is spine* concept across health care systems. Delays often occur not because of surgical indecision, but due to prehospital triage, interfacility transfer, imaging access, and operating room availability.[13] Over the next decade, system-level interventions including standardized care pathways, regionalized SCI networks, real-time decision support, and education of frontline providers will be essential to ensure that evidence-based timing targets translate into real-world neurologic benefit.

In addition to surgical timing, increasing attention has been directed toward the adequacy of decompression at the dural level. Expansion duroplasty is currently being evaluated in clinical trials to determine its additive benefit when combined with standard bony decompression in acute SCI.[14] In a 2025 systematic review, duraplasty was associated with reductions in intraspinal pressure, improvements in spinal cord perfusion pressure, and American Spinal Injury Association Impairment Scale grade conversion in selected patients, although the overall evidence base remains small and heterogeneous.[15] In this context, the ongoing multicenter phase III DISCUS trial is evaluating decompression with versus without expansile duroplasty in acute severe cervical SCI, with neurologic recovery, safety, and mechanistic physiologic endpoints as primary outcomes.[14] The results of DISCUS are expected to play a pivotal role in defining whether dural expansion should become an integral component of effective decompression strategies in acute SCI.

Diagnostics and Phenotyping in the Management of Degenerative Cervical Myelopathy

Patients with DCM can present with heterogeneous symptoms—from classic hand numbness, dexterity loss, and gait imbalance, to subtle findings—which often leads to misattribution (eg, to carpal tunnel syndrome) and diagnostic delays.[16] Although MRI and the modified Japanese Orthopaedic Association (mJOA) score remain central to clinical decision-making, they lack sensitivity for early disease and fail to identify patients at risk of rapid neurologic deterioration.[5] A major future challenge is to identify whether subgroups of patients classified as having mild DCM by mJOA scoring are at heightened risk of rapid neurologic decline and should be considered for early surgical treatment rather than observation.

One promising strategy is the standardization of patient assessment through quantitative analysis of MRI images using artificial intelligence–based models. Compared with conventional automated segmentation tools, these models learn relevant features directly from data and are more robust to noise and anatomic variability, enabling more reliable medical image segmentation.[17] In spine research, the Spinal Cord Toolbox developed by Cohen-Adad and colleagues has been widely adopted and validated across multiple studies.[18,19] Such approaches could help identify high-risk patients among those with mild symptoms and inform optimal timing of intervention.[20]

In addition, quantitative MRI techniques—diffusion tensor imaging, tractography, functional MRI—and electrophysiological measures (eg, motor evoked potentials [MEPs] or somatosensory evoked potentials [SSEPs]) show promise in detecting microstructural damage and dysfunction that elude standard MRI.[21] Such metrics could enable earlier diagnosis, objective disease staging, and monitoring of deterioration. Likewise, emerging molecular biomarkers are under investigation: for example, elevated serum neurofilament light chain and inflammatory markers (interleukin-6, etc.) have been identified in DCM patients and may have diagnostic or prognostic utility.[22] In the next decade, integrating these advances is expected to facilitate timely diagnosis and personalized phenotyping of DCM, ultimately improving clinical decision-making and outcomes.

Neuroprotection and Neuromodulation in the Management of Spinal Cord Injury

Management of acute SCI is increasingly tailored to the injury phase. In the acute phase, the priority is neuroprotection, preserving vulnerable spinal tissue by mitigating secondary injury cascades. Pharmacologic neuroprotectants like riluzole, a sodium-glutamate antagonist originally for amyotrophic lateral sclerosis (ALS), are also being used. The recent Riluzole in Acute Spinal Cord Injury Study (RISCIS), demonstrated that riluzole was associated with a more favorable composite outcome than placebo at 6 months, with potentially larger effects in selected subgroups.[23] Importantly, these findings highlight the need for phase 4 prospective *real-world* studies to evaluate effectiveness across broader, heterogeneous populations, refine patient selection, and assess outcomes that matter most to patients. Beyond riluzole, a recent systematic review of randomized controlled trials evaluated a wide range of neuroprotective interventions including corticosteroids, erythropoietin, ion-channel modulators, anti-inflammatory agents, as well as growth factors and found that, despite promising signals, evidence remains inconclusive due to small sample sizes, heterogeneous designs, and outdated trials.[24] The review underscores 2 key priorities: adequately powered multicenter studies to identify responsive patient subgroups and outcome frameworks that capture patient-meaningful functional gains, as even modest motor improvements can substantially enhance independence and quality of life. Looking ahead, these insights point toward a future in which neuroprotection is delivered through precise, phase-specific strategies that integrate pharmacologic therapies with optimized surgical timing, physiologic management, and individualized patient selection.

In the subacute/chronic phase of SCI, neuromodulation is emerging as a key strategy to restore neuroplasticity and residual network integrity. Neuromodulatory interventions aim to modulate excitability within spared descending and propriospinal pathways, facilitating functional connectivity and motor relearning.

A recent landmark study demonstrates that epidural electrical stimulation (EES), particularly when combined with intensive rehabilitation, can restore voluntary locomotion even in patients with severe or motor-complete SCI.[25] Mechanistic experiments integrating single-nucleus RNA sequencing and spatial transcriptomics in animal models identified a specific subpopulation of excitatory spinal interneurons that are essential for recovery.[26] These findings indicate that EES promotes activity-dependent remodeling of spinal locomotor circuits, rather than acting through simple neuronal excitation. Emerging evidence also supports deep brain stimulation (DBS) as a complementary neuromodulatory approach for SCI. A recent study demonstrated that DBS targeting the lateral hypothalamus immediately augmented walking in animal models and, in a pilot clinical study, improved locomotor function in 2 participants with chronic incomplete SCI, with gains that persisted even after stimulation was turned off.[27] In parallel, brain–computer interface and brain–spine interface technologies are advancing rapidly. A landmark proof-of-concept study established a fully implanted digital bridge between cortical recordings and epidural spinal stimulation, enabling an individual with chronic tetraplegia to stand and walk naturally in community settings.[28] Although these approaches remain in early-phase clinical testing with small cohorts, they represent a paradigm shift toward direct neural bypass strategies for functional restoration after SCI.

Over the next decade, neuromodulation research will increasingly focus on circuit-specific targeting, informed by molecular and transcriptomic maps of the injured spinal cord. Identifying neuronal populations that govern not only locomotion but also autonomic and upper-limb functions may enable more precise, indication-specific stimulation strategies.[29] Ultimately, combining neuromodulation with regenerative, genetic, or cell-based therapies may allow durable reconstitution of spinal circuits and expand benefits beyond assistive stimulation toward true neurologic repair.

Stem Cell-Based Therapy to Regenerate the Injured Spinal Cord

Early stem cell–based strategies for SCI were motivated by the limited capacity for spontaneous repair due to several inhibitory modulators and progressive secondary injury.[30] Preclinical studies demonstrated that transplanted cells, particularly neural stem/progenitor cells, could promote remyelination, axonal growth, and circuit plasticity in animal models.[31] Contemporary clinical trials have confirmed the feasibility and long-term safety of intramedullary neural stem cell transplantation, including human fetal–derived neural stem cells across cervical and thoracic SCI.[32–34] However, consistent clinical efficacy has not yet been demonstrated, with observed neurologic improvements being modest, variable, and often underpowered. Key limitations include heterogeneous injury profiles, insensitive outcome measures, nonstandardized rehabilitation protocols, and transplantation strategies that do not actively promote lesion bridging or circuit formation.[30,31]

Future progress will depend on shifting from proof-of-concept safety trials toward biologically informed, efficacy-driven strategies. This includes the use of more effective and regionally specified cell types, integration with bioengineering approaches to remodel lesions and stabilize functional circuits, improved immune modulation, and patient-specific trial designs.[35–37] Ultimately, stem cell therapies are expected to evolve into individualized, multimodal interventions that complement standard acute care and rehabilitation rather than replace them.

Future Directions in Clinical Trial Design and Outcome Assessment

Progress in SCI therapeutics has exposed fundamental limitations in the design of conventional clinical trials. Recent expert commentary has emphasized the need for innovative approaches incorporating adaptive and platform trial designs, biomarker-informed patient stratification, and multidimensional outcome assessment frameworks such as the global statistical test.[38] These strategies are particularly well suited to heterogeneous conditions such as SCI and DCM, where meaningful recovery spans neurologic, functional, and quality-of-life domains. Over the next decade, alignment of trial methodology with biological mechanism and patient-centered outcomes will be critical for translating promising therapies into clinical practice.

SUMMARY

Spinal cord compression disorders remain major causes of neurologic disability despite advances in surgical and perioperative care. Early surgical decompression is now firmly established as a cornerstone of acute SCI management; however, future gains will depend on the effective translation of the time is spine concept into real-world clinical practice. Emerging strategies such as expansile duroplasty aim to further optimize decompression. In DCM, AI-based imaging, electrophysiology, and molecular biomarkers may enable earlier diagnosis and more precise surgical decision-making. Neuroprotection and neuromodulation are reshaping SCI management across injury phases, moving from generalized interventions toward precision, circuit-level therapies. Stem cell–based approaches are transitioning from feasibility and safety toward biologically informed, multimodal strategies that may ultimately complement surgery and rehabilitation to enable durable neurologic repair. In parallel, advances in clinical trial design and outcome assessment, which include adaptive trial frameworks and multidimensional, patient-centered endpoints, will be essential to ensure that emerging therapies are effectively translated into clinical practice.

CLINICS CARE POINTS

- Perform surgical decompression within 24 hours whenever feasible in adults with acute spinal cord injury.
- In patients with suspected degenerative cervical myelopathy, progressive hand dysfunction, gait imbalance, or neurological deterioration should prompt early specialist assessment and MRI.
- Neuroprotective drugs, neuromodulation, and stem cell–based therapies remain investigational.

DECLARATION OF AI AND AI-ASSISTED TECHNOLOGIES IN THE WRITING PROCESS

During the preparation of this work, the authors used GPT-5.2 (OpenAI) to assist with English language editing. After using this tool/service, the authors reviewed and edited the content as needed and take full responsibility for the content of the publication.

ACKNOWLEDGMENTS

M.G. Fehlings would like to acknowledge support from the Robert Campeau Family Foundation/Dr C.H. Tator Chair in Brain and Spinal Cord Research at UHN.

DISCLOSURE

The authors have no conflicts to declare.

REFERENCES

1. Fehlings MG, Rabin D, Sears W, et al. Current practice in the timing of surgical intervention in spinal cord injury. Spine 2010;35:S166.
2. Fehlings MG, Vaccaro A, Wilson JR, et al. Early versus delayed decompression for traumatic cervical spinal cord injury: results of the surgical timing in acute spinal cord injury study (STASCIS). PLoS One 2012;7:e32037.
3. Badhiwala JH, Wilson JR, Witiw CD, et al. The influence of timing of surgical decompression for acute spinal cord injury: a pooled analysis of individual patient data. Lancet Neurol 2021;20:117–26.
4. Ahuja CS, Wilson JR, Nori S, et al. Traumatic spinal cord injury. Nat Rev Dis Primers 2017;3:17018.
5. Badhiwala JH, Ahuja CS, Akbar MA, et al. Degenerative cervical myelopathy — update and future directions. Nat Rev Neurol 2020;16:108–24.
6. Ouchida J, Nakashima H, Ito S, et al. Recent progress in surgical treatment of cervical spine myelopathy – a narrative review. J Clin Orthop Trauma 2025;68:103074.
7. Fehlings MG, Tetreault LA, Wilson JR, et al. A clinical practice guideline for the management of patients with acute spinal cord injury and central cord syndrome: recommendations on the timing ($\leq$24 hours versus >24 hours) of decompressive surgery. Glob Spine J 2017;7:195S–202S.

8. Quddusi A, Pedro KM, Alvi MA, et al. Early surgical intervention for acute spinal cord injury: time is spine. Acta Neurochir 2023;165:2665–74.
9. Fehlings MG, Tetreault LA, Hachem L, et al. An update of a clinical practice guideline for the management of patients with acute spinal cord injury: recommendations on the role and timing of decompressive surgery. Glob Spine J 2024;14: 174S–86S.
10. Jug M, Kejžar N, Vesel M, et al. Neurological recovery after traumatic cervical spinal cord injury is superior if surgical decompression and instrumented fusion are performed within 8 hours versus 8 to 24 hours after injury: a single center experience. J Neurotrauma 2015;32:1385–92.
11. Mattiassich G, Gollwitzer M, Gaderer F, et al. Functional outcomes in individuals undergoing very early (<5h) and early (5–24h) surgical decompression in traumatic cervical spinal cord injury: analysis of neurological improvement from the Austrian spinal cord injury study. J Neurotrauma 2017;34:3362–71.
12. Hachem LD, Zhu M, Aarabi B, et al. A practical classification system for acute cervical spinal cord injury based on a three-phased modified Delphi process from the AOSpine spinal cord injury knowledge forum. Glob Spine J 2024;14:535–45.
13. Wilson JR, Voth J, Singh A, et al. Defining the pathway to definitive care and surgical decompression after traumatic spinal cord injury: results of a Canadian population-based cohort study. J Neurotrauma 2016;33:963–71.
14. Saadoun S, Grassner L, Belci M, et al. Duroplasty for injured cervical spinal cord with uncontrolled swelling: protocol of the DISCUS randomized controlled trial. Trials 2023;24:497.
15. Azad TD, Kartal A, Shafi M, et al. Duraplasty in acute spinal cord injury: a systematic review. Eur Spine J 2025;34:4891–9.
16. Davies BM, Mowforth OD, Smith EK, et al. Degenerative cervical myelopathy. BMJ 2018;360:k186.
17. Khaniabadi SM, Ibrahim H, Huqqani IA, et al. Comparative review on traditional and deep learning methods for medical image segmentation, 2023. IEEE 14th Control Syst Grad Res Colloq (ICSGRC) 2023;45–50. https://doi.org/10.1109/icsgrc57744.2023.10215402.
18. Leener BD, Lévy S, Dupont SM, et al. SCT: spinal cord toolbox, an open-source software for processing spinal cord MRI data. Neuroimage 2017;145: 24–43.
19. Valošek J, Bédard S, Keřkovský M, et al. A database of the healthy human spinal cord morphometry in the PAM50 template space. Imaging Neurosci 2024;2. https://doi.org/10.1162/imag_a_00075. imag–2–00075.
20. Bédard S, Valošek J, Seif M, et al. Normalizing spinal cord compression measures in degenerative cervical myelopathy. Spine J 2025;25:1951–63.
21. Martin AR, Tetreault L, Nouri A, et al. Imaging and electrophysiology for degenerative cervical myelopathy [AO spine RECODE-DCM research priority number 9]. Glob Spine J 2022;12:130S–46S.
22. Vedantam A, Rahman M, Salam S, et al. Serum protein biomarkers for degenerative cervical myelopathy: a prospective study. J Neurosurg Spine 2025;42: 718–26.
23. Fehlings MG, Pedro KM, Alvi MA, et al. The sodium-glutamate antagonist riluzole improves outcome after acute spinal cord injury: results from the RISCIS randomised controlled trial analysed using a global statistical analytic technique. EBioMedicine 2025; 118:105863.
24. Serag I, Abouzid M, Elmoghazy A, et al. An updated systematic review of neuroprotective agents in the treatment of spinal cord injury. Neurosurg Rev 2024;47:132.
25. Wagner FB, Mignardot J-B, Goff-Mignardot CGL, et al. Targeted neurotechnology restores walking in humans with spinal cord injury. Nature 2018;563: 65–71.
26. Kathe C, Skinnider MA, Hutson TH, et al. The neurons that restore walking after paralysis. Nature 2022;611:540–7.
27. Cho N, Squair JW, Aureli V, et al. Hypothalamic deep brain stimulation augments walking after spinal cord injury. Nat Med 2024;30:3676–86.
28. Lorach H, Galvez A, Spagnolo V, et al. Walking naturally after spinal cord injury using a brain–spine interface. Nature 2023;618:126–33.
29. Samejima S, Khorasani A, Ranganathan V, et al. Brain-computer-spinal interface restores upper limb function after spinal cord injury. IEEE Trans Neural Syst Rehabil Eng 2021;29:1233–42.
30. Zipser CM, Cragg JJ, Guest JD, et al. Cell-based and stem-cell-based treatments for spinal cord injury: evidence from clinical trials. Lancet Neurol 2022;21:659–70.
31. Hosseini SM, Borys B, Karimi-Abdolrezaee S. Neural stem cell therapies for spinal cord injury repair: an update on recent preclinical and clinical advances. Brain 2023;147:766–93.
32. Curtis E, Martin JR, Gabel B, et al. A First-in-Human phase I study of neural stem cell transplantation for chronic spinal cord injury. Cell Stem Cell 2018;22: 941–50.e6.
33. Levi AD, Okonkwo DO, Park P, et al. Emerging safety of intramedullary transplantation of human neural stem cells in chronic cervical and thoracic spinal cord injury. Neurosurgery 2017;82:562–75.
34. Curt A, Hsieh J, Schubert M, et al. The damaged spinal cord is a suitable target for stem cell transplantation. Neurorehabilitation Neural Repair 2020; 34:758–68.
35. Kadoya K, Lu P, Nguyen K, et al. Spinal cord reconstitution with homologous neural grafts enables

robust corticospinal regeneration. Nat Med 2016;22: 479–87.

36. Khazaei M, Ahuja CS, Nakashima H, et al. GDNF rescues the fate of neural progenitor grafts by attenuating notch signals in the injured spinal cord in rodents. Sci Transl Med 2020;12. https://doi.org/10.1126/scitranslmed.aau3538.

37. Sugai K, Nakamura M, Okano H, et al. Stem cell therapies for spinal cord injury in humans: a review of recent clinical research. Brain Spine 2025;5: 104207.

38. Pedro KM, Fehlings MG. Progress and future directions in spinal cord injury trials. Lancet Neurol 2025; 24:3–5.

9780443474002